CLINICAL CASES®
Critical Care

AF759527

Eugene C. Toy, MD
Vice Chair of Academic Affairs
Program Director of Obstetrics and Gynecology Residency
The Methodist Hospital-Houston
Clinical Professor of Obstetrics and Gynecology
University of Texas
Medical School at Houston
John S. Dunn Senior
Academic Chief of Obstetrics and Gynecology
St. Joseph Medical Center
Houston, Texas

Terrence H. Liu, MD, MPH
Professor of Clinical Surgery
University of California San Francisco School of Medicine
San Francisco, California
Program Director
University of California, San Francisco East Bay Surgery Residency
San Francisco, California
Attending Surgeon, Alameda County Medical Center
Oakland, California

Manuel Suarez, MD, FACCP
Director of Intensive Care Unit and Pulmonary Departments
Assistant Clinical Professor of Internal Medicine
Pulmonary and Critical Care
Larkin Community Hospital
South Miami, Florida
Assistant Clinical Professor of Internal Medicine, Pulmonary and Critical Care
Affiliate Dean of Clinical Medicine
Administrative Director of Medical Education and Institutional Educational Officer
Westchester General Hospital
Miami, Florida
Assistant Clinical Professor of Medicine
Lake Erie College of Osteopathic Medicine
Bradenton, Florida
at Westchester General Hospital
Miami, Florida

Mc Graw Hill Education

McGraw Hill Education (India) Private Limited
NEW DELHI

McGraw Hill Education Offices
New Delhi New York St Louis San Francisco Auckland Bogotá Caracas
Kuala Lumpur Lisbon London Madrid Mexico City Milan Montreal
San Juan Santiago Singapore Sydney Tokyo Toronto

McGraw Hill Education (India) Private Limited

Clinical Cases®: Critical Care

Notice

Medicine is an ever-changing science. As new research and clinical experience broaden our knowledge, changes in treatment and drug therapy are required. The authors and the publisher of this work have checked with sources believed to be reliable in their efforts to provide information that is complete and generally in accord with the standards accepted at the time of publication. However, in view of the possibility of human error or changes in medical sciences, neither the authors nor the publisher nor any other party who has been involved in the preparation or publication of this work warrants that the information contained herein is in every respect accurate or complete, and they disclaim all responsibility for any errors or omissions or for the results obtained from use of the information contained in this work. Readers are encouraged to confirm the information contained herein with other sources. For example and in particular, readers are advised to check the product information sheet included in the package of each drug they plan to administer to be certain that the information contained in this work is accurate and that changes have not been made in the recommended dose or in the contraindications for administration. This recommendation is of particular importance in connection with new or infrequently used drugs.

McGraw Hill Education (India) Edition 2014

RZZYCRQURYXBL

Reprinted in India by arrangement with The McGraw Hill Companies, Inc., New York

Sales territories: India, Pakistan, Nepal, Bangladesh, Sri Lanka and Bhutan

Library of Congress Cataloging-in-Publication Data

Toy, Eugene C.
Case files. Critical care/Eugene C. Toy, Manuel Suarez, Terrence H. Liu.
p. ; cm
Critical care
Includes bibliographical references and index.
ISBN-13: 978-0-07-176857-3 (pbk. : alk. paper)
ISBN: 10: 0-07-176857-2
1. Suarez, Maneul, 1957 II. Liu, Terrence H. III. Title. IV. Title: Critical care.
[DNLM: 1. Critical Care—Methods—Case Reports. 2. Critical Care—Methods—Problems and Exercises. 3. Problem Solving—Case Reports. 4. Problem Solving—Problems and Exerecises. WX 18.2]
RC86.7
616.02'8—dc23 2013014969

ISBN-13: 978-93-392-1435-7
ISBN-10: 93-392-1435-8
Published by McGraw Hill Education (India) Private Limited
P-24, Green Park Extension, New Delhi 110 016, and printed at
Rajkamal Electric Press, Kundli-131028, Haryana

DEDICATION

To the Honorable Representative Lois W. Kolkhorst of Brenham, Texas, whose courage, vision, and dedication to Texas is like a fiery torch, giving light and warmth in the cold and darkness;

To the Texas Neonatal ICU and the Perinatal Advisory Councils of which Representative Kolkhorst championed and breathed life;

To the brilliant, unselfish, and talented members of these two Councils, whose noble goals are to improve health care for the pregnant women and newborns of Texas;

To David Williams and Matt Ferrara, two tireless state staff members, who are the heart and soul of the Councils;

To the pregnant women and newborns of the Great State of Texas, to whom I have devoted my energies, passion, talents, and professional career.

—ECT

To all the staff, medical students, residents, and colleagues that I have had the pleasure to teach and be involved with.

To the people of St Vincent and the Grenadines, my friend the Governor General Sir Dr. Frederick N. Ballantyne, my mentor Dr. Edward S. Johnson and my tutor Dr. James T. Barrett, and especially to Dr. Eugene C. Toy, who made this wonderful project possible.

To the memory of my parents Manuel and Teresa Suarez who gave me all and to the two moons of my life, my daughters Alexia Teresa Suarez and Melanie Nicole Suarez.

—MS

DEDICATION

To the Honourable [illegible] W[illegible] of [illegible], whose courage, vision and dedication to [illegible] steadfastly in the good and the [illegible].

[illegible] Representatives [illegible] honour, [illegible] and [illegible].

To the [illegible] [illegible] [illegible] [illegible] for the interest of [illegible] and [illegible] of [illegible].

To [illegible] and [illegible]

To the [illegible] devoted [illegible] wisdom, talents, and [illegible].

To all the [illegible] students, [illegible] and colleagues that I [illegible] pleasure to teach and to [illegible] with.

[illegible] who [illegible] this [illegible].

To the [illegible] of my parents [illegible] and [illegible] the two [illegible] of my life [illegible] and [illegible] in the [illegible].

[illegible]

CONTENTS

CONTRIBUTORS

James T. Barrett, PhD
Professor Emeritus
Department of Molecular Microbiology and Immunology
School of Medicine
University of Missouri
Columbia, Missouri
Approach to Meningitis/Encephalitis

Jeremy S. Bleicher, DO, MPH
Chief Resident of Internal Medicine
Larkin Community Hospital
South Miami, Florida
Approach to Airway Management, Respiratory Failure

Adrian Garcia, MD
Internal Medicine and Pediatrics
Metrohealth Medical Center
Cleveland, Ohio
Approach to Status Epilepticus

Firas Harb, MD
President
American Medical Clinicals
Naperville, Illinois
Approach to Transfer of Critically Ill Patient

Grady H. Hendrix, MD
Professor of Medicine and Cardiology
Medical University of South Carolina
Charleston, South Carolina
Approach to Cardiac Arrthymias

Edward S. Johnson, MD
Director of Infection Control and The Travelers Resource
Clara Maass Medical Center
Belleville, New Jersey
Approach to Immunosuppressed Patients

Katarzyna Jurecki, MD
Resident, Obstetrics and Gynecology
Crozer-Keystone Health System
Upland, Pennsylvania
Approach to Acute Cardiac Failure

Agon Kajmolli, MD
Henry Ford Hospital
Wayne State Medical School
Detroit, Michigan
Approach to Altered Mental Status

Gabriel Labbad, MD
Resident, Obstetrics and Gynecology
Jamaica Hospital Medical Center
Jamaica, New York
Approach to Ethics/Do Not Resuscitate/Organ Donation

Lindsey M. McAlpin, MD
Resident, Obstetrics and Gynecology
Florida State University – Pensacola
Pensacola, Florida
Approach to Scoring and Prognosis
Approach to Imaging in Critical Care
Approach to Antimicrobial Use in the ICU
Approach to Acute Kidney Injury
Approach to Acute Liver Failure

Peter Salerno, DO
Chief Resident, Internal Medicine
Larkin Community Hospital
South Miami, Florida
Approach to Stroke

Jenna Sassie
Medical Student
Class of 2013
University of Texas Medical School at Houston
Houston, Texas
Approach to Endocrinopathies in the ICU Patient
Approach to Multiogan Dysfunction
Approach to Pain Control and Sedation

Jose David Suarez, MD
Assistant Clinical Professor
NOVA School of Medicine
Davie, Florida
Faculty, Larkin Family Medicine Residency Program
South Miami, Florida
Designated Institutional Officer
Larkin Psychiatry Program
South Miami, Florida
Approach to Early Awareness of Critical Illness

Allison L. Toy
Senior Nursing Student
Scott & White School of Nursing
Temple, TX
Primary Manuscript Reviewer

Safi Zaidi, MD
Ross University School of Medicine
North Brunswick, New Jersey
Approach to Acid Base Abnormalities Part 1
Approach to Acid Base Abnormalities Part 2

ACKNOWLEDGMENTS

The curriculum that evolved into the ideas for this series was inspired by Philbert Yau and Chuck Rosipal, two talented and forthright students, who have since graduated from medical school. It has been a tremendous joy to work with my excellent coauthors, especially Dr. Manny Suarez, who exemplifies the qualities of the ideal physician—caring, empathetic, and avid teacher, and who is intellectually a giant. It was on the island of St. Vincent and the Grenadines, while reviewing the curriculum of the fledgling Trinity School of Medicine, that Manny and I conceived about the idea of this book, a critical care book for students. I also enjoy collaborating with Dr. Terry Liu, my longtime friend and colleague whose expertise and commitment to medical education is legendary. I am greatly indebted to my editor, Catherine Johnson, whose exuberance, experience, and vision helped to shape this series. I appreciate McGraw-Hill's believing in the concept of teaching through clinical cases, and I would like to especially acknowledge Cindy Yoo for her editing expertise and Catherine Saggese and Anupriya Tyagi for the excellent production. It has been amazing to work together with my daughter Allison, who is a senior nursing student at the Scott and White School of Nursing; she is an astute manuscript reviewer and already in her early career she has a good clinical acumen. I appreciate the excellent support team at St. Joseph: Linda Bergstrom, Lisa Martinez, and Vanessa Yacouby. At Methodist, I appreciate Drs. Judy Paukert, Tim Boone, Marc Boom, and Alan Kaplan who have welcomed our residents; Carolyn Ward, a talented administrator, who holds the department together. Without my dear colleagues, Drs. Konrad Harms, Priti Schachel, and Gizelle Brooks-Carter, this book could not have been written. Most of all, I appreciate my ever-loving wife Terri, and our four wonderful children, Andy, Michael, Allison, and Christina, for their patience and understanding.

Eugene C. Toy

INTRODUCTION

Mastering the cognitive knowledge within a field such as critical care is a formidable task. It is even more difficult to draw on that knowledge, procure and filter through the clinical and laboratory data, develop a differential diagnosis, and, finally, to make a rational treatment plan. In critical care, a detailed understanding of hemodynamics, cardiovascular and pulmonary medicine, and pharmacology are important. Sometimes, it is prudent to initiate therapy for significant derangements rather than finding out the precise underlying disorder. For instance, in a patient with respiratory failure, therapy to increase oxygenation and ventilation is initiated while simultaneously determining the etiology. It is done through a more precise understanding of the pathophysiology that allows for rational and directed therapy. The critical care setting does not allow for much error. A skilled critical care physician must be able to quickly assess the patient's situation and produce an efficient diagnostic and therapeutic plan.

These skills the student learns best at the bedside, guided and instructed by experienced teachers, and inspired toward self-directed, diligent reading. Clearly, there is no replacement for education at the bedside, especially because in "real life," delay in correct management leads to suboptimal outcome. Unfortunately, clinical situations usually do not encompass the breadth of the specialty. Perhaps the best alternative is a carefully crafted patient case designed to stimulate the clinical approach and the decision-making process. In an attempt to achieve that goal, we have constructed a collection of clinical vignettes to teach diagnostic or therapeutic approaches relevant to critical care medicine.

Most importantly, the explanations for the cases emphasize the mechanisms and underlying principles, rather than merely rote questions and answers. This book is organized for versatility: it allows the student "in a rush" to go quickly through the scenarios and check the corresponding answers, and it allows the student who wants thought-provoking explanations to obtain them. The answers are arranged from simple to complex: the bare answers, an analysis of the case, an approach to the pertinent topic, a comprehension test at the end, clinical pearls for emphasis, and a list of references for further reading. The clinical vignettes are placed in a systematic order to better allow students to gain an understanding of the pathophysiology and mechanisms of disease. A listing of cases is included in Section III to aid the student who desires to test his/her knowledge of a certain area, or to review a topic, including basic definitions. Finally, we intentionally did not use a multiple-choice question format in the opening case scenarios, because clues (or distractions) are not available in the real world.

SECTION I

How to Approach Clinical Problems

Part 1 Approaching the Patient

Part 2 Approach to Clinical Problem Solving

Part 3 Approaching Reading

Part 1. Approaching the Patient

The transition from the textbook or journal article to the clinical situation is one of the most challenging tasks in medicine. Retention of information is difficult; organization of the facts and recall of a myriad of data in precise application to the patient is crucial. The purpose of this text is to facilitate in this process. The first step is gathering information, also known as establishing the database. This includes taking the history (asking questions), performing the physical examination, and obtaining selective laboratory and/or imaging tests. Of these, the historical examination is the most important and useful. Sensitivity and respect should always be exercised during the interview of patients.

CLINICAL PEARL

► The history is the single most important tool in obtaining a diagnosis. All physical findings, laboratory, and imaging studies are first obtained, and then interpreted, in the light of the pertinent history.

HISTORY

1. **Basic information:**
   a. **Age, gender, and ethnicity:** These should be recorded because some conditions are more common at certain ages; for instance, pain on defecation and rectal bleeding in a 20-year-old may indicate inflammatory bowel disease, whereas the same symptoms in a 60-year-old would more likely suggest colon cancer.
2. **Chief complaint:** What is it that brought the patient into the hospital or office? Is it a scheduled appointment, or an unexpected symptom? The patient's own words should be used if possible, such as, "I feel like a ton of bricks are on my chest." The chief complaint, or real reason for seeking medical attention, may not be the first subject the patient talks about (in fact, it may be the last thing), particularly if the subject is embarrassing, such as a sexually transmitted disease, or highly emotional, such as depression. It is often useful to clarify exactly what the patient's concern is; for example, they may fear their headaches represent an underlying brain tumor.
3. **History of present illness:** This is the most crucial part of the entire database. The questions one asks are guided by the differential diagnosis based on the chief complaint. The duration and character of the primary complaint, associated symptoms, and exacerbating/relieving factors should be recorded. Sometimes, the history will be convoluted and lengthy, with multiple diagnostic or therapeutic interventions at different locations. For patients with chronic illnesses, obtaining prior medical records is invaluable. For example, when

extensive evaluation of a complicated medical problem has been done elsewhere, it is usually better to first obtain those results than to repeat a "million-dollar workup." When reviewing prior records, it is often useful to review the primary data (eg, biopsy reports, echocardiograms, serologic evaluations) rather than to rely upon a diagnostic label applied by someone else, which then gets replicated in medical records and by repetition acquires the aura of truth, when it may not be fully supported by data. Some patients will be poor historians because of dementia, confusion, or language barriers; recognition of these situations and querying of family members is useful. When little or no history is available to guide a focused investigation, more extensive objective studies are often necessary to exclude potentially serious diagnoses.

4. **Past history:**
   a. **Any illnesses** such as hypertension, hepatitis, diabetes mellitus, cancer, heart disease, pulmonary disease, and thyroid disease should be elicited. If an existing or prior diagnosis is not obvious, it is useful to ask exactly how the condition was diagnosed; that is, what investigations were performed. Duration, severity, and therapies should be included.
   b. **Any hospitalizations and emergency room visits** should be listed with the reason(s) for admission, intervention, and the location of the hospital.
   c. **Transfusions** with any blood products should be listed, including any adverse reactions.
   d. **Surgeries:** The year and type of surgery should be recorded and any complications documented. The type of incision and any untoward effects of the anesthesia or the surgery should be noted.
5. **Allergies:** Reactions to medications should be recorded, including severity and temporal relationship to the medication. An adverse effect (such as nausea) should be differentiated from a true allergic reaction.
6. **Medications:** Current and previous medications should be listed, including dosage, route, frequency, and duration of use. Prescription, over-the-counter, and herbal medications are all relevant. Patients often forget their complete medication list; thus, asking each patient to bring in all their medications—both prescribed and nonprescribed—allows for a complete inventory.
7. **Family history:** Many conditions are inherited, or are predisposed in family members. The age and health of siblings, parents, grandparents, and others can provide diagnostic clues. For instance, an individual with first-degree family members with early onset coronary heart disease is at risk for cardiovascular disease.
8. **Social history:** This is one of the most important parts of the history which includes the patient's functional status at home, social and economic circumstances, and goals and aspirations for the future. These are often critical in determining the best way to manage a patient's medical problem. Living arrangements, economic situations, and religious affiliations may provide important clues for

puzzling diagnostic cases, or suggest the acceptability of various diagnostic or therapeutic options. Marital status and habits such as alcohol, tobacco, or illicit drug use may be relevant as risk factors for the disease.

9. **Review of systems:** A few questions about each major body system ensure that problems will not be overlooked. The clinician should avoid the mechanical "rapid-fire" questioning technique that discourages patients from answering truthfully because of fear of "annoying the doctor."

PHYSICAL EXAMINATION

The physical examination begins as one is taking the history, by observing the patient and beginning to consider a differential diagnosis. When performing the physical examination, one focuses on body systems suggested by the differential diagnosis, and performs tests or maneuvers with specific questions in mind; for example, does the patient with jaundice have ascites? When the physical examination is performed with potential diagnoses and expected physical findings in mind ("one sees what one looks for"), the utility of the examination in adding to diagnostic yield is greatly increased, as opposed to an unfocused "head-to-toe" physical.

1. **General appearance:** A great deal of information is gathered by observation, as one notes the patient's body habitus, state of grooming, nutritional status, level of anxiety (or perhaps inappropriate indifference), degree of pain or comfort, mental status, speech patterns, and use of language. This forms your impression of "who this patient is."

2. **Vital signs:** Temperature, blood pressure, heart rate, and respiratory rate. Height and weight are often placed here. Blood pressure can sometimes be different in the 2 arms; initially, it should be measured in both arms. In patients with suspected hypovolemia, pulse and blood pressure should be taken in lying and standing positions to look for orthostatic hypotension. It is quite useful to take the vital signs oneself, rather than relying upon numbers gathered by ancillary personnel using automated equipment, because important decisions regarding patient care are often made using the vital signs as an important determining factor.

3. **Head and neck examination:** Facial or periorbital edema and pupillary responses should be noted. Funduscopic examination provides a way to visualize the effects of diseases such as diabetes on the microvasculature; papilledema can signify increased intracranial pressure. Estimation of jugular venous pressure is very useful to estimate volume status. The thyroid should be palpated for a goiter or nodule, and carotid arteries auscultated for bruits. Cervical (common) and supraclavicular (pathologic) nodes should be palpated.

4. **Breast examination:** Inspect for symmetry, skin or nipple retraction with the patient's hands on her hips (to accentuate the pectoral muscles), and also with arms raised. With the patient sitting and supine, the breasts should then be palpated systematically to assess for masses. The nipple should be assessed for discharge and the axillary and supraclavicular regions should be examined for adenopathy.

5. **Cardiac examination:** The point of maximal impulse (PMI) should be ascertained for size and location, and the heart auscultated at the apex as well as at the base. Heart sounds, murmurs, and clicks should be characterized. Murmurs should be classified according to intensity, duration, timing in the cardiac cycle, and changes with various maneuvers. Systolic murmurs are very common and often physiologic; diastolic murmurs are uncommon and usually pathologic.
6. **Pulmonary examination:** The lung fields should be examined systematically and thoroughly. Wheezes, rales, rhonchi, and bronchial breath sounds should be recorded. Percussion of the lung fields may be helpful: hyperresonance may indicate tension pneumothorax, while dullness may point to a consolidated pneumonia or a pleural effusion.
7. **Abdominal examination:** The abdomen should be inspected for scars, distension, and discoloration (example: the Grey-Turner sign of flank discoloration indicates intra-abdominal or retroperitoneal hemorrhage). Auscultation of the bowel can identify normal versus high-pitched, and hyperactive versus hypoactive sounds. The abdomen should be percussed, including assessing for liver and spleen size, and for the presence of shifting dullness (indicating ascites). Careful palpation should begin initially away from the area of pain, involving one hand on top of the other, to assess for masses, tenderness, and peritoneal signs. Tenderness should be recorded on a scale (eg, 1 to 4 where 4 is the most severe pain). Guarding, whether it is voluntary or involuntary, should be noted.
8. **Back and spine examination:** The back should be assessed for symmetry, tenderness, and masses. The flank regions are particularly important to assess for pain on percussion, which might indicate renal disease.
9. **Genitalia:**
   a. **Females:** The pelvic examination should include an inspection of the external genitalia, and with the speculum, evaluation of the vagina and cervix. A pap smear and/or cervical cultures may be obtained. A bimanual examination to assess the size, shape, and tenderness of the uterus and adnexa is important.
   b. **Males:** An inspection of the penis and testes is performed. Evaluation for masses, tenderness, and lesions is important. Palpation for hernias in the inguinal region with the patient coughing to increase intra-abdominal pressure is useful.
10. **Rectal examination:** A digital rectal examination is generally performed for individuals with possible colorectal disease or gastrointestinal bleeding. Masses should be assessed, and stool for occult blood should be tested. In men, the prostate gland can be assessed for enlargement and for nodules.
11. **Extremities:** An examination for joint effusions, tenderness, edema, and cyanosis may be helpful. Clubbing of the nails might indicate pulmonary diseases such as lung cancer or chronic cyanotic heart disease.

12. **Neurological examination:** Patients who present with neurological complaints usually require a thorough assessment, including examination of the mental status, cranial nerves, motor strength, sensation, and reflexes.
13. **Skin:** The skin should be carefully examined for evidence of pigmented lesions (melanoma), cyanosis, or rashes that may indicate systemic disease (malar rash of systemic lupus erythematosus).

LABORATORY AND IMAGING ASSESSMENT

1. **Laboratory:**
   a. Complete blood count (CBC) to assess for anemia and thrombocytopenia.
   b. Chemistry panel is most commonly used to evaluate renal and liver function.
   c. For cardiac conditions, the electrocardiogram (EKG), rhythm strip, and/or cardiac enzymes are critically important.
   d. For pulmonary disorders, the oxygen saturation level and/or arterial blood gas findings provide excellent information.
   e. Lipid panel is particularly relevant in cardiovascular diseases.
   f. Urinalysis is often referred to as a "liquid renal biopsy," because the presence of cells, casts, protein, or bacteria provides clues about underlying glomerular or tubular diseases.
   g. Gram stain and culture of urine, sputum, and cerebrospinal fluid, as well as blood cultures are frequently useful to isolate the cause of infection.
2. **Imaging procedures:**
   a. Chest radiography is extremely useful in assessing cardiac size and contour, chamber enlargement, pulmonary vasculature and infiltrates, and the presence of pleural effusions.
   b. Ultrasonographic examination is useful for identifying fluid–solid interfaces, and for characterizing masses as cystic, solid, or complex. It is also very helpful in evaluating the biliary tree, kidney size, and evidence of ureteral obstruction, and can be combined with Doppler flow to identify deep venous thrombosis. Ultrasonography is noninvasive and has no radiation risk, but cannot be used to penetrate through bone or air, and is less useful in obese patients.

CLINICAL PEARL

- Ultrasonography is helpful in evaluating the biliary tree, looking for ureteral obstruction, and evaluating vascular structures, but has limited utility in obese patients.

   c. Computed tomography (CT) is helpful in possible intracranial bleeding, abdominal and/or pelvic masses, and pulmonary processes, and may help delineate the lymph nodes and retroperitoneal disorders. CT exposes the patient to radiation and requires the patient to be immobilized during the procedure. Generally, CT requires administration of a radiocontrast dye, which can be nephrotoxic.

d. Magnetic resonance imaging (MRI) identifies soft-tissue planes very well and provides the best imaging of the brain parenchyma. When used with gadolinium contrast (which is not nephrotoxic), MR angiography (MRA) is useful for delineating vascular structures. MRI does not use radiation, but the powerful magnetic field prohibits its use in patients with ferromagnetic metal in their bodies (for example, many prosthetic devices).
e. Cardiac procedures:
    i. **Echocardiography:** Uses ultrasonography to delineate the cardiac size, function, ejection fraction, and presence of valvular dysfunction.
    ii. **Angiography:** Radiopaque dye is injected into various vessels and radiographs or fluoroscopic images are used to determine the vascular occlusion, cardiac function, or valvular integrity.
    iii. **Stress treadmill tests:** Individuals at risk for coronary heart disease are asked to run on a treadmill. This increases oxygen demands on the heart. Meanwhile, the patient's blood pressure, heart rate, presence of chest pain, and EKG are monitored. Nuclear medicine imaging of the heart can be added to increase the sensitivity and specificity of the test. Individuals who cannot run on the treadmill (such as those with severe arthritis), may be given medications such as adenosine or dobutamine, which causes a mild hypotension to "stress" the heart.

Part 2. Approach to Clinical Problem Solving

There are typically 4 distinct steps to the systematic solving of clinical problems:

1. Making the diagnosis
2. Assessing the severity of the disease (stage)
3. Rendering a treatment based on the stage of the disease
4. Following the patient's response to the treatment

MAKING THE DIAGNOSIS

Introduction

There are 2 ways to make a diagnosis. Experienced clinicians often make a diagnosis very quickly using **pattern recognition**, that is, the features of the patient's illness match a scenario the physician has seen before. If it does not fit a readily recognized pattern, then one has to undertake several steps in diagnostic reasoning:

1. The first step is to **gather information with a differential diagnosis in mind**. The clinician should start considering diagnostic possibilities after recording the chief complaint and present illness. This differential diagnosis is continually refined as information is gathered. Historical questions and physical examination tests

and findings are all pursued tailored to the potential diagnoses one is considering. This is the principle that "you find what you are looking for." When one is trying to perform a thorough head-to-toe examination, for instance, without looking for anything in particular, one is much more likely to miss findings.

2. The next step is to try to move from subjective complaints or nonspecific symptoms to focus on objective abnormalities in an effort to **conceptualize the patient's objective problem with the greatest specificity one can achieve.** For example, a patient may come to the physician complaining of pedal edema, a relatively common and nonspecific finding. Laboratory testing may reveal that the patient has renal failure, a more specific cause of the many causes of edema. Examination of the urine may then reveal red blood cell casts, indicating glomerulonephritis, which is even more specific as the cause of the renal failure. The patient's problem, then, described with the greatest degree of specificity, is glomerulonephritis. The clinician's task at this point is to consider the differential diagnosis of glomerulonephritis rather than that of pedal edema.

3. The last step of the diagnostic process is to **look for discriminating features** of the patient's illness. This means the features of the illness, which by their presence or their absence most narrow the differential diagnosis. This is often difficult for junior learners because it requires a well-developed knowledge base of the typical features of disease, so the diagnostician can judge how much weight to assign to the various clinical clues present. For example, in the diagnosis of a patient with a fever and productive cough, the finding by chest x-ray of bilateral apical infiltrates with cavitation is highly discriminatory. There are few illnesses besides tuberculosis that are likely to produce that radiographic pattern. A negatively predictive example is a patient with exudative pharyngitis who also has rhinorrhea and cough. The presence of these features makes the diagnosis of streptococcal infection unlikely as the cause of the pharyngitis. Once the differential diagnosis has been constructed, the clinician uses the presence of discriminating features, knowledge of patient risk factors, and the epidemiology of diseases to decide which potential diagnoses are most likely.

CLINICAL PEARL

There are 3 steps in diagnostic reasoning:

1. Gathering information with a differential diagnosis in mind.
2. Identifying the objective abnormalities with the greatest specificity.
3. Looking for discriminating features to narrow the differential diagnosis.

Once the most specific problem has been identified, and a differential diagnosis of that problem is considered using discriminating features to order the possibilities, the next step is to consider using diagnostic testing, such as laboratory, radiologic, or pathologic data, to confirm the diagnosis. Quantitative reasoning in the use and interpretation of tests were discussed in the previous section. Clinically, the timing and effort with which one pursues a definitive diagnosis using objective data depends on several factors: the potential gravity of the diagnosis in question, the clinical state of the patient, the potential risks of diagnostic testing, and the potential benefits or harms of empiric treatment. For example, if a young man is admitted to the hospital with bilateral pulmonary nodules on chest x-ray, there are many possibilities including metastatic malignancy, and aggressive pursuit of a diagnosis is necessary, perhaps including a thoracotomy with an open-lung biopsy. The same radiographic findings in an elderly bed-bound woman with advanced Alzheimer dementia who would not be a good candidate for chemotherapy might be best left alone without any diagnostic testing. Decisions like this are difficult, require solid medical knowledge, as well as a thorough understanding of one's patient and the patient's background and inclinations, and constitute the art of medicine.

Assessing the Severity of the Disease

After ascertaining the diagnosis, the next step is to characterize the severity of the disease process; in other words, it is describing "how bad" a disease is. There is usually prognostic or treatment significance based on the stage. With malignancy, this is done formally by cancer staging. Most cancers are categorized from stage I (localized) to stage IV (widely metastatic). Some diseases, such as congestive heart failure, may be designated as mild, moderate, or severe based on the patient's functional status, that is, their ability to exercise before becoming dyspneic. With some infections, such as syphilis, the staging depends on the duration and extent of the infection, and follows along the natural history of the infection (ie, primary syphilis, secondary, latent period, and tertiary/neurosyphilis).

Treating Based on Stage

Many illnesses are stratified according to severity because prognosis and treatment often vary based on the severity. If neither the prognosis nor the treatment were affected by the stage of the disease process, there would not be a reason to subcategorize as to mild or severe. As an example, a man with mild chronic obstructive pulmonary disease (COPD) may be treated with inhaled bronchodilators as needed and advice for smoking cessation. However, an individual with severe COPD may need around-the-clock oxygen supplementation, scheduled bronchodilators, and possibly oral corticosteroid therapy.

The Treatment Should Be Tailored to the Extent or "Stage" of the Disease

In making decisions regarding treatment, it is also essential that the clinician identify the therapeutic objectives. When patients seek medical attention, it is generally because they are bothered by a symptom and want it to go away. When physicians institute therapy, they often have several other goals besides symptom relief, such as prevention of short- or long-term complications or a reduction in mortality. For example, patients with congestive heart failure are bothered by the symptoms of edema and dyspnea. Salt restriction, loop diuretics, and bedrest are effective at reducing these symptoms. However, heart failure is a progressive disease with a high mortality, so other treatments such as angiotensin-converting enzyme (ACE) inhibitors and some β-blockers are also used to reduce mortality in this condition. It is essential that the clinician know what the therapeutic objective is, so that one can monitor and guide therapy.

CLINICAL PEARL

- ► The clinician needs to identify the objectives of therapy: symptom relief, prevention of complications, or reduction in mortality.

Following the Response to Treatment

The final step in the approach to disease is to follow the patient's response to the therapy. The "measure" of response should be recorded and monitored. Some responses are clinical, such as the patient's abdominal pain, or temperature, or pulmonary examination. Obviously, the student must work on being more skilled in eliciting the data in an unbiased and standardized manner. Other responses may be followed by imaging tests, such as CT scan of a retroperitoneal node size in a patient receiving chemotherapy, or a tumor marker such as the prostate-specific antigen (PSA) level in a man receiving chemotherapy for prostatic cancer. For syphilis, it may be the nonspecific treponemal antibody test rapid plasma reagent (RPR) titer over time. The student must be prepared to know what to do if the measured marker does not respond according to what is expected. Is the next step to retreat, or to repeat the metastatic workup, or to follow-up with another more specific test?

Part 3. Approach to Reading

The clinical problem-oriented approach to reading is different from the classic "systematic" research of a disease. Patients rarely present with a clear diagnosis; hence, the student must become skilled in applying the textbook information to the clinical setting. Furthermore, one retains more information when one reads with a purpose. In other words, the student should read with the goal of answering specific questions. There are several fundamental questions that facilitate **clinical thinking**. These questions are:

1. What is the most likely diagnosis?
2. What should be your next step?
3. What is the most likely mechanism for this process?
4. What are the risk factors for this condition?
5. What are the complications associated with the disease process?
6. What is the best therapy?
7. How would you confirm the diagnosis?

CLINICAL PEARL

- Reading with the purpose of answering the 7 fundamental clinical questions improves retention of information and facilitates the application of "book knowledge" to "clinical knowledge."

WHAT IS THE MOST LIKELY DIAGNOSIS?

The method of establishing the diagnosis was discussed in the previous section. One way of attacking this problem is to develop standard "approaches" to common clinical problems. It is helpful to understand the most common causes of various presentations, such as "the most common causes of pancreatitis are gallstones and alcohol." (See the *Clinical Pearls* at end of each case.)

The clinical scenario would entail something such as:

A 28-year-old man presents to the emergency room with abdominal pain, nausea and vomiting, and an elevated amylase level. What is the most likely diagnosis?

With no other information to go on, the student would note that this man has a clinical diagnosis of pancreatitis. Using the "most common cause" information, the student would make an educated guess that the patient has either alcohol abuse or gallstones. "The ultrasonogram of the gallbladder shows no stones."

CLINICAL PEARL

- The two most common causes of pancreatitis are gallstones and alcohol abuse.

Now, the student would use the phrase "patients without gallstones who have pancreatitis most likely abuse alcohol." Aside from these 2 causes, there are many other etiologies of pancreatitis.

WHAT SHOULD BE YOUR NEXT STEP?

This question is difficult because the next step may be more diagnostic information, or staging, or therapy. It may be more challenging than "the most likely diagnosis," because there may be insufficient information to make a diagnosis and the next step may be to pursue more diagnostic information. Another possibility is that there is enough information for a probable diagnosis and the next step is to stage the disease. Finally, the most appropriate action may be to treat. Hence, from clinical data, a judgment needs to be rendered regarding how far along one is on the road of:

Make a diagnosis → stage the disease → treat based on stage → follow response

Frequently, the student is "taught" to regurgitate the same information that someone has written about a particular disease, but is not skilled at giving the next step. This talent is learned optimally at the bedside, in a supportive environment, with freedom to make educated guesses, and with constructive feedback. A sample scenario may describe a student's thought process as follows.

1. **Make the diagnosis:** "Based on the information I have, I believe that Mr Smith has stable angina *because* he has retrosternal chest pain when he walks 3 blocks, but it is relieved within minutes by rest and with sublingual nitroglycerin."
2. **Stage the disease:** "I don't believe that this is severe disease because he does not have pain lasting for more than 5 minutes, angina at rest, or congestive heart failure."
3. **Treat based on stage:** "Therefore, my next step is to treat with aspirin, β-blockers, and sublingual nitroglycerin as needed, as well as lifestyle changes."
4. **Follow response:** "I want to follow the treatment by assessing his pain (I will ask him about the degree of exercise he is able to perform without chest pain), perform a cardiac stress test, and reassess him after the test is done."

In a similar patient, when the clinical presentation is unclear or more severe, perhaps the best "next step" may be diagnostic in nature such as thallium stress test or even coronary angiography. The **next step** depends upon the **clinical state of the patient** (if unstable, the next step is therapeutic), the **potential severity** of the disease (the next step may be staging), or the **uncertainty of the diagnosis** (the next step is diagnostic).

Usually, the vague question, "What is your next step?" is the most difficult question, because the answer may be diagnostic, staging, or therapeutic.

WHAT IS THE LIKELY MECHANISM FOR THIS PROCESS?

This question goes further than making the diagnosis, but also requires the student to understand the underlying mechanism for the process. For example, a clinical scenario may describe an "18-year-old woman who presents with several months of severe epistaxis, heavy menses, petechiae, and a normal CBC except for a platelet count of $15,000/mm^3$." Answers that a student may consider to explain this condition include immune-mediated platelet destruction, drug-induced thrombocytopenia, bone marrow suppression, and platelet sequestration as a result of hypersplenism.

The student is advised to learn the mechanisms for each disease process, and not merely memorize a constellation of symptoms. In other words, rather than solely committing to memory the classic presentation of idiopathic thrombocytopenic purpura (ITP) (isolated thrombocytopenia without lymphadenopathy or offending drugs), the student should understand that ITP is an autoimmune process whereby the body produces IgG antibodies against the platelets. The platelets-antibody complexes are then taken from the circulation in the spleen. Because the disease process is specific for platelets, the other 2 cell lines (erythrocytes and leukocytes) are normal. Also, because the thrombocytopenia is caused by excessive platelet peripheral destruction, the bone marrow will show increased megakaryocytes (platelet precursors). Hence, treatment for ITP includes oral corticosteroid agents to decrease the immune process of antiplatelet IgG production, and, if refractory, then splenectomy.

WHAT ARE THE RISK FACTORS FOR THIS PROCESS?

Understanding the risk factors helps the practitioner to establish a diagnosis and to determine how to interpret tests. For example, understanding the risk factor analysis may help manage a 45-year-old obese man with sudden onset of dyspnea and pleuritic chest pain following an orthopedic surgery for a femur fracture. This patient has numerous risk factors for deep venous thrombosis and pulmonary embolism. The physician may want to pursue angiography even if the ventilation/perfusion scan result is low probability. Thus, the number of risk factors helps categorize the likelihood of a disease process.

CLINICAL PEARL

- When the pretest probability of a test is highly likely, based on risk factors, even with a negative initial test, more definitive testing may be indicated.

WHAT ARE THE COMPLICATIONS TO THIS PROCESS?

A clinician must understand the complications of a disease so that one may monitor the patient. Sometimes the student has to make the diagnosis from clinical clues and then apply his/her knowledge of the sequelae of the pathological process. For example, the student should know that chronic hypertension may affect various end organs, such as the brain (encephalopathy or stroke), the eyes (vascular changes), the kidneys, and the heart. Understanding the types of consequences also helps the clinician to be aware of the dangers to a patient. The clinician is acutely aware of the need to monitor for the end-organ involvement and undertakes the appropriate intervention when involvement is present.

WHAT IS THE BEST THERAPY?

To answer this question, the clinician needs to reach the correct diagnosis, assess the severity of the condition, and weigh the situation to reach the appropriate intervention. For the student, knowing exact dosages is not as important as understanding the best medication, the route of delivery, mechanism of action, and possible complications. It is important for the student to be able to verbalize the diagnosis and the rationale for the therapy. A common error is for the student to "jump to a treatment," like a random guess, and therefore is given "right or wrong" feedback. In fact, the student's guess may be correct, but for the wrong reason; conversely, the answer may be a very reasonable one, with only one small error in thinking. Instead, the student should verbalize the steps so that feedback may be given at every reasoning point.

For example, if the question is, "What is the best therapy for a 25-year-old man who complains of a cough, fever, and a 2-month history of 10 lb weight loss?" The incorrect manner of response is for the student to blurt out "trimethoprim/sulfa." Rather, the student should reason it out in a way similar to this: "The most common cause of a cough and fever and weight loss in a young man is either HIV infection with *Pneumocystis jiroveci* pneumonia or malignancy such as lymphoma. Therefore, the best treatment for this man is either antimicrobial therapy such as with trimethoprim/sulfa, or chemotherapy after confirmation of the diagnosis."

CLINICAL PEARL

- ▶ Therapy should be logical and based on the severity of disease. Antibiotic therapy should be tailored for specific organisms.

HOW WOULD YOU CONFIRM THE DIAGNOSIS?

In the previous scenario, there is a wide differential diagnosis involving the man with a weight loss, fever, and cough, but two common disorders are *Pneumocystis carinii* pneumonia (PCP) or malignancy. Chest radiograph, or CT imaging of the chest, with possible Gallium scanning may be helpful. Knowing the limitations of diagnostic tests and the manifestations of disease aid in this area.

Summary

1. There is no replacement for a careful history and physical examination.
2. There are 4 steps to the clinical approach to the patient: making the diagnosis, assessing severity, treating based on severity, and following response.
3. Assessment of pretest probability and knowledge of test characteristics are essential in the application of test results to the clinical situation.
4. There are 7 questions that help bridge the gap between the textbook and the clinical arena.

REFERENCES

Bordages G. Elaborated knowledge: a key to successful diagnostic thinking. *Acad Med.* 1994;69(11): 883-885.

Hall JB, Schmidt GA, Wood LDH. An approach to critical care. In: *Principles of Critical Care.* 3rd ed. New York, NY: McGraw-Hill; 2005:P3-10.

Gross R. *Making Medical Decisions.* Philadelphia, PA: American College of Physicians; 1999.

Marino PL, Sutin KM. *The ICU Book.* 3rd ed. Philadelphia, PA: Lippincott Williams & Wilkins; 2007.

Mark DB. Decision-making in clinical medicine. In: Fauci AS, Braunwald E, Kasper KL, et al, eds. *Harrison's Principles of Internal Medicine.* 17th ed. New York, NY: McGraw-Hill; 2008:16-23.

SECTION II

Clinical Cases

CASE 1

Just prior to being discharged from the hospital, a patient on the general medicine ward began to display abnormal "vital signs." The patient is a 55-year-old man who was admitted 3 days prior for renal colic and hydronephrosis. His respiratory rate (RR) is 25 breaths/minute, blood pressure (BP) is 84 mm Hg/46 mm Hg, temperature is 101°Fahrenheit (F), and heart rate (HR) is 130 beats/minute with a regular rhythm. His oxygen saturation (O_2 sat) is 80% on ambient air (RA). The patient is confused and answers questions slowly but correctly. A rapid response team (RRT) is called to initiate goal-directed treatment.

- What is the most likely diagnosis?
- How would one gauge the severity of the patient's condition?
- What are the next steps in treatment and what should be done within the first hour of this patient's presentation?

ANSWERS TO CASE 1: Early Awareness of Critical Illness

Summary: A 55-year-old man admitted for renal colic and hydronephrosis is now showing signs of sepsis, and septic shock with multiorgan involvement. The focus of the infection is the urinary tract and that should determine the antibiotic choices. The presence of tachycardia, tachypnea, hypotension, hypoxemia, and low urine output combined with a decreased mental status are all responses to sepsis. **Cancel discharge, administer a fluid bolus of 20 mL/kg of normal saline, start rapid response team measures, and transfer the patient to the ICU.**

- **Most likely diagnosis:** The most likely diagnosis is sepsis, with systemic inflammatory response syndrome (SIRS) and multiple organ dysfunction (MOD) likely caused by obstructive pyelonephritis.
- **Assessment of severity:** An early warning score based on deviations of vital signs is a good objective way to assess severity of potentially critically ill patients. This patient's instability indicates a need for immediate medical attention.
- **Next steps in treatment:** The first interventions to be considered are addressing the severe hypoxemia, aggressive hydration to restore blood pressure, improve tachycardia, and increase cardiac and urine output.
- **Management priority during the first hour:** Administer the correct antibiotic(s) with coverage for the most common pathogens. Goal-directed treatment should follow the surviving sepsis guidelines. The obstructed, infected ureter/kidney should be drained.

ANALYSIS

Objectives

1. To recognize the early signs of critical illnesses.
2. To be familiar with the treatment strategies to correct abnormal vital signs and early goal-directed therapy.

Considerations

The patient described in this scenario was about to be discharged from the hospital. The nurse called regarding abnormal vital signs, which were dramatically altered from normal. The hypotension, tachycardia, hypoxemia, and confusion are very worrisome. For instance, the oxygen saturation of 80% likely correlates to an oxygen partial pressure of 45 mm Hg, which is incompatible with life. Thus, the first intervention is oxygen! This hospital has a rapid response team, which is a multidisciplinary team that assesses patients quickly when there are potential critical illnesses. The rapid response team then uses an efficient protocol regarding its objective evaluation of the patient's clinical status. A delay in assessment, recognition, or therapy could lead to adverse consequences, including death.

APPROACH TO:

Early Recognition of Critical Illness

Early awareness of a critical illness is crucial in order to reduce its morbidity and mortality. The mortality rate is about 5% among all hospitalized patients but increases to 15% in patients admitted to an intensive care unit (ICU). In cases of sepsis and acute lung injury, the death rate can approach 50%. Critical care is extremely costly and ICU costs represent about 15% of all hospital expenses. The recently developed rapid response teams or medical emergency teams which consist of a group of clinicians and nurses, brings critical care expertise to the bedside. Their early intervention with IV fluids and antibiotics for hospitalized patients who show early signs of sepsis with hemodynamic deterioration, such as tachycardia, low blood pressure, low urine output, fever, and changes in mental status has markedly lowered both morbidity and mortality.

Rapid response teams. Earlier detection of a patient's clinical deterioration provides a great opportunity to prove Ben Franklin's adage that "an ounce of prevention is worth a pound of cure." Rapid response teams are aimed at intervening as soon as possible before the patient's condition deteriorates and help ensure optimal outcome. Since most patients in this situation require respiratory care, respiratory therapists (RTs) have been considered key team members, and most hospitals have already implemented these teams with an RT member. In addition, a critical care nurse, a physician, a physician's assistant, and/or pharmacist are all important members of the team. Their expertise has drastically reduced both the incidence of cardiac arrests and subsequent deaths. It has also decreased the number of days in an ICU, hospital days, and the number of in-patient deaths. This has resulted in an increase in the number of patients who are discharged in a functional state.

Scoring systems utilizing routine observations and vital signs taken by the nursing and ancillary staff are used to evaluate the possible deterioration of patients. This deterioration is frequently preceded by a further decline in physiological parameters. Furthermore, a failure of the clinical staff to recognize this failure in respiratory or cerebral function will put patients at risk of cardiac arrest. Suboptimal care prior to admission to an ICU leads to increased mortality. Because of resource limitations, the number of patients that can be monitored and treated in an ICU is limited. The selection of patients who might benefit most from critical care is crucial. The early identification of in-patients at risk of deterioration based on measurements of physiological parameters will reduce the number of pre-ICU resuscitations required.

Early awareness score (EWS). The EWS is a tool for bedside evaluation based on **5 physiological parameters: systolic blood pressure (BP), pulse rate (PR), respiratory rate (RR), temperature, and response of the central nervous system (CNS).** The purpose of RRTs is to use protocols, which will recognize deteriorating hemodynamics as quickly as possible. This treatment can be initiated before the MD or intensivist arrives who may then give further individualized orders.

Precautions to prevent aspiration such as elevation of the head of the bed to 30° to 45° should be instituted whenever there is a change in mental status, or increased risk of aspiration, provided the current blood pressure allows this. The patient should

Table 1–1 • HEMODYNAMIC INSTABILITY	
Instability Indicated by 1 or More of the Following	**Inadequate Perfusion Indicated by 1 or More of the Following**
Hypotension	+ Lactic acidosis, >2 mmol
Tachycardia unresponsive to treatment	+ New abnormal capillary refill (>3 seconds)
Orthostatic vital sign changes	+ Reduced urine output
Multiple IV fluid boluses required to maintain adequate blood pressure or perfusion	+ New altered mental status
IV inotropic or vasopressor medication to maintain adequate blood pressure or perfusion	+ Cool, mottled extremities, body.

be transferred to the ICU for further treatment and provided continuous monitoring and goal-directed therapy based on the surviving sepsis guidelines. Cardiac arrest has been associated with the failure to correct physiological derangement in oxygenation (breathing), hypotension (blood pressure), and mental status (see Table 1–1). These features may be apparent up to 8 hours prior to eventual cardiac arrest. The introduction of the rapid response system has accelerated an early referral to the ICU and in many cases has avoided an ICU admission when the patient has a good early response and reaches clinical stability quickly.

VITAL SIGNS

Respiratory rate. The respiratory rate varies with age, but the normal reference range for an adult is 12 to 20 breaths/minute. The respiratory rate is an indicator of potential respiratory dysfunction. An elevated RR >25 to 30 breaths/minute is a poor prognostic factor in patients with pneumonia, congestive heart failure (CHF), and other illnesses such as chronic obstructive pulmonary disease (COPD).

Blood pressure. Blood pressure (BP) is measured by 2 readings; a high systolic (ventricular contraction) pressure and the lower diastolic (ventricular filling) pressure. A BP (mm Hg) of 120 systolic over 80 diastolic is considered normal. The difference between the systolic and diastolic pressure is called the pulse pressure (PP). A low or narrow PP suggests significant intravascular volume loss. If the pulse pressure is extremely low, <25 mm Hg, the cause may be a decreased low stroke volume as in CHF or shock. A narrow pulse pressure value is also caused by aortic stenosis and cardiac tamponade. **There is no absolute natural or "normal" value for BP, but rather a range of values. When excessively elevated, these values are associated with an increased risk of stroke and heart disease. Blood pressure is usually taken at the arms but may also be taken at the lower level of the legs, this is called segmental BP and evaluates blockage or arterial occlusion in a limb.**

Pulse. The pulse is the result of the physical expansion of the artery. The pulse rate is usually measured at the wrist or at the ankle and is recorded as beats/minute. The pulse is commonly taken at the radial artery. If the pulse cannot be taken at the wrist, it may be taken at the elbow (brachial artery), at the neck against the carotid artery (carotid pulse), behind the knee (popliteal artery), or in the foot (dorsalis pedis or posterior tibial arteries). The pulse rate can also be measured by listening directly to the heartbeat using a stethoscope. An irregular pulse with regular skips is very suggestive of atrial fibrillation. Rates <60 or rates >100 are defined as bradycardia and tachycardia, respectively. When there is a rapid, regular pulse, sinus tachycardia and supraventricular tachycardia should be considered.

Temperature. An elevated temperature is an important indicator of illness, especially when preceded by **chills**. Systemic infection or inflammation is indicated by the presence of a fever (temperature >38.5°C or sustained temperature >38°C), or a significant elevation of the temperature above the individual's normal temperature. Fever will increase the heart rate by 10 beats/minute with every Fahrenheit (F) degree above normal. **Temperature depression (hypothermia)**, <95°F, should also be evaluated since it is an ominous sign for severe disease and is more threatening than hyperthermia. Body temperature is maintained through a balance of the heat produced by the body and the heat lost from the body. Antipyretics should not be withheld. The patient should be made comfortable and fluid repletion should be used to counter the fever induced fluid losses. The absence of fever does not indicate the absence of infection. High spiking fevers in the 104°F to 105°F range are less likely septic and may represent a drug allergy or blood transfusion reaction. Fever and other vital signs are keys to the diagnosis of the systemic inflammatory response syndrome (SIRS). See Table 1–2.

Sepsis is defined as **SIRS** in response to a **confirmed infectious process. Severe sepsis** is defined as **sepsis with organ dysfunction, hypoperfusion, or hypotension. Septic shock** is defined as **sepsis-induced hypotension or hypoperfusion abnormalities despite adequate fluid resuscitation.**

The fifth vital sign. The phrase "fifth vital sign" usually refers to **pain** or the **oxygen saturation measurement.** Pupil size, equality in pupil size, and reactivity to light can also be used as a vital signs. Many emergency medical service (EMS) agencies use pulse oximetry and blood glucose levels as vital signs in addition to pulse rate, respiratory rate, and blood pressure. A **pulse oximetry saturation of 90% to 92% represents a P_{AO_2} near 60 mm Hg** and should be the minimal goal of O_2 supplementation. The 90% O_2sat point represents the elbow of the hemoglobin dissociation curve, whereas below this number there is rapid hemoglobin desaturation; above this number there is little gained in O_2 carrying capacity of the hemoglobin.

PROTOCOL-BASED CARE

Protocols are decision-making tools in which differential interventions are applied based on explicit directions and regular patient assessments. Whether implemented by physicians, nonphysician providers, or nurses, protocols serve to standardize care practices, reduce unnecessary variation in care, and aid in the implementation of evidence-based therapies. Protocols have been associated with improvements in the quality of critical care. These include protocols for sedation, weaning from mechanical ventilation, lung protective ventilation in acute lung injury, early adequate resuscitation in severe sepsis, and moderate glucose control in post–cardiac surgery patients.

Protocol-based care offers a unique opportunity to improve the care of patients who do not have access to an intensivist. Nurses, pharmacists, and respiratory therapists can

Table 1–2 • SYSTEMIC INFLAMMATORY RESPONSE SYNDROME (SIRS, 2 OR MORE OF THE FOLLOWING)

Temperature >38.0°C (100.4°F) or <36.0°C (96.8°F)
Heart rate >90 beats/minute
Respiratory rate >20 breaths/minute or pCO_2 <32 mm Hg
Leukocyte count >12,000/μL or <4000/μL, or >10% band forms

implement protocols successfully. Hospitalists specializing in acute care should be able to provide necessary physician services in the ICU and make minute-to-minute decisions governed by protocols. Protocols are not superior to major decisions made by a qualified intensivist or physician. In settings with optimal physician staffing, protocols have not consistently resulted in improved outcomes; however, few ICUs are staffed with the trained intensivists and multidisciplinary clinicians necessary to provide such optimal care. The evidence suggests that outcomes are improved when routine care decisions are standardized and taken out of the hands of individuals.

There are a myriad of laboratory data that can be obtained quickly to aid in the diagnosis and treatment of patients. Electrocardiography, arterial blood gas, electrolytes levels, O_2 saturation, cardiac enzyme analyses, echocardiography, CT scanning and ultrasound, are all examples of such tests. The proper evaluation of the patient's physical condition and vital signs will enable a quick and correct application of the proper treatment. The **differential diagnosis of a patient's problems should immediately identify the most catastrophic but reversible and treatable events.**

The current gold standard for the organization of critical care services is the incorporation of an intensivist in the multidisciplinary care team. The intensivist is responsible for overseeing the multidisciplinary, collaborative team of nurses, clinical pharmacists, respiratory therapists, and nutritionists. Intensivist-led multidisciplinary care is endorsed as a key to successful evidence-based practice for the management of critically ill patients.

CLINICAL CASE CORRELATION

- **See also Case 2 (transfer of critically ill patients), Case 3 (scoring systems and patient prognosis), and Case 4 (monitoring).**

COMPREHENSION QUESTIONS

1.1 A 71-year-old woman is brought to the ICU from a nursing home because of confusion, fever, and flank pain. On physical examination, her temperature is 38.5°C (101.3°F), blood pressure is 82/48 mm Hg, heart rate is 123 beats/minute, and respiration rate is 30 breaths/minute. Dry mucous membranes, costovertebral angle tenderness, poor skin turgor, and an absence of edema are noted on physical examination. The leukocyte count is 15,600/μL; urinalysis shows 50 to 100 leukocytes and many bacteria per high power field. The patient has an anion-gap metabolic acidosis and high lactic acid level. Antibiotic therapy is started. Which of the following is most likely to improve the survival of this patient?

A. Aggressive fluid resuscitation
B. 25% albumin infusion
C. Hemodynamic monitoring with a pulmonary artery catheter
D. Maintaining hemoglobin above 12 g/dL
E. Maintaining P_{CO_2} below 50 mm Hg

1.2 A 29-year-old man underwent an elective laparoscopic gall bladder surgery which was uneventful. The evening after surgery, the nurse is alarmed due to the patient's complaint of abdominal pain and a 3 gm/dL drop from his preoperative hemoglobin level, HR of 130 beats/minute, BP of 80/40 mm Hg, and urine output of 120 cc over the past 8 hours.

Which of the following is the most likely diagnosis?

A. Septic shock
B. Hemorrhagic shock
C. Cardiogenic shock
D. Pulmonary embolism
E. Anaphylactic shock

ANSWERS TO QUESTIONS

1.1 **A.** Aggressive fluid resuscitation with resolution of lactic acidosis within the first 6 hours has a beneficial effect on the survival of patients with severe sepsis. This patient has severe sepsis presumptively from pyelonephritis. The timing of resuscitation influences survival. Early goal-directed therapy that included interventions delivered within the first 6 hours to maintain a central venous oxygen saturation of >70% and to effect a resolution of lactic acidosis resulted in higher survival rates than more delayed resuscitation attempts. Crystalloid is given much more frequently than colloid, and there are no data to support routinely using colloid in lieu of crystalloid. Blood transfusions may be part of the resuscitation effort for anemic patients in shock. In stable ICU patients who are not in shock, a transfusion threshold of 7 g/dL of hemoglobin is an acceptable conservative approach, but this does not apply to the treatment of patients with severe sepsis, where having a hematocrit <30% is reason for transfusion.

1.2 **B.** This patient has hypotension and tachycardia and also oliguria. The urine output is <0.5 cc/kg/h. This constellation of findings in a postoperative patient is most consistent with hemorrhagic shock, or hypovolemic shock. There is likely to be an intra-abdominal vascular injury unless proven otherwise. The first steps in treating this patient should include placement of 2 large bore IVs, infusion of normal saline rapidly, and rapid assessment for intraabdominal hemorrhage and its surgical correction if confirmed.

CLINICAL PEARLS

- Early recognition of changes in the vital signs and the mental status are critical to the early detection of patient deterioration and the prevention of cardiac arrest.
- Continuous or bedside spot monitoring of oxygen saturation is now considered the fifth vital sign and provides accurate pulse readings and PaO_2 approximation (ABG, Svo_2 sat).
- The phrase "fifth vital sign" can refer to pain or O_2 saturation as a vital sign.
- Protocol-driven rapid response teams have significantly decreased the mortality and morbidity of in-patients and significantly reduced cardiac arrests in the hospital setting.
- Oxygen saturation via oxymetry of 90% is equivalent to a PaO_2 of 60 mm Hg, the elbow of the hemoglobin dissociation curve, and the acceptable minimum in O_2 saturation.
- Fever and other vital signs are keys to the diagnosis of the systemic inflammatory response syndrome (SIRS) and can be caused by sepsis as well as noninfectious causes.

REFERENCES

Clifford S, Deutschman MS. *Evidence-Based Practice of Critical Care*. Philadelphia, PA: Saunders; 2010.

Loscalzo J. *Harrison's Pulmonary and Critical Care Medicine*. New York, NY: McGraw-Hill; 2010.

Rhodes A, Bennett ED. Early goal-directed therapy: an evidence-based review. *Crit Care Med.* 2004; 32:S448-S450.

Rubenfeld GD, Caldwell E, Peabody E, et al. Incidence and outcomes of acute lung injury. *N Engl J Med.* 2005;353:1685-1693.

Toy E, Simon B, Takenaka K, Liu T, Rosh A. *Case Files Emergency Medicine*. 2nd ed. New York, NY: McGraw-Hill/Lange Medical Books, 2013.

CASE 2

A 55-year-old black man presents to the intensive care unit (ICU) with an acute anterior ST segment elevation myocardial infarction (STEMI). Consultation with a cardiologist indicates that the best treatment is percutaneous coronary angiography (PTCA). An alternative is the possible insertion of coronary artery stents with backup open cardiac bypass surgery, which is available at a transfer facility 30 minutes away. At the current facility, tissue plasminogen activator (TPA) is the only treatment option available. On arrival the patient was given 325 mg of aspirin, started on a heparin infusion, and nitroglycerin intravenous infusion, supplemented with a loading dose of clopidogrel. This occurred within 1 hour of symptoms.

- ▶ What are the key conditions that must be stabilized and secured when transferring a critically ill patient between facilities?
- ▶ What is involved in intra-hospital (within the same facility) transportation (IHT) of the critically ill patient?
- ▶ What other arrangements should be performed prior to interhospital transfer?

ANSWERS TO CASE 2:
Transfer of the ICU Patient

Summary: This 55-year-old man presents with a STEMI of acute onset and needs transfer for a PTCA with possible stenting, which is not available at the present facility. Transfer under acceptable transportation guidelines to a facility, which has PTCA, should be the best choice for his medical treatment and offers the best possible outcome.

- **Key conditions needing stabilization:** Stabilize the patient's vital signs, begin indicated emergency therapy, and arrange transfer to a new facility with the same treatments and personnel available in the ICU. Personnel experienced in transferring critically ill patients should be incorporated into the transfer.
- **IHT of the critically ill:** (1) Transport the patient safely with documented appropriate reason for leaving the ICU. (2) The same monitoring that the patient was receiving in the ICU must continue during the patient's transportation and his stay outside the ICU.
- **Other arrangements prior to arrival at the new facility:** (1) Prearrange acceptance prior to arrival at the accepting facility. (2) Activation of key personnel is important to avoid an interruption in patient care. (3) An agreement regarding optimal transfer methods should be reached. The fastest and safest route of transfer is the best choice. (4) The transport method chosen should have all equipment needed to enable a safe transfer.

ANALYSIS

Objectives

1. Describe how to assess the benefits and risks of transferring the critically ill patient.
2. Discuss the modalities of inter-hospital transfer the their advantages and disadvantages.
3. Describe the key requirements for transfer of the critically ill patient.
4. List the adverse effects of intra and inter-hospital transfer of ICU patients.

Considerations

Before transfer is attempted, it must be demonstrated that there is a clear benefit in the treatment available at the receiving facility compared to the current facility. The patient in this scenario is a 55-year-old with an ST elevation myocardial infarction, and he would be best served by a PTCA, which is unavailable at his current hospital. After assuring stabilization and the absence of life-threatening conditions or arrhythmias, he can be transferred with appropriate monitoring and personnel. The accepting institution is 30 minutes away which is a reasonable distance for transport. Communication and coordination are key to a successful transfer.

APPROACH TO: Transferring the Critically Ill Patient

Providing appropriate care during transport to and from the ICU presents a major challenge. Critical care transport has become a common occurrence. The centralization of therapeutic specialties and an expanding number of diagnostic and therapeutic options outside of the ICU are major causes of this necessity. Bringing improved diagnostic testing and medical-surgical services to the patient reduces the adverse effects that accompany transportation outside the ICU. Infection rates are also lower in patients who are transported less often in the ICU setting. Most instances of critical care transport occur within the hospital itself. **Nevertheless, critical care transport is a high-risk undertaking, regardless of the setting.** Adequate planning, proper equipment, and appropriate staffing can minimize the transportation risks. Inter-hospital transport of the critically ill patient presents more problems than in-house transport because of the distance, different hospital settings, and inability for prior planning. Guidelines of personnel needs such as physicians, nurses, and paramedics have come from these experiences. Alternative advantages and disadvantages in transport by air or ground are also necessarily weighed. Specific treatments such as pre-transfer tracheal intubation and other advanced life support conditions may be required (Table 2–1).

Significant physiologic disturbances occur frequently in patients during their IHT including variations in heart rate, BP, or O_2 saturation. However, physiologic variability is also common in critically ill patients in stationary circumstances, occurring in 60% of such patients compared with 66% in transported patients. An appropriately

Table 2–1 • HOSPITAL TRANSFER TERMINOLOGY

Terminology	Description
Clinical transfer	A patient is transferred to another hospital for tertiary care or facilities that are not available within the host hospital
Nonclinical transfer	A patient is transferred from a hospital due to insufficient bed capacity
Readmission	A patient is transferred back to the referring hospital when a suitable bed becomes available
Critically ill patient	A patient at risk of or showing signs of deterioration and who requires transfer to an area providing higher levels of care for any form of organ support (Level 2 or Level 3 patients)
Level 2	Level 2 patients require detailed observation or intervention including support for a single failing organ system or postoperative care. In addition, those patients stepping down from a higher level of care are classified as Level 2 patients
Level 3	Level 3 patients require advanced respiratory support alone or basic respiratory support together with support of at least 2 organ systems. This level includes all complex patients requiring support for MOD

trained transport team can safely manage these physiologic changes, but even so, serious adverse events do occur. Cardiac arrest rates of 1.6% have been noted during IHT. Reduction in the PAO_2/FIO_2 ratio occurred in patients when transported while using a transport ventilator and severe changes (ie, >20% reduction from baseline) were common. These changes persisted for >24 hours in 20% of transportees. Out-of-unit transport was an independent risk factor for ventilator-associated pneumonia (VAP). IHT is also one of the factors associated with unplanned extubation in the mechanically ventilated patient. Compared to matched controls of patients not requiring transport, IHT individuals had a higher mortality rate (28.6% vs 11.4%) and a longer length of stay in the ICU. The increase in mortality was not directly attributable to complications of the transport, and reflected a higher severity of illness in patients who required transportation. Serious adverse events did, however, occur in 6% of all transports. See Table 2–2 which follows.

Transport problems were the cause of complications. Rechecking the patient and equipment and assurance of skilled assistance prior to transfer were important preventative measures.

Transport from the operating room to the ICU. Hemodynamic variability is more common in patients being transferred from the operating room to the ICU than those transported for diagnostic procedures outside the ICU. This is probably related to the patient's emergence from anesthesia. Accurate and complete information is important in these transfers. Ideally, both the medical team (surgeon and anesthesiologist) and nursing team should communicate important information to the ICU team. A directed form to ensure that proper information is transmitted can be useful. Likewise, a clear understanding of which physician will be responsible for what aspect of the patient's care is vital.

Risk and benefit of IHT. Studies suggest that IHT is important in many circumstances. Diagnostic testing made available through IHT has been found to result in treatment changes in up to 39% of patients. Radiologic studies in ICU patients can help in directing important changes in the therapy.

Management of transport. Studies have shown that ventilators used in transport are known to reduce variability in blood gas parameters when compared with manual bagging. Nevertheless, manual bagging with a tidal volume monitor was shown to be superior to mechanical ventilation (MV). No significant variations in blood gas parameters were noted in transport patients who received

Table 2–2 • PREDICTIVE ADVERSE EVENTS DURING INTRA-HOSPITAL TRANSPORT BY RISK FACTORS

1. Pre-transport secondary insults in head-injured patients	2. FIO_2 levels higher than 50% are predictive of respiratory deterioration on transport
3. High injury severity score, age >43 years	4. The number of intravenous pumps and infusions
5. High therapeutic interventions severity score (TISS) but not Acute Physiology and Chronic Health Evaluation scoring system (APACHEII) score	6. The time spent outside the unit has been shown to correlate with the number of technical mishaps

manual ventilation when under supervision by a respiratory therapist. Changes in blood gas parameters correlate with hemodynamic disturbances like arrhythmias and hypotension. Capnometry ($ETCO_2$) monitoring clearly reduces $PACO_2$ variability in adults. In children, less than one-third of patients undergoing manual ventilation without $ETCO_2$ monitoring had ventilator parameters within the intended range.

Hypothermia. Active warming during transport prevents hypothermia, which is common in trauma patients undergoing IHT. The use of specially trained transport teams was associated with much lower complications than historical controls. The presence of physicians during transport was not clearly correlated with a reduced risk for mishap.

Interhospital transfer. The benefits to the patient of the higher care at another facility should be weighed against the considerable risks of the transport process.

Adverse effects. The interhospital transport of critically ill patients is associated with an increased morbidity and mortality during and after the journey. Even with specialist mobile intensive care teams, the mortality before and during transport is substantial (2.5%) despite a low incidence of preventable deaths during transport (0.02%-0.04%). Others have reported an even higher intertransport mortality rate and have found that 24% to 70% of such incidents are avoidable. Physiologic derangements occur during 25% to 34% of adult and 10% to 20% of neonatal and pediatric transports. In **adults**, these disturbances are **most often respiratory or cardiovascular, the most common being arterial desaturation,** a reduced PAO_2/FIO_2 ratio (hypoxemia), arterial hypotension and tachycardia, respectively. The long-term outlook for critically ill patients who require interhospital transport is poorer than for those who do not require transport. **Transported patients have a higher ICU mortality and longer ICU stays than do controls.** Studies have found a 4% increase in mortality in the transferred group despite adjustments for diagnosis. It is unclear whether this resulted from the loss of time or unaccounted confounding variables, which resulted in an increased mortality as a result of an increase in the severity of the patient's illness.

Prediction of adverse events. The prediction of patient deterioration during interhospital transport has proven difficult. The APACHE II, TISS, and rapid acute physiology score (RAPS) systems do not correlate with events in adults, and the pediatric risk of mortality (PRISM) score has proven similarly unreliable in children. The variables that predict deterioration in adults include **older age, high FIO_2 requirements, multiple injury, and inadequate stabilization**.

Planning of the transport. The importance of planning and preparing for IHT cannot be overstated. Poor plans lead to an increased incidence of adverse events and mortality. In an audit of transfers to a neurosurgical center, 43% of patients were found to have inadequate injury assessment and 24% of individuals received inadequate resuscitation. Deficiencies in assessment and resuscitation before transfer were identified in all patients who died. Guidelines have been developed to address this issue in many jurisdictions, but inadequate assessment and resuscitation remain a problem. Some found that the application of national guidelines led to only modest improvements in patient care, with an incidence of hypoxia and hypotension that remains unacceptably high.

Selection of personnel. A **minimum of 2 people** in addition to the vehicle operators should accompany a critically ill patient during transport. The team leader can be a nurse or physician depending on clinical and local circumstances. It is imperative that the team leader has adequate training in transport medicine and advanced cardiac life support (ACLS). Adequately trained nurses and physicians are acceptable in transporting critically ill children. Appropriately staffed and equipped specialist retrieval teams are superior to impromptu teams in transferring critically ill adults and children, and have recorded up to an 80% reduction in critical incidents during pediatric interhospital transport.

Mode of transport. The choice among the 3 options of ground, helicopter, and fixed wing transport is affected by 3 main factors: distance, patient status, and weather conditions. A retrospective review of adult transfers demonstrated no difference in mortality or morbidity between patients transferred by air versus ground transportation. A prospective cohort study revealed that air transport is faster than ground transport, and for transfers of <225 km, helicopter transport is faster than by fixed wing. Severely injured patients undergoing interhospital transport had a reduced mortality when carried by air compared to surface transport.

Equipment and monitoring. Comprehensive lists of equipment and medications needed for the transport of critically ill patients should be identical to that in an ICU environment. The transport ventilators used in intra-hospital transfers create less ventilatory fluctuation than hand ventilation (Ambu bagging). However, when compared to standard ICU ventilators, transport ventilators were inferior in delivering set tidal volume (V_t) and had a tendency to trap gas. Extra care in ventilatory monitoring is warranted when changing from an ICU to a transport ventilator. Arterial blood gas (ABG) analysis during interhospital transfer allows for an early identification and treatment of changes in gas exchange and metabolic parameters.

Pre-hospital personnel, pre-hospital time, and receiving care facility. When compared with EMT pre-hospital care, physician pre-hospital management of trauma patients have shown to reduce trauma related deaths. Physicians tend to treat patients more aggressively than EMTs. When pre-hospital care is delayed more than 60 minutes, severely injured patients are at higher risk for death, increased length of hospital stay, and complications. There is a reduction in mortality for severely injured trauma patients when they are transferred directly to a Level I trauma center. Patients treated primarily in Level I trauma centers had lower 1-year mortality rates than patients treated elsewhere. Subgroup analysis suggested that the mortality benefit was primarily confined to the more severely injured patients.

CLINICAL CASE CORRELATION

- See also Case 1 (Early Awareness of Critical Illness), Case 3 (Scoring Systems and Patient Prognosis), and Case 4 (Monitoring).

COMPREHENSION QUESTIONS

2.1 Following a night of heavy alcohol consumption, a 29-year-old man ran down a hallway and collided with a double-paned window, crashing through it and falling 7 stories to the ground, landing feet first. He was initially unconscious at the scene. Upon arrival at the ICU, the patient's vital signs were: blood pressure 118/68 mm Hg, pulse 94 beats/minute, respirations 21 breaths/minute, and oxygen saturation 100% on 10 L of O_2 via face mask. On regaining consciousness, he became extremely combative, complaining of severe pain from the fractures in his lower extremities. He was intubated using rapid-sequence intubation. Despite the successful placement of an endotracheal tube, the patient was noted to have intermittently poor oxygen saturation observed on pulse oximetry. His breath sounds were decreased bilaterally and a large amount of crepitus was appreciated throughout the neck and anterior chest wall. A portable chest radiograph was significant for bilateral pneumothoraxes, managed with the insertion of chest tubes. What is the next best step?

A. Stabilize the patient at the bedside.

B. Get a CT scan of the thorax.

C. Get a CT scan of the abdomen.

D. Transport the patient to a nearby facility with more capability of services.

E. Complete all diagnostic imaging to help prioritize treatment.

2.2 A 16-year-old boy presents to the ED of a small rural hospital after being extricated from a house fire with approximately 40% total body surface area burns. The patient is breathing spontaneously and maintaining 100% saturation on 10 L/min by nasal cannula. His sputum is noted to be black (carbonaceous). The current facility does not have MV capacity or a burn center with a barometric pressure chamber. The patient's blood carbon monoxide level is 40%. He is awake and easily arousable. Vital signs, CBC, electrolytes are normal. ECG and chest x-ray are normal. The family requests transfer to a better-equipped facility. The next most appropriate step in the management of this patient is:

A. Check a carboxyhemoglobin level.

B. Give 100% FIO_2 and transfer to nearest facility with burn center care capabilities.

C. Monitor the patient closely for respiratory distress.

D. Take the patient to the operating room for immediate debridement and grafting.

E. Transfer the patient to a burn center via ambulance or helicopter.

ANSWERS TO QUESTIONS

2.1 **A.** Stabilization in the ED and ICU is necessary to prepare the patient for safe transport for subsequent testing. No transfer of the patient is advised except when needed for an operative procedure or until the patient is stabilized. Bilateral pulmonary contusions and a large amount of air in the mediastinum and anterior chest wall extending into the neck have been controlled with the bilateral chest tubes. There is no need for interhospital transfer. Later, the patient improved quickly and was transferred out of the surgical ICU. The patient continued to do well on the floor and was discharged home on hospital day 7.

2.2 **B.** Stabilization in the ED and ICU is key to a safe transport to a hospital that can treat burn victims and carbon monoxide poisoning where MV is available. While this patient will most likely require transfer to a hospital equipped to handle burn victims, the first step is to stabilize the patient. Despite his 100% oxygen saturation, the presence of carbonaceous sputum is an ominous sign and should be considered an indication that the patient may require intubation and MV. Other signs and symptoms that indicate a burn victim will require intubation include hoarseness, wheezing, stridor, burns inside the nose or the mouth or face, or a carboxyhemoglobin level >10% and carbon monoxide level >20%. The good neurological status suggests that the carboxyhemoglobin and carbon monoxide levels are much decreased with 2 hours on high flow O_2. Decompensation may need intubation for upper airway obstruction secondary to edema. Once intubated and stable, patient should be transferred via fastest route available to a hospital with a burn center, accompanied by skilled personnel and all the necessary equipment for a safe transfer.

CLINICAL PEARLS

- Transport of the critically ill patients has become a necessary and important part of clinical practice.
- Physiologic derangements during transport are seen slightly more frequently than in the stationary ICU patient.
- Transport risk can be reduced by appropriate planning, including arranging for trained transport personnel, and achieving pre-transport patient stabilization.
- Trained, experienced teams are essential in interhospital transport of the critically ill patient.
- The pre-hospital interventions associated with improved outcome are (1) helicopter transport of severely injured patients; (2) presence of a physician on the pre-hospital transport team; (3) a short injury-to-hospital time of less than 60 minutes; and (4) transfer directly to a Level I trauma center.
- Correct transfer of the most severely injured critically ill patients has shown long-term benefit, evaluated at 1 year post transfer.

REFERENCES

Deutschman CC, Neligan PJ. *Evidence Based Practice of Critical Care, Expert Consult*. Philadelphia: Saunders Publishers; 2011.

Hurst JM, Davis K, Johnson DJ, et al. Cost and complications during in-hospital transport of critically ill patients: A prospective cohort study. *J Trauma*. 1992;33:582-585.

Koppenberg J, Taeger K. Inter-hospital transport: transport of critically ill patients. *Curr Opin Anaesthesiology*. 2002;15:211-215.

CASE 3

A 78-year-old man was admitted to the intensive care unit (ICU) for exacerbation of congestive heart failure (CHF). During the first 2 days of his ICU stay, his clinical condition further deteriorated, and he subsequently required intubation and mechanical ventilation. At a patient care conference with family members, his family members inquired about his prognosis and your assessment of his chances for recovery with meaningful survival.

- What can be used to predict recovery or death in this patient?
- What are the types of prognostic systems to determine severity of conditions in the ICU?

ANSWERS TO CASE 3:
Scoring Systems and Patient Prognosis

Summary: A 78-year-old man is admitted to the ICU for CHF exacerbation. By day 2 in the ICU, the patient has shown signs of continued deterioration and is placed on mechanical ventilation. The family is hoping that you can help them understand his potential for meaningful recovery.

- **Predicting outcome:** A variety of models are available for disease severity stratification and outcomes prognostication. These models are necessary for quality control and management in the ICU. Although these systems are helpful for outcomes prediction in various populations of ICU patients, the models generally are not intended to be used for outcomes prediction in individual patients.
- **Prognostic systems available for severity determination in the ICU:** ICU scoring systems are generally categorized into 4 groups: (1) General risk-prognostic scores (eg, acute physiology and chronic health evaluation [APACHE], APACHE II, APACHE III, APACHE IV, mortality prediction model [MPM], simplified acute physiology score [SAPS II and III]). (2) Disease- and organ-specific prognostic scores (eg, Glasgow coma score [GCS], Child-Pugh classification, model for end-stage liver disease [MELD] score, risk, injury, loss, and end-stage kidney [RIFLE] classification for acute kidney injury [AKI], heart failure scores). (3) Organ dysfunction scores (eg, sepsis-related organ failure score [SOFA], multiple-organ dysfunction score [MODS], logistic organ dysfunction system [LODS]). (4) Trauma scoring (eg, injury severity score [ISS], revised trauma score [RTS]).

ANALYSIS

Objectives

1. Learn the various scoring systems that are applicable to patient populations in the ICU.
2. Learn the applicability and limitations of prognostic systems in clinical practice.

Considerations

As critical care providers, we are frequently approached by patients' families to provide them with our opinion or "best guess" regarding what will happen to their loved ones. In these situations, it is important to help the family understand that there are no tools that would allow anyone to reliably predict the clinical course and outcome of an individual patient. However, several models are available to estimate the probability of in-hospital mortality and 1-year mortality in hospitalized heart failure patients, and these models may help provide some insight regarding what event could transpire during his ICU and hospital stay (Table 3–1). These heart failure outcome predictive models take into account a variety of clinical and

Table 3–1 • HEART FAILURE PROGNOSTIC MODELS

Study	Patient Population	Variables	Outcomes	Reference
AHA-GWTG-HF (2010)	Hospitalized patients	Scoring system based on 7 clinical factors collected at admission (age, SBP, HR, serum sodium, BUN, COPD, patient race)	In-hospital mortality stratification based on number of points	*Circ Cardiovasc Qual Outcomes.* 2010;3:25-32.
OPTIMIZE-HF (2008)	Hospitalized patients	Age, HR, SBP, sodium, creatinine, LV function, and HF as the reason for admission were factors used to develop a nomogram for outcomes prediction	In-hospital mortality prediction based on nomogram	*J Am Coll Cardiol.* 2008;52: 347-356.
EFFECT (2003)	Hospitalized patients	Age, SBP, respiratory rate, BUN, serum sodium, comorbidities (CVA, COPD, cirrhosis, dementia, or cancer)	30-day and 1-year mortality calculation based on points	*JAMA.* 2003;290: 2581-2587.
Seattle Heart Failure Model (2006)	Outpatients and hospitalized patients	Age, gender, AHA classification, weight, LVEF, SBP, medications, diuretic doses, laboratory data, and ventricular assist devices use were variables that help determine prognosis	1-, 2-, and 3-year survival	*Circulation.* 2006;113:1414-1433.

SBP, systolic blood pressure; HR, heart rate; HF, heart failure; COPD, chronic obstructive pulmonary disease; CVA, cerebral vascular accident; LVEF, left ventricular ejection fraction.

laboratory variables such as patient age, comorbid conditions, vital signs, laboratory values such as serum sodium and BUN, and the presence of left ventricular dysfunction. For this patient, we can enter the pertinent data into one or more of these risk-prediction models and calculate his probabilities of in-hospital and long-term survival. Ultimately, it is our responsibility as ICU care providers to remind the patient's family that the projected probabilities are our best estimation based on prior observations of cohorts of heart failure patients, and the projections may or may not hold true for our patient.

APPROACH TO:
Scoring Systems and Patient Prognosis

DEFINITIONS

GENERAL RISK-PROGNOSTICATION SYSTEMS: These systems were developed based on the assumption that acute disease severity can be measured by the patients' characteristics and degree of abnormality of various physiologic variables. The general risk-prognostication systems include the APACHE II model introduced in 1985 and is one of the most commonly applied prognostic systems of this type in the ICU. These systems are designed to help determine outcomes in populations and are useful for quality assurance and outcome assessment in cohorts of patients. *These scoring systems can provide good estimate of the number of patients who are predicted to die in a population of similar patients; however, these systems cannot be used to predict exactly which of the patients will die.*

DISEASE- AND ORGAN-SPECIFIC PROGNOSTIC SCORES: These are scoring systems used to quantify single-organ failure or disease-specific outcomes. Examples of these include the GCS, Child-Pugh classification, MELD, RIFLE classification, and the variety of heart failure predictive models discussed earlier. Unlike the general risk-prognostic scores, these scoring systems are reasonably accurate for organ-specific risk prognostication and are commonly applied for clinical decision-making.

ORGAN DYSFUNCTION SCORING SYSTEMS: There are several scoring systems that are used to quantify and monitor the progression of patients with multiple organ dysfunction syndromes. These include sepsis-related organ failure score (SOFA), multiple-organ dysfunction score (MODS), and logistic organ dysfunction system (LODS). These systems are not only useful at the bedside for clinical decision-making, but are also useful for quality assurance and outcome assessment in cohorts of patients.

TRAUMA SCORES: There are 2 commonly used scoring systems for trauma patients. These include the revised trauma score (RTS) and the injury severity score (ISS). The RTS is based on 3 physiological parameters (GCS, systolic blood pressure, and respiratory rate), whereas the ISS is an anatomy-based scoring system quantifying the number and severity of injuries in 6 distinct body regions (head, face, chest, abdomen, extremity, and external). The RTS is a useful system for the serial assessment of trauma patients, particularly during the initial assessment phase. The ISS is more useful for quality assurance and outcomes assessment in cohorts of patients, and this scoring system is not used for clinical decision-making.

CLINICAL APPROACH

Quantitative assessment of disease severity and prognostication of outcomes in the ICU have become increasingly important. From the standpoint of individual patient care, the ability to accurately assess the severity of illness and accurately determining the level of function of specific organs are very helpful in clinical decision-making and the determination of medical resources that the individual patient may require. Scoring systems that have become integral parts of day-to-day care of patients in the ICU include the **GCS, MODS, MELD, and SOFA.** The major reasons that these scoring systems have gained popularity in direct patient care are that these scores can be easily calculated by care providers and the calculations are reproducible between observers. The drawback of using any scoring system for outcome prognostication is that while all scoring systems are useful to indicate when a patient's condition is improving or deteriorating and help project probabilities of clinical outcomes, the scores are in no way predictive of individual outcomes. As all scoring systems are mathematical models, usefulness of each model is influenced by its *discrimination* and *calibration*.

The **discrimination** of a predictive model measures the ability to distinguish patients who would have one outcome versus another (eg, live or die). **Discrimination is most commonly expressed by a receiver operating curve (ROC). The ROC plots the sensitivity of a test (y-axis) against 1 specificity (x-axis). The area under the ROC (aROC) represents the combined performance of the model.** A perfect model has aROC of 1; whereas an aROC of 0.5 suggests that the model is no better than chance alone. Most predictive models that are useful have an aROC≥ 0.7, an aROC >0.8 is considered good, and an aROC of >0.9 is considered excellent. With further discrimination, the curve will have a more vertical initial rise followed by a more horizontal extension (Figure 3–1).

The **calibration** of a scoring system is a measurement of its accuracy at different levels of risk. The calibration of a system can be examined using **goodness-of-fit statistics**, which looks at the difference between the observed frequency and the expected frequency for a wide range of groups of patients. The Hosmer-Lemeshow test is a statistical goodness-of-fit test for logistical regression models used to test

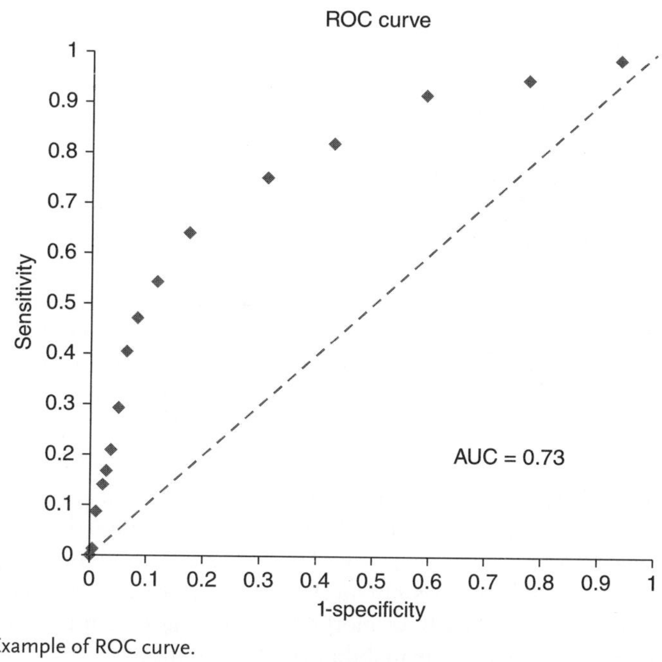

Figure 3–1. Example of ROC curve.

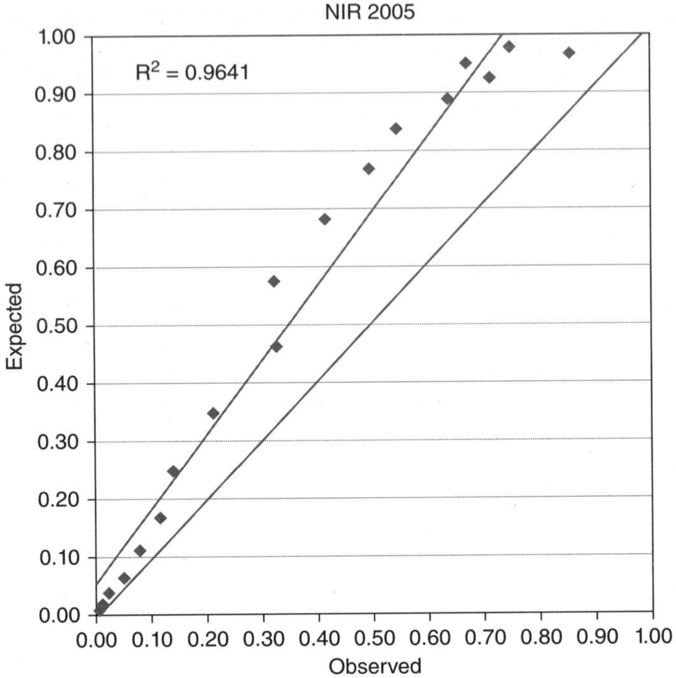

Figure 3–2. An example of goodness-of-fit curve. (In this example, the observed outcomes are closer to the expected outcome in the low-risk cohorts in comparison to the cohorts in the higher risk groups.)

whether the expected outcomes match the observed outcomes in various population subgroups. A *P*-value can be calculated, and if it is large then the model is well calibrated or fits the data well (Figure 3–2).

APPLICATIONS OF SCORING SYSTEMS

Organ-specific prognostic scores are frequently used to follow an ICU patient's progress and guide clinical decisions. These systems are easy to use and have good interobserver reproducibility. Most available scoring systems will provide good outcome estimates in a population of patients; however, they are not designed to predict outcomes for individual patients. Mortality prediction using serial severity scores have been evaluated by a number of groups. These results have demonstrated that with the assessment of serial scores such as APACHE II and APACHE III, the specificity of the predictive models can be improved. The values of most scoring systems are for the evaluation of ICU performance and for the determination of patient eligibility for enrollment in clinical trials (see Table 3–2). When scoring systems are used for ICU performance evaluation, it is important that choice of model for outcome prediction is appropriate. For example, an ICU with a lower actual mortality compared with the expected mortality does not necessarily indicate that the care is better. Multiple factors can influence ICU mortality including case-mix, admission and discharge policies, and resource availability (such as staffing).

Table 3–2 • GENERAL RISK-PROGNOSTIC SYSTEMS FOR MORTALITY PREDICTION

	Year Intro-duced	Origin of System	Age of Population (y)	aROC of Original Report	Parameters	Applications
APACHE II	1985	United States	>16	0.86	17 variables selected by panel of experts: age, physiologic status, acute conditions, and chronic disease processes	Research, benchmarking for quality improvement
APACHE III	1991	United States	>16	0.90	26 variables selected based on multiple logistic regression: age, chronic conditions and acute conditions	Research, benchmarking for quality improvement; sequential application to monitor clinical progress
APACHE IV	2006	United States	>16	0.88	Improved over APACHE III in that it can be used to provide for ICU length of stay prediction, which can provide benchmarks for comparison of ICU efficiency and resource	Research, benchmarking for quality improvement; sequential application to monitor clinical progress
SAPS II	1993	Europe and North America	>18	0.86	17 variables developed from multiple logistic regression based on data collected during the first 24 hours of ICU admission	Research, benchmarking for quality improvement; sequential application to monitor clinical progress

(*Continued*)

Table 3–2 • GENERAL RISK-PROGNOSTIC SYSTEMS FOR MORTALITY PREDICTION (CONTINUED)

	Year Introduced	Origin of System	Age of Population (y)	aROC of Original Report	Parameters	Applications
SAPS III	2005	Multinational	>16	0.85	Modified from SAPS II. 20 variables are divided into 3 subscores relating to patient characteristics prior to ICU admission, circumstances for ICU admission, and derangements that occurred during the first hour after admission	Research, benchmarking for quality improvement; sequential application to monitor clinical progress
MPM II 0	1993	North America and Europe	>18	0.82	A score at admission; 5 admission variables	Research; benchmarking for quality improvement
MPM II 24	1993	North America and Europe	>18	0.84	A second score at 24 hours after admission; include 8 additional variables	Research; benchmarking for quality improvement

aROC, area under receiver operating curve; APACHE, acute physiology and chronic health evaluation; SAPS, simplified acute physiology score; MPM, mortality prediction model; ROC, receiver operating curve.

CLINICAL CASE CORRELATION

- **See also Case 1 (Early Awareness of Critical Illness), Case 2 (Transfer of Critically Ill Patients), and Case 4 (Monitoring).**

COMPREHENSION QUESTIONS

3.1 A fourth year medical student is beginning the ICU rotation and is assigned to research the applicability of various scoring systems to clinical usefulness. There are several patients in the ICU including those with trauma, stroke, sepsis, and heart disease. Which of the following scoring system has been found to directly correlate with change in a patient's condition and is most useful for bedside decision-making?

A. Injury severity score (ISS)

B. Revised trauma score (RTS)

C. Multiple organ dysfunction score (MODS)

D. APACHE II

E. APACH III

3.2 Which of the following is an organ-specific scoring scheme rather than a general-risk prognostication scoring system?

A. APACHE II

B. SAPS II

C. MPM II

D. APACHE III

E. GCS

3.3 An ICU director is initiating a new quality improvement process for a general medical-surgical ICU. Which of these scoring systems is most useful for maintenance of quality control in this unit?

A. MODS

B. ISS

C. MELD score

D. RIFLE

E. APACHE III

ANSWERS TO QUESTIONS

3.1 **B.** The revised trauma score (RTS) is a physiologic scoring system. This is based on the patient's GCS, systolic blood pressure, and respiratory rate. A drop in RTS of ≥2 during the early post-injury observational period generally indicates a worsening condition and would require reassessment of the patient. The ISS is an anatomy-based trauma scoring system that is most useful when assessing population outcomes and quality management of trauma services. The MODS is a scoring system to document the severity of organ dysfunction. It is used to direct care, when there is a pattern of change that is unexpected. It is however not as useful as the RTS in direct decision-making in the ICU. The APACHE II and APACHE III scores are general prognostication scores that are mainly applied for quality management. Some groups have shown that serial measurements of APACHE II and III scores can be used for individual outcome prognostication.

3.2 **E.** The Glasgow coma score is not a general-risk prognostication scoring system; whereas, all the other scoring systems listed are general-risk prognostication scores.

3.3 **E.** In a combined medical-surgical ICU population, the APACHE III scoring system would be the most useful for outcome prognostication and quality control. The MODS score is an organ dysfunction scoring system that may not capture all the patient outcomes in a mixed ICU population. Similarly, ISS is for trauma severity grading. The MELD and RIFLE are organ-specific scoring systems for liver and kidney injury quantification, and these scoring systems would not capture all the important variables that might influence outcome.

CLINICAL PEARLS

- Most general-risk prognostic scoring systems are designed for population risk-prognostication and lack specificity for individual risk prognostication.
- Some of the disease-specific scoring systems are useful for bedside decision-making, and these include GCS, RIFLE, and MELD scores.
- THE APACHE score is probably the most commonly used system in the general ICU. The higher the score, the greater the mortality: APACHE II score of 25 = predicted mortality of 50%, and a score of over 35 = predicted mortality of 80%.
- The RIFLE score applies to acute kidney injury and can be remembered since RIFLE begins with "R" for "Renal."
- The MELD score is used to assess liver failure, the "LD" of MELD means "Liver Disease."
- The RTS score is useful for bedside decision making of trauma patients. It is weighed heavily toward the GCS (significant head trauma) and significant physiological problems (SBP and RR).

REFERENCES

Capuzzo M, Moreno RP, Le Gall J-R. Outcome prediction in critical care: the simplified acute physiology score models. *Curr Opin Crit Care*. 2008;14:485-490.

Gartman EJ, Casserly BP, Martin D, Ward NS. Using serial severity scores to predict death in ICU patients: a validation study and review of the literature. *Curr Opin Crit Care*. 2009;15:578-582.

Strand K, Flaatten H. Severity scoring in the ICU: a review. *Acta Anesthesiol Scan*. 2008;52:467-478.

Vicent J-L, Bruzzi de Carvalho F. Severity of illness. *Semin Resp Crit Care Med*. 2010;31:31-38.

Vincent J-L, Moreno R. Clinical review: scoring systems in the critically ill. *Critical Care*. 2010;14:207-215.

CASE 4

A 55-year-old man with a long-standing history of coronary artery disease is admitted to the ICU with hypotension following a 24-hour episode of intermittent chest pain. While on an IV nitroglycerin drip, he is free of chest pain. On the second hospital day, he suddenly develops chest pain, shortness of breath, and a change in mental status. A catheter is placed in his pulmonary artery and provided the following hemodynamic readings: central venous pressure (CVP) 12 mm Hg (0-5 mm Hg), pulmonary artery pressure (PAP) 40/15 mm Hg (20-25/5-10 mm Hg), pulmonary capillary occlusion "wedge" (PCW) pressure 18 mm Hg (6-12 mm Hg), and cardiac output (CO) 3.0 L/min (4-8 L/min). On physical examination his temperature is 38.2°C, heart rate 140 beats/minute, blood pressure 75/45 mm Hg, and respiration rate 35 breaths/minute. The jugular venous pressure is difficult to assess. Auscultation of the lungs reveals bilateral rales. The cardiac examination reveals a regular rhythm, a normal S_1 and accentuated S_2, and a new S_3 gallop. The legs are noted to have bilateral pitting edema to the level of the knees, and palpation reveals cool extremities and weak pulses.

- ▶ What is the most likely diagnosis?
- ▶ What are the best next steps in treatment of this patient?

ANSWERS TO CASE 4:
Hemodynamic Monitoring

Summary: This 55-year-old man with coronary artery disease has an acute decompensation in his status. The data from the hemodynamic monitoring (HM) reveal evidence for cardiogenic shock (CS), with hypotension, hypoperfusion, decreased mental status, and cool extremities. There is a new S_3 gallop. The PAC data indicates a volume overload with an elevated central venous and PCW pressure.

- **Most likely diagnosis: Cardiogenic shock based on** elevated pulmonary capillary wedge pressure is elevated with low cardiac output.
- **Best treatment steps:** Begin cardiac inotropes; optimize IV fluids according to CO and PCWP. Begin therapy with afterload reducing agents and then adjust therapy guided by the PAC and CO readings. An aortic balloon pump may also be indicated.

ANALYSIS

Objectives

1. To understand the goals of hemodynamic monitoring.
2. To appreciate the various forms available for acute hemodynamic monitoring.
3. To be able to interpret data from hemodynamic monitoring.

Considerations

This is a 55-year-old man with unstable angina requiring a nitroglycerin drip. On the second hospital day, he suddenly decompensates and is noted to be in cardiogenic shock. His BP is low, cardiac output low, and he has developed pulmonary edema. The most likely cause is cardiac pump failure. He is in need for quick reversal of organ hypoperfusion with fluids and vasopressors, including the possible use of an intra-aortic balloon pump to bridge him to a definitive intervention such as open heart surgery with coronary artery bypass. At this juncture, the patient is critically ill, and timely and accurate diagnosis and intervention are critical to his survival. Invasive hemodynamic monitoring helps optimize fluid and vasopressor/inotropic intervention.

APPROACH TO:
Hemodynamic Monitoring

HEMODYNAMIC MONITORING GOALS

The goal of HM is to evaluate the vital signs needed to **maintain adequate tissue perfusion**. HM can be accomplished by noninvasive (preferred) or invasive means. Continuous monitoring allows an early recognition of poor tissue perfusion based on low blood flow. Invasive PAC provides data on systemic, pulmonary arterial and venous pressures, and measurements of CO (cardiac output). Since the flow of blood into organs cannot be measured directly, normal BP and, more specifically, mean arterial pressure (MAP >60 mm Hg and urine output) are used as indirect indicators of adequate tissue perfusion. In the ICU, **hypotension has been identified as the most common cause of hemodynamic instability.** Assuming that the CVP and PAOP are adequate estimates of the volume of the systemic and pulmonary circulation, respectively, one can create a working relationship between CVP and PAOP, and CO or stroke volume (SV). This can be plotted in a Starling curve, pointing to the optimum range of end diastolic volume and CO for each patient. Misleading readings can occur with abnormal pressure/volume relationship (compliance) of the RV or LV, increased intrathoracic pressure (PEEP, auto PEEP, intra-abdominal pressure), and valvular heart disease (mitral stenosis).

CVP is often used as the sole guide to monitor hemodynamic function. Techniques such as echocardiography, transesophageal echocardiography, Doppler, and volume-based monitoring can be used. No single monitoring technique has been demonstrated to improve patient outcome. **Assuring the veracity of the data is key to the correct interpretation.** Time is crucial for an early diagnosis of a hemodynamic catastrophe and the early detection and application of effective therapy. Trends of data information are more reliable than single data points.

Monitors

Critically ill patients require continuous monitoring to diagnose and manage their complex medical conditions. This is most commonly achieved by using direct pressure monitoring systems. PaP measurements are much less commonly used today than previously. Monitoring central venous pressure (CVP) and intra-arterial blood pressure (BP) are common approaches to evaluate hemodynamic functioning. Most facilities use noninvasive monitoring of hemodynamic functions of BP and other basic vital signs.

Continuous Vital Signs

Modern electronic devices continually monitor up to 5 vital signs (heart rate, respiration rate, skin temperature, oxygen saturation, and blood pressure). The data is entered into a 5-point index that is constantly on display. Nursing staff can review these vital signs and the patient status index regularly to identify patients experiencing distress. This improves the prospect to stabilize the patient and initiate goal-directed therapy to recover from these abnormalities. This should lead to fewer unplanned admissions to ICUs and minimize cardiac arrests occurring out-of-intensive care units, thereby significantly improving cost and life savings.

Monitoring of Cardiac Function

The assessment of ventricular function is based on the measurement of both blood volume and pressure. The ejection fraction (EF) as left ventricular dp/dt_{max} has been widely accepted as an index of the contractile performance of the left ventricle. Measurement of left ventricular dp/dt_{max} is a satisfactory index of ventricular contractility.

ECG Monitoring

All ICU patients have continuous ECG monitoring. The diagnosis of arrhythmias and the commencement of rapid treatment is a goal of hemodynamic monitoring. The waveform display is arranged to monitor Leads I, II, or V, whichever provide the **tallest QRS complex.** Alarms must be set and placed in the "on position" at all times. High and low alarm settings are assessed and documented in the graphic record. Upper and lower alarm limits are selected for each individual patient. The rhythm strip is for rhythm interpretation; for the evaluation of morphology a 12-lead ECG is needed.

Intra-arterial Blood Pressure Monitoring

Intra-arterial BP monitoring is used to obtain direct and continuous BP measurements in ICU patients who have hypertension or hypotension. Arterial blood gas measurements and blood sampling can be obtained repeatedly. If no collateral circulation exists and the cannulated artery becomes occluded, ischemia and infarction of the area distal to that artery could occur. To check collateral circulation to the hand, use the Allen test to evaluate the radial and ulnar arteries or use an ultrasonic Doppler to evaluate any of the arteries. In the Allen test, the radial and ulnar arteries are compressed simultaneously. The Allen test confirms the presence of collateral circulation. If this collateral circulation is not confirmed, arterial blood gases (ABGs) using that site should be avoided. The preparation of sites for arterial lines and their subsequent care are the same as for CVP catheters. **Complications in the use of arterial lines include local obstruction with distal ischemia, external hemorrhage, massive ecchymosis with compartmental syndrome, dissection, air embolism, blood loss, pain, arteriospasm, and infection.** Blood pressure readings are more commonly obtained by automatic self-inflating cuff devices. Under most circumstances these produce comparable blood pressure results when compared to arterial lines. BP cuffs should be avoided on arms with shunts to avoid occlusion.

To Catheterize or Not to Catheterize?

In the past, the pulmonary artery balloon tip thermodilution catheter (PAC) has been the gold standard for evaluating the circulatory function of patients in the ICU. A higher mortality rate has been reported in patients in whom a PAC was inserted. A PAC-based hemodynamic management is successful in improving patient outcome in instances of planned major surgery. This benefit has not been translated to the ICU patient. PAC-based monitoring has its limitations, the most significant being the misinterpretation of the data being produced even by well-trained intensivists and cardiologists. PAC monitoring provides measurements of PaP, pulmonary capillary wedge pressure (PCWP or PAOP), and right atrial pressure. Flow variables such as CO and mixed venous O_2 (Svo_2) are also measured. Calculations of systemic and pulmonary vascular resistance (SVR, PVR), right ventricular stroke work, and left ventricular stroke work (LVSW) are obtained. There was no significant difference regarding outcome or postoperative complications whether managed with a CVP or a PAC (see Table 4–1).

Table 4–1 • HEMODYNAMIC CHANGES WITH VARIOUS DISORDERS

		Right Atrial (mmHg)	Right Ventricle Systolic (mmHg)	Right Ventricle Diastolic (mmHg)	Pulmonary Artery Systolic (mmHg)	Pulmonary Artery Diastolic (mmHg)	Pulmonary Capillary Wedge (mmHg)	Cardiac Index (L/min)/m²	Systemic Vascular Resistance (dyne × s)/cm⁵
Normal values		<6	<25	0-12	<25	0-12	<6-12	2.5	(800-1600)
Myocardial Infarction without pulmonary edema		—	—	—	—	—	13 (5-18)	2.7 (2.2-4.3)	—
Pulmonary edema		No Δ/ Increased	No Δ/Increased	No Δ/Increased	**Increased**	**Increased**	**Increased**	No Δ / Decreased	Increased
Cardiogenic shock	**Left ventricular failure**	No Δ/ Increased	No Δ/Increased	No Δ/Increased	No Δ/ Increased	**Increased**	**Increased**	**Decreased**	No Δ/Increased
	Right ventricular failure	**Increased**	Decreased/ No Δ/Increased	**Increased**	Decreased/ No Δ/ Increased*	Decrease/ No Δ/ Increased*	Decrease/ No Δ/ Increased*	**Decreased**	**Increased**
Cardiac tamponade		**Increased**	No Δ/Increased	**Increased**	No Δ/ Increased	No Δ/ Increased	No Δ/ Increase	Decreased	Increased
Acute mitral regurgitation		No Δ/ Increased	Increased	No Δ/Increased	**Increased**	**Increased**	**Increased**	No Δ/ Decreased	No Δ/Increased
Ventricular septal rupture		Increased	No Δ/Increased	Increased	No Δ/ Increased	No Δ/ Increase	No Δ/ Increased	Increased Pulm BF⁺ Decreased System BF⁺	No Δ/Increased
Hypovolemic shock		Decreased	No Δ/Decreased	No Δ/Decreased	Decreased	Decreased	Decreased	Decreased	Increased
Septic shock		Decreased	No Δ/Decreased	No Δ/Decreased	Decreased	Decreased	Decreased	Increased	Decreased

***Different subsets of diseases have different values**

⁺Pulm BF = pulmonary blood flow; System BF = systemic blood flow.

Central Venous Catheter

PAC has not improved survival or organ function and has been associated with more complications than CVP-guided therapy. Newer CVP catheters provide a continuous recording of O_2 saturation, which helps in **maintaining venous O_2sat goals at >70% to 75%.** CVP catheters should be placed with guidance from ultrasound. PIC lines are also an option as a central line.

PAOP does not always reflect left ventricular end diastolic volume (LVEDV). The CVP and PAOP parallel each other closely in patients with EF >50%. In EF <40%, the correlation between the CVP and PAOP decreases due to changes in myocardial compliance caused by myocardial hypertrophy or a stiff LV. Patients with PAC placement receive more fluid in the first 24 hours and have an increased incidence of renal failure and thrombocytopenia than with CVP use. A line infection is one of the most important risks. Complications arose in approximately 20% of the instances in which a catheter was left in place for more than 6 days.

Mixed Venous Oxygen Saturation

Continuous monitoring of venous oxygen saturation (Svo_2) by reflectometry immediately detects trends and abrupt changes in the oxygen supply-to-demand ratio. Svo_2 has been promoted as an indicator of changes in CO. **Normal values for Svo_2 range from 70% to 75%.** A linear correlation has been demonstrated between the CO and Svo_2. Svo_2 reflects the overall oxygen reserve of the whole body. A normal Svo_2 value does not rule out an impaired oxygen supply to individual organs. The pulmonary artery carries blood from all vascular beds of the body; thus, Svo_2 represents the amount of oxygen in the systemic circulation that is left after passage of the blood through the tissues. Svo_2 thus serves as a measure of global oxygenation. The determinants of Svo_2 are SAO_2, systemic VO_2, CO, and Hb.

$$\mathbf{Svo_2 = (SAO_2 - VO_2)/(1.39 \times Hb \times CO)}$$

An increase in VO_2 and a decrease in Hb, CO, and arterial oxygenation will result in a decrease of Svo_2. Interpretation of Svo_2 values might be difficult in conditions where DO_2/VO_2 relationships are altered. Arterial-venous microcirculatory shunting in sepsis may increase Svo_2 tissue oxygenation while regional tissue dysoxia is present.

Monitoring of the Right Ventricle

The right ventricle is responsible for accepting venous blood and pumping it through the pulmonary circulation. Circulatory homeostasis depends on an adequate function and synchronization of both ventricles. Changes in the dimensions of one ventricle influence the geometry of the other. Monitoring of CVP has demonstrated its value in judging right ventricular function. Moreover, the use of RVEDV and RVEF is unaffected by arbitrary and poorly reproducible zero points for pressure transducers. RVEF by thermodilution measurements is easy to perform.

Measurement of Extravascular Lung Water and Intrathoracic Blood Volume

Depressed left ventricular performance increases hydrostatic pressure in the pulmonary circulation, influencing fluid flux across a damaged pulmonary microvascular membrane. Extravascular lung water (EVLW) can be measured at the bedside using a double-dye technique with indocyanine green. Intrathoracic blood volume appears to be a more reliable indicator of preload than cardiac filling pressure.

Echocardiography

Assessing global and regional LVF is the domain of echocardiography, via either transthoracic echocardiography (TTE) or transesophageal echocardiography (TEE). Two-dimensional echocardiography provides significant information including left ventricular cavity size, fractional shortening, and abnormalities in regional wall motion. Two-dimensional colored echocardiography enables a quantification of shunts, CO, and provides a noninvasive assessment of concomitant valvular disease. The **presence and extent of ischemic heart disease is determined by monitoring segmental wall motion.** These abnormalities are indirect markers of myocardial perfusion that can persist for prolonged periods in the absence of infarction. TEE provides more accurate information on ventricular size than standard TTE. End diastolic volume (LVEDV) is a better predictor of myocardial performance than PAOP. Echocardiography is the first diagnostic method which should be used when suspicion of aortic dissection, endocarditis, or pulmonary embolism with hemodynamic instability are believed to exist. Hypovolemia, left ventricular failure, global systolic function, and the size of both ventricles can be rapidly identified using TTE/TEE. Valvular abnormalities and functionally important heart disease can be readily determined.

Monitoring of Organ Perfusion and Microcirculation

Monitoring of tissue oxygenation and organ function in the clinical setting is based on measuring variables of global hemodynamics, pulse oximetry, capillary refill, urine output, or by the use of indirect biochemical markers. These parameters remain insensitive indicators of dysoxia and are considered poor surrogates for measuring O_2 at the tissue levels. The net balance between cellular O_2 supply and O_2 demand determines the status of tissue oxygenation. Regional tissue dysoxia can persist despite the presence of adequate systemic blood flow, pressure, and arterial oxygen content.

Oxygen Delivery and Oxygen Consumption

Total body perfusion and oxygenation relies on an adequate arterial oxygen saturation (SaO_2), appropriate hemoglobin (Hb) concentration, and cardiac output. The total amount of oxygen delivered to the peripheral tissue per minute (DO_2) can be calculated as $DO_2 = CO \times CaO_2$, with $CaO_2 = (Hb \times 1.39 \times SaO_2)$. In steady state conditions, the uptake of oxygen from the arterial blood (VO_2) represents the sum of all oxidative metabolic reactions in the body. VO_2 can be measured by analysis of the expired gas or calculated from CO and arterial and mixed venous blood samples. The VO_2/DO_2 is the oxygen extraction ratio. VO_2/DO_2 dependency occurs when the increase in oxygen extraction can no longer fully compensate for the fall in DO_2. The relationship between DO_2 and VO_2 can therefore be used to assess the adequacy of tissue oxygenation. The determination of DO_2 and VO_2 requires right heart catheterization to measure CO.

Blood Lactate Level

Arterial blood lactate levels in critically ill patients have proven very useful. Lactate is formed from pyruvate by the cytosolic enzyme lactate dehydrogenase. A lactate concentration >2 mmol/L is generally considered a biochemical indicator of inadequate oxygenation. Circulatory failure with impaired tissue perfusion is the most common cause of lactic acidosis. Mechanisms other than impaired tissue oxygenation may cause an increase in blood lactate, including an activation of glycolysis, a reduction in pyruvate dehydrogenase activity, or liver failure. The complex process of tissue lactate production and its utilization mandates an understanding of the usefulness and limitations of blood lactate levels. Elevated lactate levels should prompt the clinician to initiate procedures for assessment of the circulatory status.

Respiratory Monitoring

Breathing waves are generated by the standard 3 ECG leads used in the ICU for ECG rhythm monitoring. A change in breathing rate disturbs the electrical triangle formed by the leads measuring respiratory rate and apneas. This method is not accurate and is predisposed to deliver incorrect data. Noninvasive monitoring of pulmonary function is most important in the mechanically ventilated patient. The respiratory system requires the generation of pressure for the inflation needed to overcome resistive and elastic properties of the lung. Resistance is located mainly in the airways. Several techniques are available to measure respiratory mechanics, but the most practical method is the rapid airway occlusion technique. This technique estimates the elastic recoil pressure of the alveoli by measuring the inspiratory plateau airway pressure (Pplat). Functional lung monitoring has questionable prognostic value and is of limited use in daily clinical practice. Bedside monitoring of static compliance and Pplat should be used routinely to detect the presence of alveolar overdistention and at least qualitatively assess the risk for volume-induced lung injury (VILI). An important factor in respiratory mechanics is intrinsic positive end-expiratory pressure (PEEPi). This is commonly measured using end-expiratory airway occlusion. PEEPi causes decreased cardiac output, alveolar overdistention, increased work of breathing, and patient-ventilator asynchrony. If neglected, PEEPi leads to an underestimation of compliance.

O_2 Saturation

The determination of O_2 saturation (O_2sat) via pulse oximeters is a valuable adjunct to clinical oxygen monitoring. When properly applied, it reliably indicates the patient's HR and arterial oxygen saturation. ECG synchronization reduces motion artifacts when the ECG R wave is detected. The **diagnosis of hypoxemia requires an arterial blood gas analysis and is commonly defined as a PaO_2 of <60 mm Hg or O_2Sat <90%.** Pulse oximetry is commonly used for assessing hypoxemia. However, this modality measures the saturation of hemoglobin and not PaO_2, reflecting oxygen dissolved in the blood, which includes both bound and unbound O_2. Thus, a patient with severe anemia may have a normal PaO_2 but a low O_2 content. Low pulse oximetry values <90% coincide with significant hypoxemia, but normal oxygen saturation does not exclude hypoxemia, especially in patients receiving a high FiO_2.

Normal PAO_2 levels are 80 to 100 mm Hg in a healthy patient. Pulse oximetry values may remain normal until PAO_2 decreases to <60 mm Hg. For this reason, the alveolar-arterial oxygen gradient should be evaluated in patients receiving a high FIO_2. A widening alveolar-arterial oxygen gradient is a sign of an increasing hypoxemia. Pulse oximetry may be unreliable in cases of severe anemia, carbon monoxide poisoning, methemoglobinemia, or peripheral vasoconstriction.

End-Tidal CO_2 Monitoring

End-tidal CO_2 monitoring is now standard in intraoperative care. This lack of bedside monitoring is particularly significant because the most common form of respiratory monitoring is normal pulse oximetry. Capnometry or end-tidal volume CO_2 ($EtCO_2$) monitoring is used to evaluate the $PACO_2$ level during surgery and in intubated patients in the ICU. In children, manual ventilation with $EtCO_2$ monitoring resulted in increased $PACO_2$ readings falling within the intended range.

Urinary Bladder Pressure

Measurement of intra-abdominal pressure (IAP) is accomplished via the use of Foley bladder balloons in critically ill patients. Monitoring IAP to avoid and detect abdominal compartment syndrome is increasingly recommended and is advocated in monitoring patients after abdominal surgery. IAP is usually estimated indirectly by measuring intrabladder pressure (IBP).

Electroencephalographic Monitoring

Continuous EEG monitoring (CEEG) is a powerful tool for evaluating cerebral function in obtunded and comatose patients. Ongoing analysis of CEEG data is a major task because of the amount of data generated and the near real-time interpretation of a patient's EEG. Methods such as the computerized detection of seizures have increasingly allowed focused reviews of EEG epochs of interest. These allow personnel and inexperienced staff to recognize significant EEG changes in a timely fashion.

Esophageal Pressure Measurement

The chest wall includes the abdomen. Abdominal pathology affects respiratory mechanics. Eesophageal pressure and airway pressure define the contribution of each of these compartments to respiratory mechanics and particularly to compliance. Supine measurements are less reliable.

Near-Infrared Spectroscopy

Near-infrared spectroscopy (NIRS) is a noninvasive way to measure oxygenated and deoxygenated Hb as well as the redox state of cytochrome 3 as an average value of arterial, venous, and capillary blood. It has been used primarily in studies of cerebral or muscle oxygenation after different types of hypoxic injuries.

CLINICAL CASE CORRELATION

- **See also Case 5 (Vasoactive Drugs), and Case 16 (Acute Cardiac Failure).**

COMPREHENSION QUESTIONS

4.1 A 45-year-old man is admitted to the ICU after a motor vehicle accident. The nurse calls to notify you of a continuous venous O_2 saturation which has been dropping steadily over the last few hours from 75% to 65%. What is the most likely cause?

A. CHF Stage 1
B. Noncompressible arterial disease
C. Peripheral venous disease
D. Systemic hypoperfusion
E. COPD

4.2 A 20-year-old pregnant woman develops a urinary tract infection with positive blood cultures. She is admitted to the ICU with a blood pressure of 88/52 mm Hg, which has persisted despite fluid challenge. Her condition deteriorates as she develops increasing respiratory distress. She appears to be developing adult respiratory distress syndrome (ARDS) and is intubated for mechanical ventilation. The resident staff inserts a right heart catheter to measure pulmonary vascular pressure. Which of the following HM findings is likely to be seen in this case?

A. Low wedge pressure, low cardiac output
B. Low wedge pressure, high cardiac output
C. High wedge pressure, low cardiac output
D. High wedge pressure, high cardiac output
E. Normal cardiac output, normal wedge pressure

ANSWERS TO QUESTIONS

4.1 **D.** Systemic hypoperfusion with increased oxygen uptake by the tissues and decreased delivery of oxygen, especially to organs with high oxygen demands decreases venous O_2 saturation. The increased difference in oxygen consumption and lower venous O_{2Sat} is a direct indicator of some form of decreased oxygen delivery, such as decreased cardiac output, severe anemia, respiratory failure (ARDS), hypoxemia, and sepsis.

4.2 **A.** In a patient with ARDS due to sepsis, one would expect the PCWP to range between normal and low and the CO to be low. Considering the gram-negative uroseptic syndrome described in this case, endotoxin from the infecting bacteria has acted as a circulating cardiosupressant. The SvO_2 measurements will direct treatment, with a goal of attaining an SvO_{2Sat} >70% to75%. Dobutamine is indicated to treat the decreased CO, which was induced by the gram-negative septic shock.

CLINICAL PEARLS

- There is no specific monitoring technique that is known to improve patient outcome.
- PAC has not been associated with improvement in patient outcomes.
- PAC is now rarely used except in selected cases.
- An MAP of 60 mm Hg is a target associated with signs of adequate urine output and MS.
- CVP and PAOP are comparable in patients with EF >50% and indicate end diastolic volume.
- Maintaining plateau alveolar pressures at <30 cm H_2O reduces alveolar strain, and barotrauma.
- PEEP is clinically titrated by measuring its effects on gas exchange and on hemodynamics.
- The mechanical characteristics of the respiratory system are compliance, resistance, and intrinsic PEEP; all can be measured using standard ventilators and bedside maneuvers.
- Monitoring esophageal pressure can help assess the extent of alveolar strain from PEEP.

REFERENCES

Loscalzo J. *Harrison's Pulmonary and Critical Care Medicine*. New York, NY: McGraw-Hill; 2010.

Pulmonary-Artery versus Central Venous Catheter to Guide Treatment of Acute Lung Injury. The National Heart, Lung, and Blood Institute Acute Respiratory Distress Syndrome (ARDS) Clinical Trials Network. *N Engl J Med*. 2006;354:2213-2224.

Summerhill EM, Baram M. Principles of pulmonary artery catheterization in the critically ill. *Lung*. 2005;183:209-219. [PMID: 16078042]

CASE 5

You are called to give orders for a 62-year-old woman admitted to the ICU in septic shock. The patient is receiving intravenous (IV) vancomycin, levofloxacin, and gentamicin for suspected urosepsis and potential pneumonia. The patient has been admitted from a skilled nursing facility. The vital signs indicate the blood pressure is 100/60 mm Hg, heart rate 120 beats/minute, respiratory rate (RR) 30 breaths/minute, with a urinary output of 20 mL/h. Two liters of normal saline was given within 1 hour without a noticeable improvement in BP or heart rate. A central venous line recorded a venous O_2 saturation of 60%.

- ▶ What is the next step in addressing the blood pressure?
- ▶ What other measures should be undertaken in this patient?

ANSWERS TO CASE 5:
Vasoactive Drugs and Pharmacology

Summary: A 62-year-old woman is in sepsis with decreased blood pressure as well as signs of decreased intravascular volume and cardiac output.

- **Next step in addressing blood pressure:** Given the low mean arterial pressure and tachycardia, the first step should incorporate efforts to increase the BP is with IV fluids, mainly normal saline, followed by proper vasopressors if the BP does not improve. The blood pressure should be supported to ensure that the blood flow to target organs is sufficient with this combination.
- **Other measures:** Appropriate maintenance of fluid and blood volume with adherence to goal-directed therapy. A pH of at least 7.20 is needed for vasopressors to be effective.

ANALYSIS

Objectives

1. To describe the indications to the use of vasopressors.
2. To understand the pharmacological mechanisms of vasopressors action.

Considerations

This 62-year-old woman is admitted to the ICU with urosepsis and possible pneumonia. The patient's hypotension and decreased urine output indicate profound septic shock. The keys to treatment, and thereby improving survival include rapidly addressing the abnormal hemodynamic parameters, early correction of the underlying cause of the sepsis. This means administration and correct antibiotics in a timely fashion (within 1 hour for hospital inpatients and up to 6 hours for outpatients).

APPROACH TO:
Fluid and Vasopressor Use

IV FLUIDS

IV fluids are usually the **first therapy for hypotension**. Fluid therapy is effective in increasing intravascular volume (IVC), which in turn increases the BP. An ideal fluid would maintain IVC without expanding the interstitial space (ISFV). Crystalloid solutions are universally used for initial volume resuscitation. In sepsis, significant tissue accumulation of resuscitation fluid occurs, which results in adverse effects. Crystalloid solutions may be isotonic, hypotonic, or hypertonic and are in universal use as primary resuscitation fluids in critical illnesses. The determination of which crystalloid to use remains controversial. Aggressive resuscitation with crystalloids induces a dramatic increase in extracellular fluid (ECF), alterations in acid–base balance, electrolyte composition, colloid balance, and coagulation. Combinations of crystalloids and colloids given together have proven effective since significantly greater tissue perfusion occurs when compared with crystalloid alone.

The volume distribution of 1 L of NaCl 0.9% would put 250 mL in the IVC and 750 mL in the ISFV. In contrast the administration of 5% albumin will increase plasma volume by 52% of the volume infused. Albumin increases the cardiac index significantly more than saline and has a significant effect on hemoglobin dilution. The tendency for crystalloids to extravasate may lead to relative hypoperfusion. There is **emerging evidence that intravenous fluids may have an indigenous proinflammatory property.** The findings in Iraq from studies on injured soldiers, who were resuscitated from a hypotensive state with low volume hypertonic saline, demonstrated an elevation in BP without an increase in inflammatory markers. **Isotonic saline, when administered in large volumes, is associated with hyperchloremic nongap acidosis.** During sepsis, there is a dramatic increase in capillary permeability. In these circumstances, up to 80% of the crystalloid solutions used cause edema which varies linearly with the volume of crystalloid that is administered.

Lactated Ringers Solution

Infusion of lactated Ringers solution is associated with the expression of adhesion molecules in lung and spleen whether or not hemorrhage has occurred. When preceded by shock, the use of lactated Ringers solution for resuscitation is associated with histologic evidence of increased pulmonary edema and inflammation. Lactated Ringers solution and other isotonic crystalloid solutions may activate inflammatory cytokines and result in cellular apoptosis, possibly increasing lung injury.

Ethyl Pyruvate

Ketone buffered IV fluids such as ethyl pyruvate may have anti-inflammatory effects. In animals, ethyl pyruvate versus lactated Ringers solution resulted in less cellular apoptosis in pulmonary tissues.

Hypertonic Saline

The osmolality of normal plasma is 280 to 295 mOsm/L. Any solution with an osmolality exceeding 310 mOsm/L is considered to be a hypertonic fluid. Hypertonic saline (HS) and sodium bicarbonate are examples of hypertonic fluids. The most commonly used concentrations of HS are 1.8%, 3%, 7.5%, and 23.4%. The higher the concentration of Na in HS, the larger the amount that stays in the IVC. The two well-defined uses of hypertonic fluid are: first, to expand the IVC in patients in hypovolemic shock, as a means of low-volume, high-impact resuscitation (eg, war victims with closed trauma). The second use is a corollary of the first use, namely for intracellular volume depletion. This second advantage is widely appreciated in neurosurgery and neuro critical care where the reduction of cerebral volume and intracranial pressure (ICP) is especially important. HS dramatically increases the osmotic pressure in the compartment into which it is injected. Water flows along the osmotic gradient into the compartment, expanding the compartment's fluid volume for several hours. HS may also increase myocardial contractility. The metabolic consequences of HS are hypernatremia, hyperosmolality, and hyperchloremic nongap acidosis.

Some studies and case reports suggest that patients have better hemodynamic profiles when given HS than when given isotonic crystalloid. No study of the pre-hospital administration of HS has shown an overall statistically significant benefit. Survival benefit has been noted for patients requiring surgery and receiving pre-hospital administration of HS plus dextran (HSD) versus an equal volume of isotonic crystalloid. Wade and colleagues reported an improved survival in patients who had suffered penetrating trauma if they were given HS. The major controversy in trauma is not the utility of HS but in the timing of its use. There are no large prospective studies on the use of HS in sepsis. Hypothetically, HS should improve overall systemic perfusion and presumably oxygen delivery, and in addition it may modulate the inflammatory response.

Albumin

Albumin is a volume expander in vials of 250 and 500 mL and is also used as a 25% solution in 50- and 100-mL vials. Albumin products contain 130 to 160 mEq of sodium per liter of solution. The 5% solution is iso-oncotic with respect to human plasma; the 25% solution is 4 to 5 times more oncotically active . Albumin solutions do not appear to alter blood coagulation. The administration of albumin is associated with a rapid but unpredictable expansion of the plasma volume. There is no evidence that the injection of albumin reduces mortality. Concerns that albumin therapy may increase mortality appear to be unfounded. Albumin is safe to use, but it is costly. There is no evidence that the administration of albumin improves patient recovery from sepsis.

Colloids

High molecular-weight solutions (colloids) are used widely as plasma substitutes. Colloid solutions remain in the intravascular space because of their large molecular size, which is associated with low membrane impermeability. Colloids may also plug leaky capillaries and increase colloid oncotic pressure (COP), thus expanding the intravascular volume (IVC). One can achieve a volume expansion equal to or greater than the volume administered, which reduces tissue edema. There is a strong argument that colloid solutions are expensive, leak into the extracellular space, and affect blood coagulation. **Blood products are discussed in another section.**

VASOPRESSOR AGENTS

Vasopressor therapy is used when hypotension, such as caused by sepsis, is unresponsive to fluid therapy. Vasopressors are used to assist in the maintenance of mean arterial pressure (MAP), whereas inotropes are used to increase cardiac output, cardiac index, stroke volume, and Svo_2. The exact MAP target in patients is uncertain because each patient autoregulates within their own individualized limits. Autoregulation in various vascular beds can be lost below a certain MAP. This could lead to conditions in which tissue perfusion becomes linearly dependent on blood pressure. The titration of norepinephrine (NE) to an MAP of 65 mm Hg is known to preserve tissue perfusion. A patient with preexisting hypertension may well require a higher MAP to maintain adequate tissue perfusion. The ideal "pressor" would

Table 5–1 • COMMON VASOACTIVE DRUGS AND THEIR ACTIONS

	Dopamine	β_1	β_2	α
Dopamine	++++	++ (Moderate dose)	++	+++ (Higher dose)
Dobutamine (β_1 agonist)	0	++++	++	+
Epinephrine (α and $\beta_{1/2}$ agonist)	0	++++	+++	+++
Norepinephrine (α and β_1 agonist)	0	++++	0	++++
Phenylephrine (pure α agonist)	0	0	0	++++

restore blood pressure while maintaining cardiac output and preferentially perfuse mainly the brain, heart, splanchnic organs, and kidneys. All vasopressors are associated with adverse effects (Table 5–1).

Dobutamine

Dobutamine is a synthetic catecholamine with primarily β_1 agonist activity, leading to increased cardiac contractility. The increase in heart rate caused by dobutamine is offset by its vasodilation effect with little net effect on blood pressure (BP). The principal use of dobutamine is in patients with refractory CHF, hypotension, or septic patients with hypoperfusion in whom vasodilators cannot be used because of their effect on blood pressure (BP). The onset of dobutamine action is 1 to 10 minutes after its administration with its peak effect being reached in 10 to 20 minutes. The usual drip rate for adults is at 2.5 to 20 μg/kg/min with a recommended maximum of 40 μg/kg/min. It is important to titrate the dosage to achieve the desired target of increased cardiac output. Vasopressors should be administered into large veins preferably via a central line. **Dobutamine has less effect on heart rate than dopamine.** Dobutamine appears particularly effective in splanchnic resuscitation, increasing pH (gastric mucosal pH), and improving mucosal perfusion when compared to dopamine. As part of an early goal-directed resuscitation protocol that combined close medical and nursing attention with aggressive fluid and blood administration, dobutamine was associated with a significant absolute reduction in the risk for mortality.

Dopamine

Dopamine has predominantly β-adrenergic effects in low-to-moderate dose ranges (up to 10 μg/kg/min). It is converted to NE in the myocardium and activates adrenergic receptors. In higher doses, its ability to sensitize α-adrenergic receptors causes vasoconstriction. **Dopamine is a mixed inotrope and vasoconstrictor.** At all dose ranges, dopamine is a potent chronotrope. Dopamine causes more tachycardia and is more arrhythmogenic than NE. Evidence suggests that dopamine does not have a net substantial effect on the kidneys. It may interfere with thyroid and pituitary function and may have an immunosuppressive effect. The use of "renal-dose" dopamine has been proven false. **Dopamine-resistant septic shock (DRSS)** has been described, defined as MAP <70 mm Hg despite administration of dopamine at 20 μg/kg/min. The incidence of DRSS was 60%, and those patients had a mortality rate of 78%, compared with 16% in the dopamine-sensitive group.

Norepinephrine

Norepinephrine (NE) has pharmacologic effects on both α_1- and β_1-adrenergic receptors. NE is used to maintain BP in hypotensive states and is a more potent vasoconstrictor than its relative phenylephrine. The usual maintenance dose is 2 to 4 μg/min. Doses as high as 0.5 to 1.5 μg/kg/min for 1 to 10 days have been used in patients with septic shock. The potential for extravasation is avoided when the administration is via a large vein. Currently, NE is considered the agent of choice for the patient requiring fluid resuscitation, although this is controversial. Both vasoconstriction and increased MAP are evident when NE is used in the normal dosage range. NE does not increase heart rate. The main beneficial effect of NE is to increase organ perfusion by increasing vascular tone. Studies that have compared NE to dopamine have favored NE in terms of overall improvement in oxygen delivery, organ perfusion, and oxygen consumption. Oxygen delivery and oxygen consumption increased in both dopamine and NE patient study groups. Norepinephrine is metabolically less active than epinephrine and reduces serum lactate levels. Norepinephrine significantly improves renal perfusion and splanchnic blood flow in sepsis, particularly when combined with dobutamine.

Epinephrine

Epinephrine has potent β_1-, β_2-, and α_1-adrenergic activity, although the increase in MAP in sepsis is mainly from an increase in cardiac output (stroke volume). There are 3 major drawbacks to using this drug: (1) epinephrine increases myocardial oxygen demand; (2) it increases serum glucose and lactate, which is largely a calorigenic effect (increased release and anaerobic breakdown of glucose); and (3) epinephrine appears to have adverse effects on splanchnic blood flow, redirecting blood to peripheral tissues as part of the fight-and-flight response. A combination of dopamine and norepinephrine enhanced gastric mucosal blood flow more than epinephrine alone. There are few data that distinguish epinephrine from norepinephrine in their ability to achieve hemodynamic goals, and epinephrine is a superior inotrope. Concern about the impact of epinephrine on splanchnic perfusion needs to be considered. Concern about the effect of increased serum lactate and hyperglycemia has limited the use of epinephrine. Hypokalemia and arrhythmia are the result of the β_2 agonist action of epinephrine, which drives potassium into the cell resulting in hypokalemia.

Phenylephrine

Phenylephrine is an almost pure α_1-adrenergic agonist with moderate potency. Although widely used in anesthesia to treat iatrogenic hypotension, it is often an ineffective agent in treating sepsis. Phenylephrine is an adrenergic agent least likely to cause tachycardia. It is a less effective vasoconstrictor than norepinephrine or epinephrine. Compared with norepinephrine, phenylephrine is more effective in reducing splanchnic blood flow, oxygen delivery, and lactate uptake. Phenylephrine may be a good therapeutic option when tachyarrhythmias limit therapy with other vasopressors.

Vasopressin

Arginine-vasopressin is an endogenous hormone that is released in response to decreases in intravascular volume and increased plasma osmolality. Vasopressin constricts vascular smooth muscle directly through V_1 receptors. It also increases the responsiveness of the vasculature to catecholamines. Vasopressin is a hormone ADH analog secreted from the posterior pituitary. It is now the first drug administered to adults in out-of-hospital asystole (cardiac arrest) with 40 units given IV as the standard dose. If spontaneous circulation is not restored in 3 minutes, then this dose is repeated or epinephrine therapy as a bolus is begun. If no IV access is available then 40 units diluted with NS to a total volume of 10 mL should be delivered endotracheally. An intra-osseous device can be used to gain IV access. Vasopressin may be used in patients with refractory shock where adequate fluid and pressor resuscitation has failed to increase BP. Vasopressin has emerged as an additive vasoconstrictor in septic patients who have become resistant to catecholamines. There appears to be a quantitative deficiency of this hormone in sepsis, and administration of vasopressin in addition to NE increases splanchnic blood flow and urinary output. Vasopressin does not increase myocardial oxygen demand significantly, and its receptors are unaffected by acidosis.

Neosynephrine

Phenylephrine and neosynephrine are selective α_1-adrenergic receptor agonists used primarily as decongestants, to dilate the pupil, and to increase BP. MI originates from the frequent or overuse of these compounds in nasal sprays. The response of blood pressure and the emergence of side effects to these compounds render them inadequate for use in the ICU. NE and phenylephrine are used more commonly in situations involving anesthesia or critical care. Phenylephrine is especially useful in counteracting the hypotensive effect of epidural and subarachnoid anesthetics. With its pure α activity it lacks inotropic or chronotropic activity, and so it elevates the blood pressure without increasing the heart rate or contractility. Reflex bradycardia may result from the elevation of blood pressure, and this effect may be useful in hypotensive patients that present with a tachyarrhythmia.

Levosimendan

Levosimendan is a calcium sensitizer. It increases the sensitivity of the heart to calcium, thereby increasing cardiac contractility without forcing a rise in intracellular calcium. The combined inotropic and vasodilatory actions result in an increased power of contraction with decreased preload and decreased afterload.

Other Vasopressors

A variety of other vasopressors are available and some of these which are in use include phosphodiesterase inhibitors, such as milrinone and enoximone. These appear to be alternatives to dobutamine as a treatment for cardiomyopathy of critical illness while restoring splanchnic blood flow.

CLINICAL CASE CORRELATION

- **See also Case 4 (Hemodynamic Monitoring), Case 16 (Acute Cardiac Failure), Case 28 (Blunt Trauma), and Case 41 (Hemorrhage, Coagulopathy).**

COMPREHENSION QUESTIONS

5.1 A 75-year-old man is brought to the ED from a nursing home because of confusion, fever, and flank pain. On physical examination, his temperature is 38.8°C (101.9°F), blood pressure is 78/46 mm Hg, heart rate is 117 beats/minute, and respiration rate is 29 breaths/minute. Dry mucous membranes, poor skin turgor, costovertebral angle tenderness but no edema is noted on physical examination. The leukocyte count is 22,000/μL; urinalysis shows 3+ leukocytes. The patient has an anion-gap metabolic acidosis and high lactic acid level. Antibiotic therapy is started. Which of the following is most likely to improve survival for this patient?

A. Fluid resuscitation and correction of BP and lactic acidosis
B. Administration of 25% albumin infusion
C. Hemodynamic monitoring with a pulmonary artery catheter
D. Maintaining hemoglobin above 12 g/dL
E. Maintaining P_{CO_2} below 50 mm Hg

5.2 You are paged by the ICU nurse at 3 AM to evaluate a 72-year-old man whose BP has dropped from 114/78 to 82/48 mm Hg in the past hour. His mucous membranes are dry. You see that the patient was admitted 6 hours ago with a temperature of 38.5°C (101.3°F), BP 118/84 mm Hg, heart rate 104 beats/minute, and respiration rate of 28 breaths/minute. His WBC on admission was 18,000/μL. The patient has been receiving normal saline at 200 mL/h for the past 6 hours. Which of the following is the best first-line pharmacological intervention most likely to improve the patient's blood pressure?

A. Epinephrine alone
B. Norepinephrine
C. Dobutamine
D. Vasopressin
E. Phenylephrine

ANSWERS TO QUESTIONS

5.1 **A.** Aggressive fluid resuscitation with IV antibiotics and resolution of lactic acidosis would have a beneficial effect on this patient's survival. The patient has severe sepsis presumptively from pyelonephritis. The timing of resuscitation matters relative to survival. Early goal-directed therapy includes interventions delivered within the first 6 hours of the patient's presentation to the hospital or within 1 hour if the patient has already been admitted. The goal is to maintain a central venous pressure of 8 to 12 cm H_2O and an oxygen venous saturation of >70%. This results in higher survival rates than more delayed resuscitation attempts. Reversal of the lactic acidosis is paramount.

5.2 **B.** This patient presents with hyperdynamic septic shock. Hyperdynamic septic shock is characterized by hypotension, low SVR, and high CI. Norepinephrine (NE) and phenylephrine are the drugs of choice for the control of hyperdynamic septic shock. NE should be used initially followed by phenylephrine if no improvement is noted. NE is a more potent vasoconstrictor than phenylephrine. Epinephrine is not a first-line treatment as a vasopressor in sepsis. High-dose dopamine is more efficacious in treating hypodynamic septic shock, characterized by hypotension, low SVR, and low CI, resulting in cold extremities. Dobutamine is used in sepsis to reverse the cardiosuppressant effect induced by the gram-negative sepsis; it does not significantly elevate BP. Vasopressin as a supplementary agent in refractory hypotension has been effective.

CLINICAL PEARLS

- Crystalloid solutions are universally used for initial volume resuscitation in sepsis and septic shock to compensate for fluid debt.
- Colloid solutions achieve hemodynamic goals faster than crystalloids with lower volumes.
- Isotonic saline, when administered in large volumes, is associated with hyperchloremic acidosis; this may affect splanchnic blood flow and may be nephrotoxic.
- Dobutamine is a potent inotrope that is a useful adjunct to fluid resuscitation in early sepsis.
- Epinephrine is a potent vasoconstrictor and inotrope. It causes an early lactic acidosis secondary to aerobic glycolysis and may reduce splanchnic blood flow.
- NE is a potent vasoconstrictor that maintains CO and restores blood flow to dependent organs.
- It is essential that patients be fluid-resuscitated before commencing vasopressor therapy.
- The goal of vasopressor support is to maintain BP in the autoregulation range of organs.
- Phenylephrine may be a good therapeutic option when tachyarrhythmia limits therapy with other vasopressors.

REFERENCES

Loscalzo J. *Harrison's Pulmonary and Critical Care Medicine*. New York, NY: McGraw-Hill; 2010.

Roberts I, Alderson P, Bunn F, et al. Colloids versus crystalloids for fluid resuscitation in critically ill patients. *Cochrane Database Syst Rev*. 2004;CD000567.

Toy S, Takenaka, LR. *Case Files Emergency Medicine*. 2nd ed, New York, NY: McGraw-Hill, Lange, 2013.

CASE 6

A 44-year-old man with a subarachnoid hemorrhage and a Glasgow coma score (GCS) of 9 is admitted to the ICU after initial assessment in the emergency department, where he was intubated and placed on a ventilator. A CT of the brain revealed a subarachnoid and an intracerebral hemorrhage. Several hours after his arrival to the ICU, the patient is noted to have increased ventilatory pressures and decreased breath sounds on the left. His O_2 saturation remains at 100%.

- What are the possible causes for the patient's change in condition?
- What imaging modalities can you use to further assess the patient's problem?

ANSWERS TO CASE 6:
Imaging in Critical Care

Summary: An intubated 44-year-old man with a subarachnoid hemorrhage develops increased ventilatory pressures and decreased left-sided breath sounds.

Possible causes for the patient's condition: Right mainstem intubation or left pneumothorax.

Confirmatory studies: Portable chest radiograph to determine whether the patient has developed a pneumothorax and/or if the endotracheal tube has advanced into the right mainstem bronchus. Bedside ultrasound can also be used to determine the presence (or absence) of visceral/parietal pleural sliding. The presence of this tissue interface would confirm a fully expanded left lung and exclude the diagnosis of left pneumothorax.

ANALYSIS

Objectives

1. To learn the values and indications of portable chest radiographs in the ICU.
2. To learn the indications and applications of bedside ultrasound in the ICU (diagnostic and procedure guidance).
3. To learn to apply echocardiography and CT scans for the management of patients in the ICU.

Consideration

This is a 44-year-old patient who is receiving positive pressure ventilation and has been recently transported from the emergency department to the CT scanner and then to the intensive care unit. Additionally, patients with traumatic brain injuries often undergo invasive procedures such as placement of central venous catheters for central venous pressure monitoring. Such events place them at risk for both malpositioning of the endotracheal tube into the right mainstem bronchus and the development of pneumothorax. Both of these conditions can present clinically with decreased left-sided breath sounds.

APPROACH TO:
Imaging in ICU Patients

DEFINITIONS

PORTABLE CHEST RADIOGRAPHY: A modality for performing chest radiographs at the patient's bedside. Patients are often supine or semi-supine for these studies. Portable radiographs are performed using antero-posterior technique, where x-ray beams penetrate from the anterior position. This orientation decreases the quality of the image and impairs detection of small pneumothoraces and hemothoraces due to the supine position. Portable x-rays are helpful for confirmation of endotracheal tube positions and infiltrates or effusions that may signify pathology.

ULTRASOUND: Tissue interfaces reflect sound waves. These "acoustic signals" can be translated into 2-dimensional images that represent the anatomy beneath the ultrasound probe. The images are displayed with those structures closest to the probe at the top of the image whereas those farthest away from the probe appear at the bottom of the image. Subcutaneous air and dense structures (eg, bones, gallstones, foreign bodies) can create artifacts that distort the ultrasound images. Body habitus and lack of skin-to-probe interface secondary to surgical dressings or wounds can also limit visibility and quality of images. Ultrasonography in the ICU is useful for diagnostic purposes (detection of pneumothorax, intraperitoneal fluid, bladder filling) or for the guidance of bedside procedures (central venous catheter placement, arterial line placement, peripheral venous catheter placement, drainage of intraperitoneal or intrapleural fluid collections).

ECHOCARDIOGRAPHY: Ultrasound that is used specifically to evaluate cardiac anatomy and function. Modern day echocardiography adds computerized functions such as color flow Doppler and waveform analysis to quantify flow patterns across (and within) anatomic regions of the heart. The addition of flow analysis and volume measurement software enhances the diagnostic range of echocardiograms. As with other forms of ultrasound, subcutaneous air, wounds, and body habitus all play a role in the quality of images obtainable in individual patients. Echocardiography is useful for the determination of cardiac performance and intravascular volume statuses, especially in patients with clinical shock.

CLINICAL APPROACH

Portable Chest Radiography in the ICU

Portable chest radiographs allow for assessment of ICU patients with acute or progressive respiratory changes. One of the major advantages of these bedside procedures is that transport during instability is avoided. Despite a reduction in image quality, bedside chest radiographs are helpful in determining many different conditions that warrant prompt intervention (Table 6–1).

Table 6–1 • PORTABLE RADIOGRAPH DIAGNOSTIC INDICATIONS
• Right mainstem intubation
• High-positioned endotracheal tube (ETT) (ie, when cuff of the ETT is at or above the vocal cords)
• Malpositioning of other medical devices (eg, feeding tubes, central lines, thoracostomy tubes)
• Pneumothorax
• Hemothorax
• Effusion
• Pulmonary edema
• Pneumonia
• Lobar collapse from mucous plugging
• Bilateral patchy infiltrates secondary to adult respiratory distress syndrome

Portable chest radiographs are less helpful in determining if respiratory decompensation is due to pulmonary embolism (PE). Patients with seemingly "normal" radiographs can have venous embolic disease as the source of their ventilation/perfusion mismatch. If the findings on portable chest films do not elucidate a cause and the patient is at risk for PE, CT angiography can be helpful to rule in or out embolic disease.

Historically, the practice of daily "routine" chest films was common in the ICU. In a recent meta-analysis, this practice was compared to the practice of only performing chest radiographs when clinically indicated (ie, "on demand"). There was no difference in mortality, ICU length of stay, or days on the ventilator between the 2 groups. Patients who received studies only when clinically indicated were exposed to less radiation and had lower hospital costs.

Bedside Ultrasound in the ICU

The advent of small, portable ultrasound machines with improved image resolution and greater depth capabilities has made bedside ultrasonography a valuable tool in the intensive care setting. In comparison to CT scans, ultrasonography does not require the transport of critically ill patients, is not associated with radiation or intravenous contrast exposure. It is more often available and can be repeated more easily than computed tomography. Accessibility and ease of use have made ultrasound an extension of the physical examination for the assessment of critically ill patients.

Ultrasound can be used for almost all anatomic regions. In the thorax, ultrasound assessment of pleural approximation can reliably rule out pneumothorax. Cardiac function can be evaluated in a number of ways, including estimates of ejection fraction and qualitative assessment of wall motion symmetry. In the abdomen, visualization of inferior vena cava diameter changes during the respiratory cycle can give an estimate of a patient's central venous volume status. The focused assessment with sonography for trauma (FAST) allows for initial and serial assessments for increases in intraperitoneal fluid that can represent ongoing hemorrhage after abdominal trauma (Table 6–2).

Ultrasound also offers therapeutic options. Real-time visualization of central venous structure during catheter insertions is associated with lower procedure-related complications and is a practice endorsed by most professional organizations. Fluid in the pericardium can more safely be sampled using ultrasound guidance for pericardiocentesis. Infectious source control can sometimes be accomplished by ultrasound-guided drainage of fluid collections in the thorax, pericardium, abdomen, or soft tissues (Figures 6–1 to 6–4).

Table 6–2 • THE FOCUSED ASSESSMENT WITH SONOGRAPHY FOR TRAUMA (FAST)
Although this method was developed to assess trauma patients in the emergency department, it offers an organized approach for assessment of the abdominal compartment in the ICU. Three of the four views taken in the FAST examination evaluate the abdomen and the nonabdominal view evaluates the patient's pericardium.
Abdominal components of FAST examination:
1. Right upper quadrant—determines fluid inferior to the liver
2. Left upper quadrant—determines fluid around the spleen
3. Suprapubic region—determines fluid in the pelvis

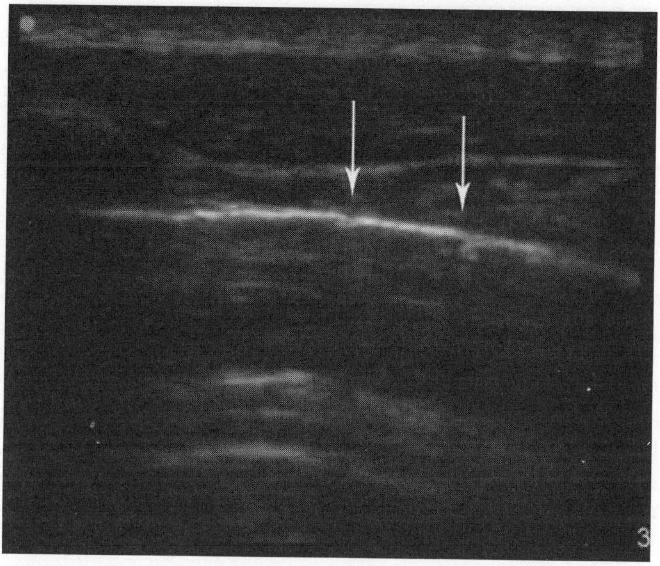

Figure 6–1. Pleural sliding to rule out pneumothorax: the bright white line represents apposition of visceral and parietal pleura. The arrows represent "comet tails" artifacts created by the interface of pleural layers. When these findings are absent, the likelihood of pneumothorax increases. (Courtesy of Arun Ngdev, M.D., Emergency Medicine Residency Program, Alameda Health System.)

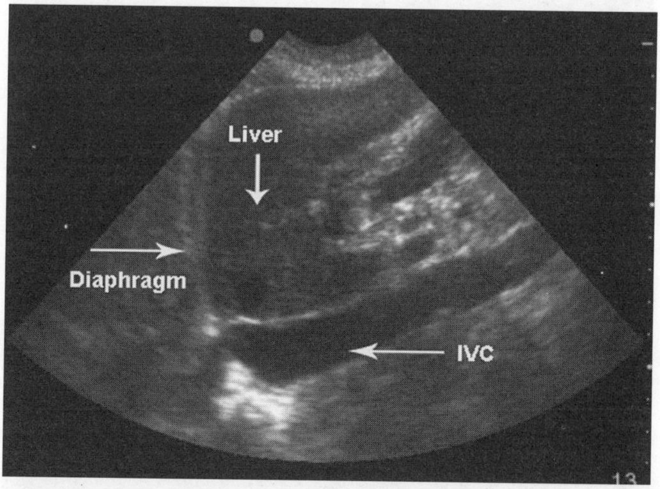

Figure 6–2. Inferior vena cava (IVC) anatomy on ultrasound. Visualization of the IVC during the respiratory cycle yields a reliable estimate of volume status. In the normovolemic state, the IVC will narrow during inspiration and distend during expiration. In severe hypovolemia, the IVC will collapse. In hypervolemia, the IVC diameter will not change throughout the respiratory cycle. (Courtesy of Arun Ngdev, M.D., Emergency Medicine Residency Program, Alameda Health System.)

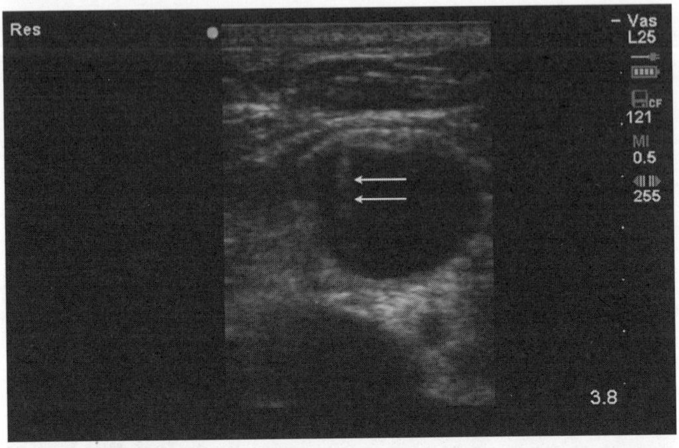

Figure 6–3. Line placement under ultrasound guidance. Real-time visualization for catheter placement: the white arrows point to a needle entering the internal jugular vein for central venous access. (Courtesy of Arun Ngdev, M.D., Emergency Medicine Residency Program, Alameda Health System.)

Learn to Apply Echocardiography and CT Scans for the Management of Patients in the ICU

When patients in the ICU are hemodynamically unstable and ongoing resuscitative efforts do not appear to correct perfusion, one must consider whether cardiac

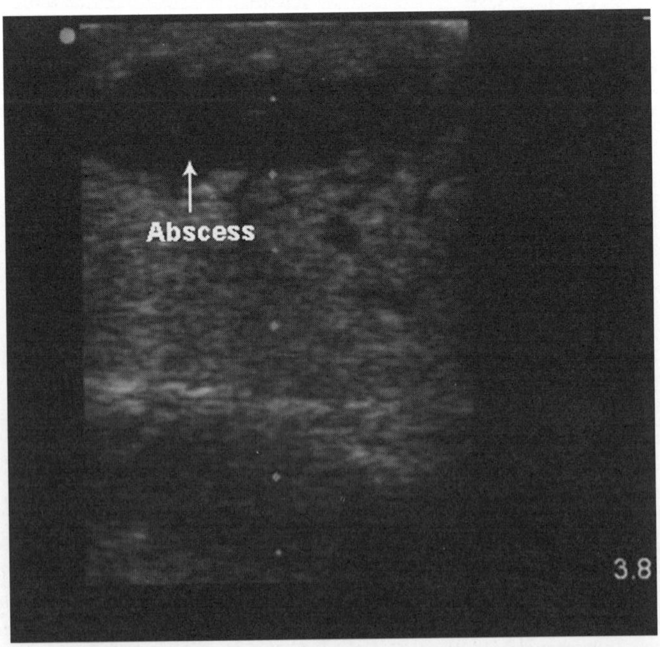

Figure 6–4. Abscess image on ultrasound. Subcutaneous abscess. (Courtesy of Arun Ngdev, M.D., Emergency Medicine Residency Program, Alameda Health System.)

dysfunction is contributing to the clinical presentation. **Bedside echocardiography offers a real-time assessment of the patient's cardiac function.** Echocardiography can be used to estimate left ventricular wall motion, ejection fractions, right heart filling volumes, and pulmonary venous pressures. Information gleaned from such assessments can direct the initiation of inotropic agents, further volume resuscitation, or addition of vasoconstrictors.

Left ventricular function: Bedside echocardiography can qualitatively assess left ventricular wall motion and estimate ventricular function. These qualitative estimates can be performed with most ultrasound machines by clinicians with basic ultrasound training. More sophisticated quantitative measurements can be performed with slightly more advanced ultrasound machines that can be found in many modern day ICUs. Such machines must be able to clearly image the endocardial layer and obtain ventricular areas or volumes during the cardiac cycle. By noting the change in measured areas or volumes of the ventricle during diastole and during systole, *fractional area change* or *ejection fraction* can be calculated.

$$\text{Fractional area change} = \frac{\text{End-diastolic area} - \text{end-systolic area}}{\text{End-diastolic area}}$$

$$\text{Ejection fraction} = \frac{\text{End-diastolic volume} - \text{end-systolic volume}}{\text{End-diastolic volume}}$$

Right ventricular function: The right ventricle is normally a compliant, thin-walled chamber with low pressures. In critical illness, however, factors such as increased pulmonary vascular resistance, left ventricular dysfunction, or marked fluid overload may alter the pressures routinely found in the right ventricle. An acute increase in right ventricular pressures leads to right ventricular dysfunction and if severe, right ventricular failure. Just as in the assessment of the left ventricle, echocardiography can assess the right ventricle qualitatively or quantitatively. Qualitative findings of right ventricular enlargement and septal "bulging" toward the left ventricle suggest severe right ventricular dysfunction. For quantitative measurements, image resolution must be adequate to assess chamber volumes and Doppler flow measurements. Whether clinicians are armed with basic skills and equipment or more advanced training with slightly more sophisticated equipment, bedside echocardiography offers an accessible, noninvasive adjunct for diagnosis of unstable, critically ill patients.

Volume status: Assessment of adequate resuscitation is crucial in the management of patients in shock. Echocardiography offers several noninvasive options for assessment of preload (ie, volume status). As mentioned previously, IVC diameter change during the respiratory cycle can reliably estimate central venous pressure (CVP). Equipment capable of measuring Doppler flow patterns can further elucidate preload by measuring flow across the mitral valve and within the pulmonary artery. Likewise, echocardiographic assessment of left ventricular volumes during the cardiac cycle can estimate left ventricle preload by measuring left ventricular end diastolic volumes. Doppler technology can be used to measure flow across the left ventricular outflow tract to estimate cardiac output.

Anatomic pathology: In addition to wall motion abnormalities, bedside echocardiography can be used to diagnose valvular vegetations, papillary muscle rupture, and ventricular aneurysms. Defects in the ventricular or atrial septum and valvular regurgitation can be visualized with flow Doppler. Increased fluid in the pericardium and its effect on filling of the ventricles during diastole will identify tamponade physiology if preload is compromised by the amount of fluid in the pericardial space. Additionally, therapy for cardiac tamponade can be initiated with ultrasound-guided pericardiocentesis.

Computed tomography: Computed tomography (CT) requires patient transport to radiology; however in some instances, the information gained is worth the risk of transport. CT arteriograms are the study of choice to diagnose pulmonary emboli. Thoracic, abdomen, and pelvic CT scans can determine sources for sepsis that are too deep for detection or obscured by artifact with bedside ultrasonography. CT scans can guide placement of percutaneous drainage catheters for source control, a key component of treatment in the septic patient.

Source identification: When patients experience clinical decline, imaging plays a key role in identifying the source of the problem (see Table 6–3). Portable radiographs and ultrasound are easily accessible and do not require IV contrast and radiation exposure. These studies can be nonspecific and in the case of ultrasound, operator-dependent. Additionally, there are regions of the abdomen, mediastinum, and cranium that are difficult to image with portable ultrasound due to the density of adjacent structures, especially bone. Computed tomography offers a more sensitive and specific way to evaluate the brain, thorax, and abdomen. CT scans can identify fluid collections, areas of active bleeding, inflammation, or edema.

When the acute decline is neurologic, noncontrast computed tomography is used to assess for intracranial pathology, such as worsening traumatic brain injuries, hemorrhagic stroke, or ischemia strokes. Noncontrast CT is less sensitive in determining

Table 6–3 • IMAGING STUDY FOR CLINICAL VARIOUS SITUATIONS

Symptoms	Diagnosis	Imaging Study
Fever, leukocytosis Hemodynamic instability	Sepsis	Portable chest radiograph (infiltrate suggests pneumonia) Ultrasound (especially for suspected biliary source) Computed tomography (full anatomic assessment possible)
Fever, leukocytosis Hemodynamic instability	Systemic inflammatory response syndrome	Computed tomography (if no new findings after source control, likely SIRS)
Altered mental status	Stroke	Noncontrast computed tomography of head
Respiratory failure	Pneumothorax Hemothorax Pneumonia Pulmonary embolism	Portable chest radiograph (pneumonia, pneumo/hemothorax) Computed tomography of the chest (chest angiogram if suspicion for PE)

ischemic strokes; however, CT perfusion imaging (when available) improves accuracy in detection of irreversible cerebral ischemia. Although magnetic resonance imaging (MRI) is the most sensitive for assessment of cerebral ischemia, this study is less feasible in critically ill patients since it requires them to be isolated in the scanning cylinder for a period of time while the study is performed. Patients who require mechanical ventilation, close monitoring, and frequent interventions are poor candidates for this diagnostic modality.

CLINICAL CASE CORRELATION

- **See also Case 13 (DVT/Pulmonary Emboli), Case 16 (Acute Cardiac Failure), and Case 28 (Blunt Trauma).**

COMPREHENSION QUESTIONS

6.1 Which of the following methods provides the safest approach for placement of internal jugular central venous catheters?

A. Using an ultrasound to mark the vein position prior to applying sterile skin prep
B. Portable chest radiograph before and after the procedure
C. Echocardiogram to visualize catheter in right atrium
D. Ultrasound imaging of vein at time of venipuncture
E. Ultrasound of lung apices during procedure to avoid pneumothorax

6.2 A 22-year-old woman has just arrived to the intensive care unit from an uneventful femur fixation in the operating room. During transport, her oxygen saturations dropped to 82%. The respiratory therapist reports that she became more difficult to ventilate with the Ambu-bag (transport ventilation device). On your preliminary examination, she has absent breath sounds on the right and her respiratory rate is 34 breaths/minute and her oxygen saturations are now 87% with an increase to 100% inspired oxygen on the ventilator. The patient's blood pressure is 115/70 mm Hg and heart rate is 110 beats/minute. Which of the following diagnostic test is most likely to be helpful?

A. Ultrasound of the abdomen
B. Computed tomography of the chest
C. Portable chest film
D. MRI of the chest
E. Nuclear medicine scan of the chest

6.3 A 67-year-old man is brought to the emergency department after being found unconscious in his backyard. On initial evaluation, he is unresponsive, his skin is ashen, extremities are cool, and he is perspiring. His blood pressure is 80/65 mm Hg, heart rate is 102 beats/minute, and he has distended neck veins. He is intubated and has bilateral breath sounds. There are several trauma resuscitations on other patients occurring simultaneously and you are given one choice of diagnostic machine to use (because all the equipment is being shared). Which instrument would you choose?

A. Portable chest radiograph machine

B. ECG machine

C. Ultrasound machine with echocardiography probe and Doppler flow

D. CT scan

E. Ultrasound with thoracic and abdomen soft tissue probe

6.4 A hospital has recently identified that transporting critically ill patients to the CT imaging has inherent hazards. Which of the following patients is most appropriate to have a CT scan?

A. A 87-year-old woman, BP 110/70 mm Hg, HR 90 beats/minute, RR 14 breaths/minute, O_{2sat} 95% with ipsilateral decreased breath sounds after central line placement.

B. A 370-lb man, with a subhepatic abscess and extensive subcutaneous emphysema. He is fully resuscitated but remains on 2 vasopressor agents and has a mean arterial pressure of 72 mm Hg.

C. A 43-year-old man on the ventilator with increased peak airway pressures, increased work of breathing, and diminished breath sounds on the left.

D. A 92-year-old woman with BP 86/48 mm Hg, HR 105 beats/minute, RR 18 breaths/minute, serum creatinine of 2.1 mg/dL, and distended neck veins.

E. A 22-year-old man, who was stabbed with a 3-in knife in the third intercostal space, lateral to the right nipple, BP 128/78 mm Hg, HR 82 beats/minute, RR 12 breaths/minute.

ANSWERS TO QUESTIONS

6.1 **D.** "Real-time" imaging of the internal jugular vein while it is being cannulated has been shown to be the safest approach when compared to the anatomic landmark technique and when compared to pre-procedure vein location marking.

6.2 **C. Chest Radiograph is most appropriate.** Although thoracic computed tomography can give valuable information on chest pathophysiology, the patient presented with acute respiratory decompensation and signs worrisome for right pneumothorax. Transport to the CT scanner in such a tenuous patient would invite catastrophe. Modalities such as bedside thoracic ultrasound to evaluate presence or absence of pleural sliding and portable chest radiograph (performed in a timely manner) could both identify a clinically significant pneumothorax. Right needle thoracostomy can be performed in patients in whom you have a high index of suspicion for pneumothorax. This procedure, when performed appropriately, is of relatively low risk and transient therapeutic benefit. Repeating auscultation once a room quiets down is quick, easy, and can help confirm presence or absence of breath sounds. The important point here is if a patient is unstable and diagnosis can be made at the bedside, it is safest not to transport the patient elsewhere for diagnostics.

6.3 **C.** The patient presents in shock with no available history. Clinical findings suggest cardiac dysfunction with severe malperfusion and distended neck veins. Although an ECG can give some information that can help rule in or out a potential infarction, a bedside echocardiogram can quickly identify anatomic and functional abnormalities such as pericardial tamponade, papillary muscle rupture, severe wall motion abnormalities, septal rupture, and so on. With echocardiography, the patient's volume status can also be estimated, as can the presence of increase pulmonary vascular pressures. In the instance of tamponade, echocardiography can be used real-time for a safer method of pericardiocentesis.

6.4 **B.** Of the patients listed, the obese man with subcutaneous emphysema will likely be technically challenging for bedside ultrasound-guided drainage of his subhepatic abscess. His body habitus and the subcutaneous air will increase artifacts and lessen the safety of the ultrasound-guided technique. CT-guided abscess drainage offers a much safer route for patients who have limited ultrasound views. Patients "A, C, and E" all have suspected pulmonary diagnoses that can be evaluated with either portable radiographs or thoracic ultrasound. Patient "D" has a likely cardiac source for her symptoms and can be evaluated with bedside echocardiography.

REFERENCES

Beaulieu Y, Marik PE. Bedside ultrasound in the ICU: Part 1. *Chest*. 2005;128:881-895.

Guillory RK, Gunter OL. Ultrasound in the surgical intensive care unit. *Curr Opin Crit Care*. 2008;14: 415-422.

McLean AS, Needham A, Stewart D, et al. Estimation of cardiac output by noninvasive echocardiographic techniques in critically ill subjects. *Anaesth Intensive Care*. 1997;25:250-254.

Oba Y, Zaza T. Abandoning daily routine chest radiography in the intensive care unit: meta-analysis. *Radiology*. 2010;255:386-395.

Vigno P, Mucke F, Bellec F, et al. Basic critical care echocardiography: validation of a curriculum dedicated to noncardiologist residents. *Crit Care Med*. 2011;39:636-642.

CASE 7

A 25-year-old male organ donor in the ICU is diagnosed as brain dead after suffering a closed head trauma in a motorcycle accident. He is intubated on an AC mode with a rate of 16 breaths/minute, V_t 450 mL, FIO_2 35%. Arterial blood gas (ABG) data are: pH 7.36, $Paco_2$ 36 mm Hg, Pao_2 150 mm Hg on fractional inspired oxygen concentration (FIO_2) of 35%. The transplant team and operation room team are alerted. The blood pressure (BP) is 110 mm Hg systolic and 60 mm Hg diastolic, heart rate (HR) is 110 beats/minute and regular; temperature is 96°Fahrenheit (F), weight 70 kg, and height 62 in. Electrolyte values are sodium (Na+) 155 mEq/L, potassium (K^+) 4 mEq/L, chloride (Cl^-) 105 mEq/L, bicarbonate (HCO_3) 20 mEq/L. His urine output is 150 mL/h.

- ▶ What are the most appropriate next steps while awaiting organ transplant?
- ▶ What is the most important parameter that impacts on organ survival?

ANSWERS TO CASE 7:
Ethics in Critical Care

Summary: This 25-year-old patient is brain dead and is an organ donor. Life support should continue while striving to maintain physiologic and laboratory variables "within normal limits" to preserve organ integrity until procurement of the organ by the transplant team.

- **Next steps while awaiting organ transplantation:** Maintain the patient/donor's physiologic parameters as close to normal as possible.
- **Most important criteria for organ survival:** Time is of the essence in this situation. Coordinate all paperwork and required testing ASAP. Decreased time equals increased cell or organ survival.

ANALYSIS

Objectives

1. To understand basic care for brain death in adult organ donor patients.
2. To understand the physiologic changes involved in organ donors.

Considerations

This unfortunate 25-year-old man suffered a motor vehicle and has been diagnosed as brain dead, presumably due to global and irreversible loss of brain stem function. This patient is a candidate to be an organ or tissue donor, which is identified based on prior wishes such as indicated in an advanced directive or an organ donor card, and based on discussion with the family. Significant emotional issues may be involved with a loved one; thus, a specially trained hospital staff member or a representative of an organ procurement organization speaking to the family can help the family through some of the difficult decisions and respecting the family's wishes. The declaration of brain death requires establishing the patient being in a coma and with no evidence of brain stem reflexes (such as breathing independently, pupil reaction to light, eye movement, or arms and legs pulling away from noxious stimuli). To produce the best outcome for organs, keeping the patient's physiological processes as normal as possible is important: BP, RR, oxgynation, and fluid/electrolyte status. A coordinated team approach is likewise optimal to help the family through the grieving process, working with the medical team, and communicating with the transplant team.

APPROACH TO:
General Organ Donor Issues

In this situation common sense judgments of critical care are applied. Guidelines generally include optimizing cardiovascular and pulmonary function, fluid and electrolyte balance, identification and treatment of infection, and the administration of hormones. The Donor Risk Index shows how these "fixed" criteria are interrelated with the variable criteria. Donor organs are influenced by the prevailing systemic physiology (eg, oxygen delivery, blood electrolyte composition, regional and systemic cytokines). General parameters of optimal care are addressed as well as individual factors that may affect a transplantable organ (see Table 7–1).

TREATMENT TIME

Minimize the time between collection and implantation of the donor organ. Specialized centers seriously dedicated to following the best practice guidelines have had a major impact in increasing satisfactory treatment. **Transplantation specialists encourage modestly elevated blood glucose levels.** Neuroglycopenia during insulin therapy ceases to be a concern in the brain-dead donor. The immunosuppressive effect induced by hyperglycemia might benefit the recipient.

Coagulopathy and Transfusion Therapy

The optimal hemoglobin and hematocrit levels for donor patients are outlined in Table 7–1. The requirement for oxygen uptake is now freed from consideration of the brain, a major oxygen-consuming organ. The reduction in cardiac output lowers oxygen delivery to transplantable organs. Items of particular concern are the inflammatory mediator burden, acute lung injury, and possible transmission of viruses to the recipient. The potential effect of a compromised immune status due to transfusion is unknown. Multiple blood transfusions usually improve transplant success. Hemorrhage is not desirable, but "intrinsic" anticoagulation may be beneficial for organ perfusion. **Infusion of the coagulation factors contained in fresh-frozen plasma and platelet concentrates** have been associated with **transfusion related acute lung injury** in critically ill medical patients (TRALI), which is indistinguishable from

Table 7–1 • RECOMMENDATIONS FOR DONOR CARE GUIDELINE PARAMETERS

Central venous pressure 4-12 mm Hg	Glucose 70-150 mg/dL
Pulmonary artery occluded pressure 8-12 mm Hg	pH 7.40-7.45
Cardiac index >2.4 L/min/m	$Paco_2$ 30-35 mm Hg
Cardiac output >3.8 L/min	PaO_2 >80-90 mm Hg
Mean arterial pressure 60 mm Hg	Hemoglobin >10 g/dL
Systolic blood pressure >90 and <120 mm Hg	Hematocrit >30%
Urine output 1-3 mL/kg/h	

ARDS. Recombinant factor VIIa represents a special concern. Although often used for off-label indications during traumatic and neurosurgical bleeding, the value of this factor has not been evaluated in donors. Platelet transfusion likewise may precipitate lung injury and release proinflammatory substances. The benefit or potential harm of supplemental platelet infusions when antiplatelet drugs have recently been used to treat thrombocytopenia remains unknown.

Body Temperature and Hormone Replacement

After brain death, most donors develop mild to moderate hypothermia, which may aid in reducing metabolism in donor organs. The harmful side effects of hypothermia include increased polyuria, alterations in coagulopathy, and dysrhythmias. Polyuria may respond to the administration of vasopressin and fluids.

Primary hypoadrenalism may result from brain death or the donor's antecedent injuries or diseases. Corticosteroids above "stress dosages" are commonly used to support lung transplantation. Supplemental mineralocorticoids may correct donor hyponatremia, but this is balanced with the high incidence of coexisting diabetes insipidus. Additional doses of corticosteroids or an IV infusion may be needed if donor care extends beyond 8 to 12 hours. More organs can be recovered when various synergistic combinations of hormones are used. Corticosteroid therapy is an exception and if it is not used for lung support, it is still given for full stress coverage, especially when hypotension persists despite adequate fluid and vasoactive drug treatment. **Thyroid hormone** therapy is widely accepted for routine administration as well as a "rescue" medication to treat hypotension that is refractory to inotropic or vasopressor agents. The recommended dose of triiodothyronine (T_3) is 2 to 3 mg per hour intravenously.

Polyuria, which commonly occurs after brain death, places organs at risk due to subsequent hypovolemia, hypotension, and hypoperfusion. Etiologies of polyuria include physiologic diuresis, residual effects of diuretics given for the treatment of intracranial hypertension, osmotic diuresis due to residual mannitol, hyperglycemia, or diabetes insipidus (DI). Polyuria from causes other than DI usually does not produce significant hypernatremia. Hypernatremia after transplantation is associated with reduced liver function. Sodium levels >155 mEq/L are the accepted maximum. Intravenous replacement with balanced salt solutions or hypotonic saline is recommended when the urine output is above 150 to 200 mL/h. Significant hyperglycemia may develop if excess dextrose and water solutions are used, and should be treated. Aqueous vasopressin may be administered in repeated intravenous boluses (5-10 U) or titrated as an infusion to treat polyuria. Desmopressin (DDAVP) is also effective as an intravenous bolus (0.5-2 micrograms) repeated as necessary to achieve the desired urine output.

Nutrition, Reperfusion, and Preconditioning

Nutrients may facilitate glycogen deposition in the liver, enhance the availability of fatty acids and glutamine useful to the heart, and provide omega-3 fatty acids or amino acids helpful for renal protection. The administration of coenzyme CoQ10 has some promise as a cardiac protectant. Studies have shown that CoQ10 lowers blood pressure slightly and potentially protects the heart against decreasing the synthesis of this enzyme in the heart, which can be depleted by Statin use.

Injury to transplanted organs occurs via the production and release of free radicals and other harmful substances at the time of organ implantation, rewarming, and reperfusion. In addition, injury is seen when significant hypotension is followed by resuscitation and improved tissue perfusion to the transplanted organ. An episode of controlled hypotension, however, may precondition some organs (especially the liver) before explantation, by increasing its tolerance to reperfusion injury after implantation. Dopamine use is not beneficial in preventing such injury.

Conclusion

Donor care is often a complex undertaking. Providing the best possible organs to awaiting recipients demands careful attention to multiple variables. The paucity of evidence-based data is a challenge to the critical care, organ procurement, and transplantation teams. "Do-not-resuscitate" (DNR) orders are ethical issues that frequently occur in the ICU. These orders should be displayed clearly on the patient's chart. If such orders are not present, the patient can be asked about their wishes for resuscitation following a cardiac arrest or life-threatening arrhythmia. Like many other medical decisions, deciding whether or not to resuscitate a patient who suffers a cardiopulmonary arrest involves a careful consideration of the potential likelihood for clinical benefit balanced with the patient's preferences for the intervention and its likely outcome. Decisions to forego cardiac resuscitation are often difficult because of real or perceived differences in these considerations.

WHEN SHOULD CPR BE ADMINISTERED?

Cardiopulmonary resuscitation (CPR) and advanced cardiac life support (ACLS) are a set of specific medical procedures designed to establish circulation and breathing in a patient. CPR and ACLS are designed to maintain perfusion to vital organs while attempts are made to restore spontaneous breathing and cardiac rhythm by bedside defibrillation. If the patient stops breathing or cardiac arrest occurs in the hospital, the standard care is to perform CPR in the absence of a valid physician's order to withhold it. Paramedics responding to an arrest in the field are required to administer CPR.

Hospitals have policies, which describe circumstances under which CPR can be withheld. Some general situations which justify withholding CPR are

- When CPR is judged to be of no medical benefit.
- When the patient with the capacity to make serious decisions clearly indicates that he/she does not want CPR, with signed documents confirming these wishes clearly written in medical rather than legal language.
- When the patient displays an impaired decision-making capacity, a surrogate can make the decisions for the patient. The surrogate can clearly indicate that the patient does not wish to receive CPR.

CPR is futile when it offers the patient no clinical benefit; in these circumstances, physicians are ethically justified in withholding resuscitation. Clearly, it is important to define what it means to "be of benefit." The distinction between merely providing measurable effects (eg, normalizing the serum potassium) and providing significant health benefits is helpful in this deliberation.

One approach to defining benefit examines the probability of an intervention leading to a desirable outcome. CPR has been prospectively evaluated in a wide variety of clinical situations. Knowledge of the probability of success with CPR could be used to determine its futility.

CPR might also seem to lack benefit when the patient's quality of life is so poor that no meaningful improvement is expected with resuscitation. Judging "quality of life" tempts prejudicial statements about patients with a chronic illness or disability. There is substantial evidence that patients with such chronic conditions often rate their quality of life much higher than would healthy people. There is probably a consensus that patients in a permanent unconscious state possess a quality of life that few would accept. Therefore, CPR is usually considered "futile" for patients in a persistent vegetative state.

There is no obligation to provide CPR when it is judged to be medically futile. Nevertheless, in keeping with the principle of autonomy, the patient and/or their family should still have a role in the decision about a do-not-resuscitate (DNR) order. In many cases, the patient/family, upon being given a caring but frank understanding of the clinical situation, will agree with the DNR order. In such cases a DNR order can be written at that time. Each hospital should have specific procedures for writing a valid DNR order. In all cases, the order must be written or cosigned by the attending physician. A decision to withhold CPR may also arise from a patient's expressed wish that CPR not be performed. If the patient understands the existing medical condition and possesses an intact decision-making capacity, then the DNR request should be honored.

Ethicists and physicians are divided over how to proceed if the family members disagree. A DNR order can only be written with full patient/family agreement. Every reasonable effort should be made to explain all details of the medical situation with involved parties, which usually will lead to a resolution of the conflict. In difficult cases, an ethics consultation can prove helpful. Nevertheless, CPR should generally be provided to such patients, even if judged futile. **The so-called "slow-codes,"** where half-hearted efforts at resuscitation are made, **are not ethically justified.** Such actions undermine the patient's rights and violate the code of physician–patient trust. In most instances, the decision to initiate or deny CPR occurs at a time when the patient is unable to participate in decision making, and their preference is unknown. There are 2 general approaches to this dilemma: Advanced directives and Surrogate decision makers.

Advanced Directive

The advanced directive is a document that details the kinds of decisions the patient would like to have made if he/she is unable to participate at the time when the critical decision must be made. This document may list or indicate specific decisions (eg, **living will**); otherwise it may designate a specific person to make health-care decisions for them (ie, **durable power of attorney for health-care and surrogate**). There is some controversy of how literally living wills should be interpreted. Preferences expressed in a living will are most compelling when they reflect long-held, consistently stable views of the patient. This can often be determined by conversations with family members, close friends, or health-care providers who have had a long-term relationship with the patient.

Table 7–2 • HIERACHY OF FAMILY RELATIONSHIPS IN SURROGATE DECISION MAKING	
1. Legal guardian with health-care decision-making authority	**4.** Individual given durable power of attorney for health-care decisions
2. Spouse	**5.** Adult children of patient (all in agreement)
3. Parents of patient	**6.** Adult siblings of patient (all in agreement)

Surrogate Decision Maker

In the absence of a written document, the law recognizes a hierarchy of family relationships in determining which family member should be the official "spokesperson." See Table 7–2.

CONCLUSIONS

Basic medical treatment should not be withheld, but established medical and ethical practices should be performed. When confronted with decisions regarding interventions with CPR, the healthcare team should demonstrate respect for personal autonomy and provide informed consent. DNR orders should not be converted into do-not-treat or do-not-rescue orders without adequate documentation from a proper source. Emergencies do not alter the standards of medical care, but the best possible care should be rendered under the circumstances, within the patient's informed consent. The standard of care is the same in sickness and in health, including medical/surgical emergencies.

CLINICAL CASE CORRELATION

- **See also Case 3 (Scoring Systems and Patient Prognosis).**

COMPREHENSION QUESTIONS

7.1 Mr H is a 24-year-old man who resides in a skilled nursing facility, where he is undergoing rehabilitation from a cervical spine injury. The injury left him as a quadriplegic. He has normal cognitive function and no problems with respiration. He is admitted to your service for treatment of pneumonia. The resident suggests antibiotics, chest physiotherapy, and hydration. The intern says "he should be a DNR, based on medical futility." In which of the following clinical scenarios does CPR intervention offer the most benefit?

A. ICU patient with acute stroke

B. Patient with metastatic cancer

C. Patient in septic shock

D. Patient with renal failure

E. Patient with severe pneumonia

7.2 An 82-year-old woman with colon cancer and liver metastases was admitted for chemotherapy. Because of her poor prognosis, she is asked about a DNR order, but she requests to be "a full code." Which is the most appropriate management of this patient?

A. Explain to the patient that her signing a DNR order means the patient will need to be placed in hospice care.

B. Emphasize to the patient with compassion that a decision should be made in the next several hours in case a cardiac arrest occurs.

C. Sharing this decision with family members is rarely helpful since guilt is often a complicating factor.

D. Discuss with the patient that DNR will not mean the patient will receive less care.

ANSWERS TO QUESTIONS

7.1 **D. Renal failure can be treated both acutely and chronically with dialysis.** The other answer choices are associated with higher medical futility, meaning that an intervention such as CPR may offer no chance of significant benefit to the patient. Interventions can be considered futile if the probability of success (discharged alive from the hospital) is <1% and/or the quality of life is below the minimum acceptable to the patient. In the scenario from this question, the patient's probability of survival after CPR is below average, based on his quadriplegia and mild pneumonia. In fact, in cases of severe pneumonia and respiratory failure survival is <1%. His quality of life is not without value. Since he is fully awake and alert, Mr H could be asked about his view of the quality of his life. A discussion about likely scenarios should he have a cardiac arrest and need CPR is important. Thereafter, Mr H can tell you if he prefers to have CPR or nothing done in the event of an arrest. No judgment about the possible utility or futility of CPR based on Mr H's current condition can be reached without a discussion. The decision about resuscitation should occur only after consulting with the patient and family members about his situation and reaching a joint decision.

7.2 **D.** This patient is elderly and has a diagnosis of metastatic cancer. Out of hospital survival would *not* be expected should this patient require CPR. Thus CPR for Ms W could be described as a "futile" effort. The patient does not meet other criteria for futility. It is important that she is of sound mind. A DNR order should not be written even if a CPR would be judged as useless unless there is patient or family concurrence. Patients must be given time to understand the seriousness of their diagnosis. Periodic readdressing the question of CPR with them and their family should be continuing. This is best done in the context of other medical decisions that occur during the patient's care. Emphasize that a DNR order *does not* mean the patient will be abandoned or receive a lower standard of care.

CLINICAL PEARLS

- A coordinated approach to the donor patient and family is crucial, to address emotional and spiritual needs, optimize the physiological parameters, and work together with the transplant team.
- While there is limited data guiding this area, expert opinion recommends a maintenance or restoration of normal physiologic and laboratory parameters.
- Cardiovascular instability often occurs during the evolution of brain death due to catecholamine surges, cytokine production, and neurovascular changes.
- Aggressive critical care interventions can correct cardiovascular instability and reverse or preserve normal organ functions, allowing transplantation to proceed.
- More research is needed to define the level of physiological variability that is acceptable in organ donors.

REFERENCES

Annas GJ. Standard of care: in sickness and in health and in emergencies. *N Engl J Med*. 2010;362: 2126-2131.

Cherniack EP. Increasing use of DNR orders in the elderly worldwide: whose choice is it? *J Med Ethics*. 2002 Oct;28(5):303-307.

Deutschman C, Neligan P. *Evidence-Based Practice of Critical Care*. Philadephia: Saunders, Elsevier; 2010.

Holmquist M, Chabalewski F, Blount T, et al. A critical pathway: guiding care for organ donors. *Crit Care Nurse* 1999;19:84-98.

Loscalzo J. *Harrison's Pulmonary and Critical Care Medicine*. New York: McGraw-Hill; 2010.

Wood KE, Becker BN, McCartney JG, et al. Care of the potential organ donor. *N Engl J Med*. 2004;351: 2730-2739.

CASE 8

You are called to manage the airway of a 22-year-old male boxer who is admitted to the ICU for inspiratory stridor after suffering from head and neck trauma during a professional boxing match earlier that evening. He is suffering from rhabdomyolysis and a concussion. He is confused about the timeline of events that night. A CT scan of his brain reveals mild cerebral edema and no evidence of intracranial bleeding. He is responsive to deep voice stimuli. He is 72 in tall and 80 kg in weight.

- What is the most important initial step in the management of this patient?
- What are other management considerations?

ANSWERS TO CASE 8:
Airway Management/Respiratory Failure

Summary: This 22-year-old boxer has inspiratory stridor, which indicates impending respiratory failure due to upper airway obstruction or collapse.

- **Most important initial management:** (1) Rapid-sequence intubation (RSI) to protect the airway; (2) avoid the use of a nasal gastric tube (NGT) since this patient has facial trauma, and there is risk of perforation of the cribriform plate by the NGT. Insertion via the mouth is the preferred option.
- **Other steps:** Chest x-ray to evaluate the trachea and correct placement of the endotracheal tube (ETT) as well as pneumothorax. If cerebral edema is present, high minute ventilation should be used to produce a respiratory alkalosis to decrease intracranial pressure (ICP). Positive end expiratory pressure (PEEP) should not be excessive to avoid increasing ICP. Propofol is indicated for induction and sedation since it lowers ICP, has anti-seizure activity, and has a rapid elimination profile allowing for accurate assessment of the CNS status.

ANALYSIS

Objectives

1. To understand the indications and contraindications for endotracheal intubation (ETI).
2. To understand alternative methods for airway control.
3. To understand the most common complications of endotracheal intubation.
4. To understand the required steps and tools for endotracheal intubation.

Considerations

This 22-year-old boxer presents with head and neck trauma and shows inspiratory stridor, which portends possible airway collapse. This requires RSI for the protection and control of the airway. A "wait and see" attitude in this patient would likely lead to devastating consequences. A nasogastric tube may be required to reduce the likelihood of aspiration of blood. Aspiration precautions were begun with elevation of the head of the bed to 45 degrees upright. Mechanical ventilation is begun on assist control (AC) mode of 22 breaths/minute with a tidal volume of 500 mL with a 100% FIO_2, and a PEEP of 5. A higher minute ventilation is prudent to decrease intracerebral pressure.

APPROACH TO:
Airway Management/Ventilator Support

INTUBATION IN CRITICAL CARE SETTINGS

The **most common indication for endotracheal intubation (ETI) is to treat hypoxic respiratory failure and hypercarbic ventilatory failure.** The initial treatment for hypoxia begins with the insertion of a low-flow nasal cannula and the delivery of about 3% per liter of FIO_2 then escalating to 100% with the use of a non-rebreather mask or high-flow O_2 therapy. Patients with impaired consciousness and an inability to protect their airway have secondary indications for ETI. One should assure that the patient does not have any documentation where endotracheal intubation and mechanical ventilation have been refused or where a do-not-intubate (DNI) or do not resuscitate (DNR) order exists. The patient's wishes or those of the family or the legal guardian should be considered prior to further invasive measures. Other secondary indications for ETI include the significant aspiration of particulate matter.

ETI may be indicated for patients requiring bronchoscopy and pulmonary lavage, those with neurological or traumatic injuries who need deep sedation and intubation to perform necessary imaging tests or diagnostic and therapeutic procedures, and for individuals with status epileptics who require deep sedation or paralysis for treatment of seizures.

Endotracheal Intubation

Endotracheal intubation (ETI) is the definitive method for control of the airway, and a common procedure for patients undergoing general anesthesia. The laryngeal mask airway (LMA), device that does not require a tube through the trachea or a laryngoscope for placement, and is an alternative for patients scheduled for shorter surgeries. The LMA is a short ETT-type tube that is surrounded and held in place by a laryngeal mask. The apex of the mask, with its open end pointing downward toward the tongue, is pushed backward toward the *uvula*. The LMA is effective as a short-term option and does not require as much expertise for placement as ETI. Those patients who may need airway control range from those scheduled to receive anesthesia to critically ill patients with multi-system disease or injuries. Emergency situations such as cardiac or respiratory arrest also require the need for ETI. It is effective in situations to protect the airway from aspiration, address inadequate oxygenation or ventilation, and for patients with existing or anticipated airway obstruction. These indications are increasingly more complicated in an era of advanced technology in oxygen delivery systems and noninvasive forms of ventilation. These forms can be divided in 3 basic categories: (1) hypoxic respiratory failure (decreased PO_2), (2) hypercarbic ventilator failure (including cardiac arrest), drug overdose (elevated PCO_2), and (3) impaired level of consciousness, requiring airway protection to prevent aspiration.

The excessive presence and inability of the patient to clear secretions are more important indicators for airway protection and ETI than is absence of the gag reflex. **The lack of a gag reflex is not a sensitive predictor for ETI for airway control.**

Checking of the gag reflex should be performed with suctioning equipment is at hand, since it may induce vomiting and cause aspiration. The accumulation of large amounts of secretions in the oral cavity, without ability to clear, is an indication for ETI. If the patient can speak, is cooperative, and responds to verbal questioning, then one should consider a trial of NIV (noninvasive ventilation), provided it does not delay an eventual ETI. The assisted ventilation provided from NIV therapy can provide additional time for the treatment of underlying medical conditions with steroids, bronchodilators, diuretics, nitrates, or other medications.

Hypoxic Respiratory Failure

Hypoxic respiratory failure or Type 1 hypoxic respiratory failure is defined as hypoxemia without hypercarbia. An impairment of oxygen exchange via the pulmonary alveolar capillary membrane (>A-a gradient) results in hypoxemia, leading to a diminished delivery of oxygen to the cells and tissues. A quick and easy way to calculate the A-a gradient is shown later. You should not have a negative A-a gradient as determined by the equation:

$$\textbf{A-a gradient} = (\mathrm{FIO_2} \times 7) - \mathrm{PAO_2} - (\mathrm{PACO_2} \times 1.2) \text{ normal is } <20 \text{ mm Hg}$$

The initial treatment of all causes of hypoxemia includes: (a) ensure a patent airway, (b) provide adequate ventilation, and (c) provide supplemental oxygen. A PAO_2 value of 60 mm Hg or an arterial oxygen saturation of 90% to 92% is often suggested as a minimal accepted value. Patients with hypoxemia will improve upon delivery of increasingly higher FIO_2, indicating VQ mismatch as the underlying pathophysiologic cause. If the hypoxemia is resistant to high FIO_2 concentration, the most likely cause is shunting (eg, ARDS).

The treatment of hypoxia begins by ensuring a patent airway for adequate ventilation and oxygenation of the patient. Trials of noninvasive ventilation (NIV) may be indicated, but this should not delay intubation and MV if needed. If the O_2 saturation fails to improve on 100% FIO_2, then ETI and MV should be undertaken so PEEP can be administered.

Hypercarbic Ventilatory Failure ($PACO_2$)

Hypercarbic ventilatory failure occurs when there is an inability to remove carbon dioxide (CO_2) from the alveoli. This condition may be the result of a primary lung disorder or secondarily associated with cardiac, neurologic, or metabolic causes.

The symptoms and signs of hypercarbia are explained by the fact that increasing $PACO_2$ results in vasoconstriction, confusion, sedation, and acidosis. Diagnosis of hypercarbia is confirmed with an ABG with a $PACO_2$ >45 mm Hg and significant acidemia secondary to the elevated $PACO_2$. The rate of change in $PACO_2$ will affect the signs and symptoms. If the change in $PACO_2$ is gradual, then the onset of symptoms such as lethargy, headache, and confusion will be more gradual. However, if the $PACO_2$ rapidly changes, then the onset of symptoms will be more pronounced. **Treatment of hypercarbic ventilator failure includes supplemental oxygenation and ensuring that the patient has a patent airway.** The treatment should be specifically directed toward the underlying etiology. If the patient's condition does not improve with the initial treatment, then increasing the minute ventilation is necessary.

Noninvasive positive pressure ventilation should be attempted first unless there is an obvious need for an ETI. The indications for progressing to ETI are ventilatory failure despite CPAP, signs of impending respiratory failure such as increasing dyspnea, tachypnea, the use of accessory breathing muscles, and low tidal volume ventilation.

Impaired Consciousness and Airway Protection

Patients with Glasgow coma scale (GCS) values of 8 or less should be intubated because of diminished levels of consciousness, continued hypoventilation, and a need for airway protection. Comatose patients have decreased respiratory drive, hypoventilation, airway obstruction and the decreased ability to clear secretions. Thirty percent of the patients with subarachnoid hemorrhage and traumatic brain injury are likely to develop pulmonary edema, severe acute adult lung injury, or ARDS. When there is concern of increased ICP and uncal herniation, hyperventilation with alkalosis has been shown to be helpful by inducing cerebral vasoconstriction. Propofol for sedation has also been shown to reduce intracranial pressure. Prolonged hyperventilation for prophylaxis of ICP should be avoided because of the risk for ischemic brain injury. Other indications for ETI include traumatic injury or swelling to the face or neck, or other obstructive airway processes.

Contraindications to Endotracheal Intubation

Because of the urgency for ventilatory support or airway control, relatively few contraindications exist for ETI. Direct laryngoscopy is contraindicated in patients with partial transection of the trachea because this can cause a complete loss of the airway. In this situation, one should consider establishing a surgical airway. If the cervical spine is unstable to bending as in RA, then strict, inline stabilization of the cervical spine is needed and must be maintained during ETI to avoid cord injury and paralysis. Of note, video-assisted ETT placement has reduced the need to hyperextend the neck during intubation.

Special Considerations

Before intubation, all the necessary equipment must be at hand. The recommended equipment includes: gloves, protective face shield, suction system, bag-valve mask attached to an oxygen source, ETT with a stylet, 10 mL syringe, ETT holder, end-tidal carbon dioxide detector, stethoscope, and laryngoscope with blade or new fiberoptic technology. The fiberoptic laryngoscope allows visual guidance of the blade and observing the insertion of the ETT past the vocal cords. The two common types of blades currently in use are the Miller straight blade and the curved MacIntosh blade. ETTs are available in different internal diameters: 7.0, 7.5, and 8 mm. In adults, the 8-mm diameter tube should be used when possible. The tracheal size is best estimated by the patient's predicted BMI and not actual BMI. The ETT are available cuffed and uncuffed varieties. The uncuffed tubes are usually for children whereas the cuffed tubes are for older children and adults. Cuffs should not be over-inflated, since they are designed as large-volume, low-pressure systems to prevent mucosal ischemia of the trachea. Pre-oxygenation, with 100% oxygen by a non-rebreather mask or a bag-valve mask is necessary to increase oxygenation in the blood; this is achieved by replacing the higher proportion of N_2 in the room air with oxygen. This is accomplished by using 100% O_2, which also increases the patient's functional reserve capacity with oxygen and increases the interval before the next desaturation. Increasing the amount of oxygenation reduces the amount of positive-pressure ventilation, which reduces the risk of aspiration of gastric contents.

Before any procedure is initiated, one should confirm that consent forms have been signed, unless it is an emergency. If it is an emergency, one should ensure that there is no order for do-not-resuscitate (DNR) or a do-not-intubate (DNI). The stylet, is normally flexible and can be reshaped, is usually placed into the ETT to maintain the natural curvature of the airway. IV access should be established and the patient's vital signs should be continuously monitored. Proper positioning the patient before intubation is important. The patient's head should be level with the lower portion of the sternum. The "sniffing" position can be accomplished by placing a pillow or folded towel beneath the patient's occiput. Alignment of the 3 axis of the oral cavity, pharynx, and larynx, which is ideal for vocal cord visualization, can be arranged by flexing the neck and extending the head. Any dentures should be removed. An assistant should perform the Sellick maneuver (applying firm pressure to the cricoid cartilage), which compresses the esophagus between the cricoid cartilage and the cervical vertebrae avoiding aspiration of the gastric content. This maneuver reduces the risk of passive aspiration of gastric contents and improves visualization of the glottis.

INTRAVENOUS ACCESS AND DRUGS FOR SEDATION AND PARALYSIS

Neuromuscular blocking agents and strong sedatives are used to improve visualization of the vocal cords and to reduce the likelihood of vomiting and aspiration. Midazolam and fenyanyl are the hypnotic agents typically used for induction. Other combinations include thiopental and ketamine. A commonly used neuromuscular blocking agent is succinylcholine. Rocuronium is a substitute when there is a contraindication for succinylcholine especially in the presence of hyperkalemia. Succinylcholine should be avoided in hyperkalemia because of the depolarization at the neuromuscular junction. Edema, obstruction, tumors, trauma, and infections can all increase the difficulty of intubation. Other situations that can make intubation more difficult are small mandible, limited neck mobility, and edematous tongue (angioedema, amyloidosis). *Neuromuscular blockers* used to paralyze the patient for MV are associated with neurological deficits and sequelae and should be avoided.

Confirmation

After the placement, the ETT should be in the mid trachea, with the ETT tip 3 to 4 cm above the carina. Bilateral breath sounds and equal expansion of the lungs should be noted. An **end-tidal carbon dioxide detector (capnography) needs to be connected to the ETT, and this monitor should change color within the first 6 breaths.** Lack of color change suggests that the ETT is not in the trachea. The ETT should be repositioned until the CO_2 monitor confirms correct endotracheal placement by changing colors. A chest x-ray is needed to verify ETT placement and ensure that the ETT is not in the right or left main stem bronchus. After successful

ETI, the tube should be secured via an ETT holder or adhesive tape. If facial hair interferes with securing the ETT, simply shave the patient.

Major complications of ETT placement include: bronchospasm, hypoxemia, hypercapnia, and death. Vomiting, bradycardia, laryngospasm, pneumonitis, and pneumonia are also seen. Some authorities recommend IV lidocaine prior to ETI to reduce ETI-induced bronchospasm. ETI and MV also are associated with increased cases of ICU delirium.

SUMMARY

The main goal of ETI and MV is to provide a patent airway for the delivery of oxygen and proper ventilation that are primary to a patient's survival. This also allows suctioning of secretions, application of PEEP, and delivery of aerosolized medications. The decision to proceed with this invasive ETI requires an understanding of the pathologic and physiologic disorders that necessitate its use. A qualitative colorimetric $EtCO_2$ monitor is commonly used to determine placement and is nearly 100% sensitive and specific for ETT placement in the trachea.

CLINICAL CASE CORRELATION

- **See also Case 3 (Scoring Systems and Patient Prognosis), Case 9 (Ventilator Management), Case 11 (Asthmatic Management), and Case 12 (Noninvasive Methods of Ventilatory Support).**

COMPREHENSION QUESTIONS

8.1 A 34-year-old man arrives in the emergency department (ED) 45 minutes after being shot in the abdomen with a .38-caliber handgun. On arrival the patient is alert, oriented to person, place, and time with blood pressure 76/50 mm Hg, pulse 140 beats/minute, respiratory rate 32 breaths/minute, and pulse oximetry of 72% initially on room air. Chest x-rays showed bilateral pneumothoraces with partial lung collapse. RSI is begun with an 8-mm ETT. Bilateral chest tubes are inserted. The patient is started on a pressure support of +10 mm Hg with 0 PEEP and FIO_2 of 100%. Additional chest x-rays and blood gas determinations are pending. Which of the following is the most reliable confirmation of the proper tracheal placement of the ETI?

A. Ease of bagging with ventilation

B. Positive color changes on a CO_2 monitor attached to the endotracheal tube

C. Auscultation by stethoscope for good breath sounds bilaterally

D. Pulse oximetry reading above 95%

E. Chest expansion with every breath

8.2 You are called to evaluate a 45-year-old white man who developed a pneumothorax after abdominal surgery. He had been intubated with an 8-mm ETT for anesthesia. He is 5'2" and weighs 60 kg. His front teeth are at the 32 cm mark on the ETT. Examination reveals good breath sounds and definite expansion of the left chest, but no breath sounds and no expansion of the right chest. What is the most likely etiology for these findings?

A. Carbon monoxide poisoning.

B. Low FIO_2 on ventilator settings.

C. Adult respiratory distress syndrome.

D. Esophageal placement.

E. Endotracheal tube is in the right main stem bronchi.

ANSWERS TO QUESTIONS

8.1 **B. The most reliable methods of confirming that the ETT is in the trachea are** seeing the ETT go through the vocal cords or noting the change in color of a CO 2 monitor connected to the ETT while the patient is being ventilated. Regardless, a chest x-ray is performed for confirmation of tube placement. Sometimes, bronchoscopy may be needed to confirm proper placement or to assist in placement of the ETT. The tip of the ETT should be 3 to 4 cm above the carina. Head flexion makes the "ETT tip go away from carina" and can cause extubation. Head extension makes the "ETT tip come closer to carina" and can selectively intubate the right main stem bronchus. Other maneuvers that are usually performed include pulse oximetry and auscultation of the lung fields; however, these measures are not as good predictors of accurate ETT placement.

8.2 **E.** The patient's ETT is placed too low, causing the right main stem to be selectively intubated because of its more direct angle versus the left main stem bronchus. The left main stem bronchus diverges at a 45-degree angle, making it less likely to be selectively intubated. A common error in intubation is esophageal placement of the ETT. Proper placement of the ETT requires confirmation visually or via a CO_2 monitor connected to the ETT. A chest x-ray to assure correct positioning of the ETT tip 3 to 4 cm above the carina should be performed.

CLINICAL PEARLS

- Clinical assessment, combined with medical experience, is the most important tool for identifying patients requiring intubation.
- Indications for ETI and MV are commonly divided into hypoxic respiratory failure, hypercarbic ventilatory failure, impaired consciousness, and a need for airway protection.
- Planned ETI in a controlled setting is always preferable to emergent airway management.
- Ventilation can be monitored by capnography, which noninvasively measures the partial pressure of carbon dioxide in the exhaled breath.
- ABG and P_{ACO_2} measurements are necessary to evaluate hypercarbic ventilatory failure because pulse oximetry values can remain near normal until ventilatory collapse occurs.
- Unlike pulse oximetry for detecting hypoxemia, bedside monitors for detecting hypercarbia are not routinely available.
- Neurologic indications for ETI for impaired consciousness and presumed airway protection may account for 20% of patients intubated in the intensive care unit (ICU).
- Auscultation is not reliable for determining the placement of the endotracheal tube.
- Patients requiring RSI usually present with increasing dyspnea, tachypnea, use of accessory breathing muscles, and low tidal volume ventilation with paradoxical breathing.

REFERENCES

Grekin P, Chin MM. Syncope, In: Toy EC, Simon BC, Takenaka KY, Baker B, Rosh AJ. Syncope. *Case Files, Emergency Medicine*, Second Edition. New York, NY: McGraw-Hill, 2009.

Loscalzo J. *Harrison's Pulmonary and Critical Care Medicine*. New York, NY: McGraw-Hill; 2010.

Orebaugh S, Snyder JV. *Direct Laryngoscopy and Tracheal Intubation in Adults*. Waltham, MA: UpToDate; 2011.

CASE 9

You are called to recommend the settings of a mechanical ventilator for a 24-year-old man who is a near-drowning victim. The patient was intubated on site by the paramedics with an 8-mm size endotracheal tube (ETT), and placed on 100% F_{IO_2} producing an O_2 saturation (SaO_2) of 92%. The patient had attended an all-night New Year's Eve party. He is arousable and responsive to deep stimuli. The chest x-ray shows bilateral interstitial infiltrates with a normal heart size and clear costophrenic angles. The ETT tip is 3 cm above the carina. His spontaneous respiratory rate is 12 breaths/minute. His blood pressure is 100/50 mm Hg, heart rate is 150 beats/minute, and temperature is 95°F (35°C). He weighs 70 kg (154 lb). He is awaiting transfer to the intensive care unit (ICU) for further treatment.

- ▶ What is the best initial mode of mechanical ventilation and settings for this patient?
- ▶ What are the most common complications of mechanical ventilation?
- ▶ What special problems are presented by near-drowning victims?

ANSWERS TO CASE 9:
Ventilator Management

Summary: This is a 24-year-old man near-drowning victim presenting with adult respiratory distress syndrome (ARDS). His HR is 150 beats/minute and blood pressure is normal.

- **Best initial mode and mechanical ventilation settings:** The goals in this patient are to achieve an adequate amount of ventilation and oxygenation while decreasing the work of breathing. Assist control (AC) mode following low-volume mechanical ventilation guidelines using 6 to 8 mL/kg as a starting tidal volume (V_t) with a goal of a plateau pressure of <30 cm H_2O would achieve these goals. Other initial settings include a rate of at least 16 breaths/minute, an FIO_2 of 100%, and a positive end expiratory pressure (PEEP) of 5 cm H_2O.
- **Most common complications of MV:** Barotrauma, aberrant (esophageal) intubation, and right main stem bronchus intubation.
- **Special problems in drowning victims:** Controlling hypothermia and addressing atelectasis.

ANALYSIS

Objectives

1. To begin with the mechanical ventilator parameters which will best assure an acceptable pH, $PACO_2$, and PAO_2 (eg, AC of 16, V_t 6-8 mL/kg, FIO_2 100%, PEEP 5 cm H_2O).
2. To switch to pressure support as soon as possible to increase patient comfort and reduce need for sedation.
3. To keep head of bed elevated at minimum of 45 degree as main key to aspiration precautions.

Considerations

The patient is a 24-year-old man near-drowning victim with ARDS. He needs rapid-sequence intubation (RSI) with MV. Because of the ARDS, a low V_t strategy of 6 to 8 mL/kg with a plateau pressure <30 mm Hg is indicated. The ETT should be sized 8 mm or more to allow fiberoptic bronchoscopy (FOB) to evaluate for any aspirated material while maintaining MV. Hypothermia may alter the patient's neurological status, which cannot be accurately evaluated until core temperature correction. When the chest x-ray shows atelectasis or pulmonary volume loss, especially with high ventilation pressures, an obstruction of the bronchi should be suspected. FOB should be considered to determine if sand or other foreign objects were aspirated.

APPROACH TO:
Mechanical Ventilation

Continuous oxymetry reading is standard in all MV patients. **The goal is to keep O_2 saturation equal or exceeding 90%, which equals a PAO_2 of 60 mm Hg.** This is a time-tested goal of oxygenation and the elbow of the hemoglobin disassociation curve. An improving or normal neurological status is a secondary predictor of a good outcome. Interestingly, most near-drowning victims suffer more from asphyxiation (pharyngeal spasm from fear of breathing under water) and dry lungs rather than aspiration of water and wet lungs. Increased levels of PEEP and 100% FIO_2 may be required to maintain this O_2sat goal (see Table 9–1). PEEP can prevent the collapse of small airways and alveoli by maintaining alveolar recruitment. PEEP further improves oxygenation and matching of ventilation with perfusion (VQ).

MECHANICAL VENTILATORS

The **most common reason for mechanical ventilation (MV) is respiratory failure due to sepsis, pneumonia, ARDS, COPD, pulmonary edema, or coma.** The objective of MV is to decrease the work of breathing and to reverse life-threatening hypoxemia, hypercarbia, and acidosis. The work of breathing is redistributed back to the systemic circulation (kidneys, heart, brain, gut). MV is delivered via an ETT or tracheostomy tube. The ETT has more dead space than a tracheostomy tube; thus the tracheostomy patient requires lower tidal volumes. The use of fiberoptic-assisted ETT is easier than direct laryngoscopy and has the added benefit of clearly seeing the ETT pass through the vocal cords into the trachea. The IV administration of lidocaine prior to intubation may decrease cardiac arrhythmia and blunt the undesired responses induced by ETT insertion into the trachea.

The MV is a machine, with adjustable variations in cycling modes between inspiration (inhalation) and expiration (exhalation). Independent variables are set and monitored by microprocessors and displayed on a monitor. MV can control many different means of delivering a positive pressure breath to the patient. This inspiration under positive pressure created by the MV totally reverses the normally negative inspiratory cycle in the spontaneously breathing patient. Some of the more common ventilator modes include: assist control (AC), synchronized intermittent ventilation (SIMV), pressure support ventilation (PSV), controlled mechanical ventilation (CMV), and pressure release ventilation (PRV).

Table 9–1 • COMMON MECHANICAL VENTILATION MODES

- Controlled mandatory ventilation (CMV)
- Assist control (AC) ventilation
- Synchronized intermittent ventilation (SIMV, IMV)
- Pressure support ventilation (PSV), pressure-controlled ventilation (PCV)
- Continuous pressure airway pressure ventilation (CPAP)
- Airway pressure release ventilation (APRV)
- JET ventilation and high-frequency ventilation (HFOV)

Tidal volume (V_t), fractional inspired concentration of oxygen (FIO_2), respiratory rate (RR), positive end expiratory pressure (PEEP), peak inspiratory pressure (PIFR), humidification, and warming of inspired air can all be controlled by the MV.

The different MV settings provide a predetermined mixture of patient-initiated (spontaneous) and MV-delivered controlled breaths (see Table 9–1 for common MV modes). The best choice is the one that delivers and meets the physiologic needs for oxygenation and ventilation while maintaining patient comfort and decreasing the need for sedation.

MVs have sensors that must be activated to deliver an MV breath. Inside the MV tubing, an artificial nose humidifies the respiratory circuit. The artificial nose reduces contamination by respiratory water-borne pathogens by eliminating water reservoirs. Upper airway heat and humidification also is achieved with the patient's own respiratory system. The respiratory circuit tubing should not be changed unless there is a reason (eg, leak). Reduced manipulation of the MV circuitry has decreased patient infection rates and contamination by resistant organisms. MV circuits are equipped with a built-in reusable suction catheter. This is a clean closed system, in which a collapsible plastic cover built in to the suction catheter allows for its reuse as needed. MV also has the flexibility to allow for the in-line delivery of aerosolized medications without disconnecting the patient from the MV.

Medications commonly used in MV include β_2 agonists, ipratropium bromide, steroids, antibiotics, and mucolytics. Invasive ventilation with MV is needed when noninvasive ventilation (NIV) fails or in situations requiring airway control. Patients intubated for respiratory failure develop respiratory muscle fatigue, and muscle retraining is required. Muscular dysfunction must be reversed. Anxiety, which is the most common treatable side effect of MV, can be minimized with pressure support MV and using patient-driven MV modes (SIMV). SIMV is associated with improved synchronization between the patient's natural breathing pattern and the MV. The respiratory demand and the amount of required ventilator support determines the mode of ventilation (see Table 9–2).

Assist control ventilation is usually the initial MV mode since delivery of a backup respiratory rate and minute ventilation is assured regardless of patient contribution. SIMV or IMV are equivalent since all IMV devices are synchronized. The main goal of MV is to supply needed ventilation and oxygenation by retraining and strengthening the respiratory system and resting the fatigued respiratory muscles. An eventual goal is to exercise the rested muscle to allow successful extubation. Extubation is considered as successful when reintubation is not required within the next 48 hours.

Daily portable chest x-rays are advised for all MV patients during the **acute** course of the disease. This aids not only in evaluating the placement of ETT, the

Table 9–2 • GENERAL PRINCIPLES TO MECHANICAL VENTILATORS AND THEIR MODES

Positive pressure breath delivery, positive intrathoracic pressure during inspiration	Can be triggered by patient, set by MV, or both	FIO_2, V_t, flow rates, PEEP, PS, IPAP, EPAP can be delivered, measured, and monitored by the MV

recognition of new infiltrates, the development of barotrauma, and the placement of central venous line, but also in detecting abnormalities of NGT or feeding tubes. The extension of the chin away from the chest can move the ETT down and selectively intubate the right main stem bronchus. In contrast, flexion of the chin toward the chest can pull the ETT up and extubate the patient if the ETT is not properly placed. The recommended placement of the tip of the ETT is 3 to 4 cm above the carina (T_4 level) to avoid these changes due to chin placement.

ASSIST CONTROL VENTILATION

In **AC, MV breaths are delivered at a preset rate and tidal volume**. If a spontaneous breath is not generated within a specified time, a mechanical breath will be delivered at a scheduled time period depending on the rate set. For example, the MV will cycle a breath every 3 seconds for set rate of 20 breaths/minute, even if no spontaneous breath occurs within that minute. The patient can only breathe and receive MV breaths above the set rate, but never below it. Lack of coordination of the patient's breathing with the MV breaths may cause significant patient discomfort and an increase in the work of breathing (see Figure 9–1 for waveform representation of different MV modes).

The goals of MV are to provide adequate minute ventilation (V_m = rate × V_t) and minimize the risk of barotrauma. In an AC mode, if the patient breathes above the set MV respiratory rate, the machine will deliver another full MV breath which can lead to an acute respiratory alkalosis. Tachypnea on the AC MV mode can lead to the stacking of MV breaths with trapping of air as the expiratory time decreases. This results in auto PEEP. Intrinsic and auto PEEP are factors of fast respiratory rates and shorter exhalation times (reverse I-E ratios). If during exhalation the pressure does not return to baseline (0), this intrinsic PEEP increases the inspiratory effort; the patient's next inspiratory effort must overcome this new baseline pressure to initiate the next spontaneous breath. Lengthening the expiratory time by decreasing the volume or rate alleviates this problem and decreases the intrinsic PEEP/auto PEEP. Disconnecting a patient from the MV circuit loses the PEEP and the alveoli that had been recruited. These alveoli will now collapse and are difficult to re-expand. Should this auto PEEP be the cause of hemodynamic deterioration, the disconnecting maneuver can be life saving. Intravascular volume should be increased with fluids and PEEP levels should be decreased.

SYNCHRONIZED INTERMITTENT MANDATORY VENTILATION

SIMV is similar to AC, except that **breaths that are spontaneously generated by the patient occur without activating an MV breath.** Breaths initiated by the patient are only in the V_t amount generated by the patient and not by the MV. Both ventilator breaths and spontaneous breaths generated by the patient can be assisted with pressure support ventilation (PSV). SIMV should not be used alone without PSV since this actually increases the work of breathing. SIMV of at least 5 cm H_2O of PS should be applied. All IMV are synchronized to keep a ventilator breath from pushing against a patient's natural or forced exhalation. This will avoid possible barotrauma and pneumothorax (PTX) secondary to increased intra bronchial pressures.

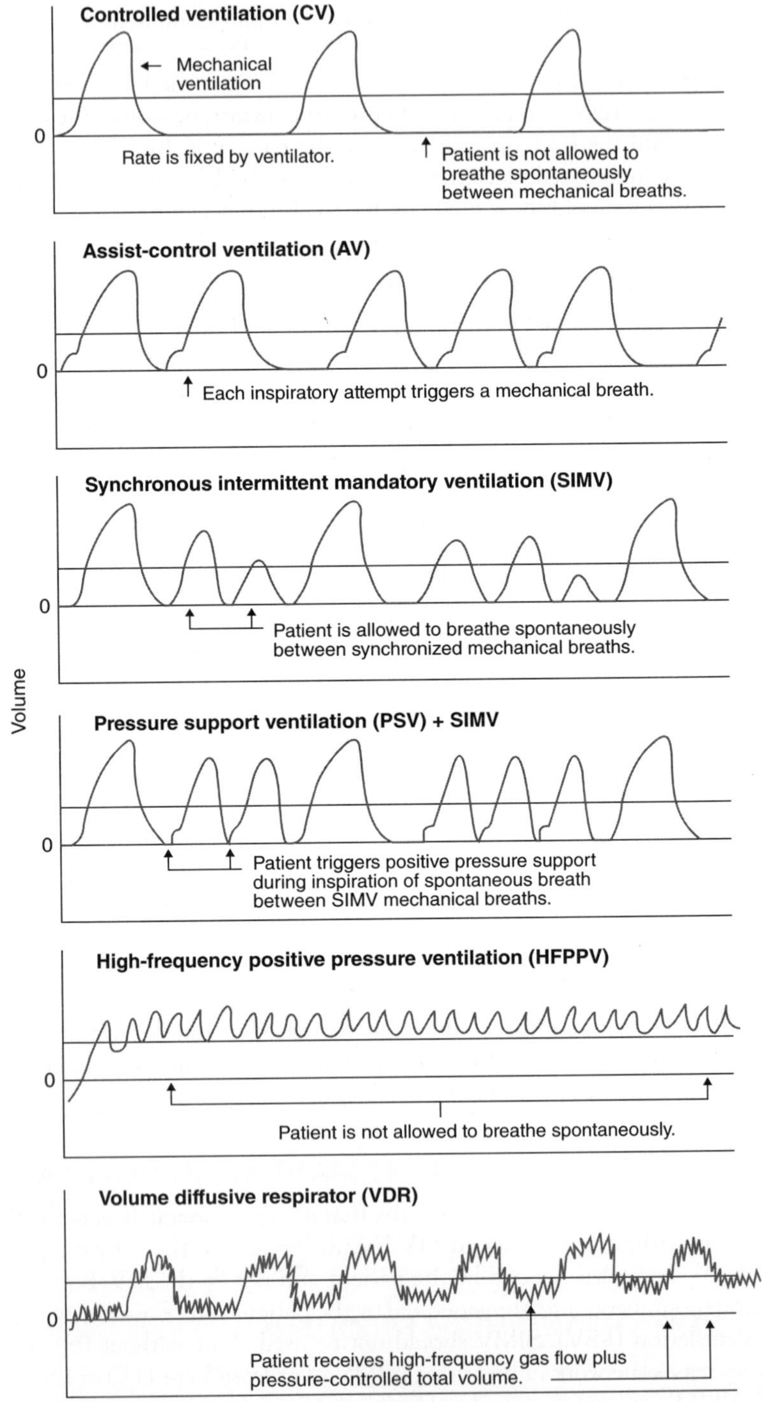

Figure 9–1. Mechanical ventilator modes. Waveforms of various mechanical ventilator modes demonstrating volume versus time. (Reproduced, with permission, from Gomella LG, Haist SA. *Clinician's Pocket Reference*. 11th ed. New York, NY: McGraw-Hill Education; 2007; Figure 20-20.)

PRESSURE SUPPORT/CONTROLLED VENTILATION

Pressure support ventilation (PSV) and pressure-controlled ventilation (PCV) were originally designed for weaning or liberating the patient from MV. These modalities should be used in combination when SIMV is used, since SIMV needs a support mode. In PSV, the patient is spontaneously breathing and each patient breath is assisted by a preset amount of "pressure support" measured in centimeter H_2O. Pressures can be set for inhalation and exhalation, as well as for continuous or intermittent application. With increased inhalation pressure, V_t increases. This effect usually reaches a maximum at pressures of 25 to 30 cm H_2O. PSV acts as an assist device that allows the patient to establish the V_t and respiratory rate at levels which are most comfortable. This mode does not require much sedation.

PCV is the same as PSV except there is a preset pressure that **must** be reached with every patient-initiated breath. PCV activates itself only if the preset pressure is not reached by the patient's own efforts. It is technically referred to as a series of ventilations that are time triggered, time cycled, and pressure limited. PSV and PCV are ideally used when low airway pressure is required as in patients with a pneumothorax, and when there are concerns of barotraumas.

CONTINUOUS POSITIVE AIRWAY PRESSURE

CPAP is the most commonly used MV support mode to reduce the need of or liberate a patient from MV. In CPAP, there is a continuous pressure so that each inspiration is assisted by a preset amount of pressure. Since CPAP is continuous, it acts as PEEP during exhalation. Ventilation on CPAP occurs on spontaneous breaths by the patient. No preset mechanical breaths occur, which leads to more patient comfort and a decreased need for sedation.

AIRWAY PRESSURE RELEASE VENTILATION

Airway pressure release ventilation (APRV) is another form of MV that allows patients to breathe spontaneously over intermittent and variable levels of CPAP. APRV may be thought of as alternating levels of CPAP with or without pressure support. APRV allows patients to breathe spontaneously over intermittent and alternating levels of CPAP. These alternating levels of CPAP are termed, at the higher level (P_{high}), which is a recruiting maneuver, and with an alternating lower set pressure (P_{low}) or PEEP, which maintains patency of the recruited airways. In an APRV, the inspiratory cycle is set by the length of the inspiratory time. For example, cycle time of 6 seconds = RR of 10 breaths/minute (60 sec/6 sec = 10 cycles). APVR works best at respiratory rates of <15 breaths/minute, preferably near 12 breaths/minute or less. Alveoli are recruited, preventing their collapse, by the continuous pressure set and maintained by APVR.

JET VENTILATION AND HIGH-FREQUENCY VENTILATION

Jet ventilation is rarely used in routine practice. Bronchopleural fistula is one condition in which high-frequency ventilation (HFOV) may assist healing by having low inflation pressures. For HFOV, the patient must be temporarily paralyzed since oxygenation is controlled by diffusion and CO_2 by ventilation. The use of paralytic agents has significant neurological sequelae in patients who eventually recovered. A small V_t is delivered at very high respiratory rates in the range of 180 to 600 breaths/minute. The HFOV or jet ventilation is an alternative mode of MV that protects the lungs. Most clinical trials on HFOV have been performed on neonates. Awareness of the injurious effects of mechanical ventilation has led to a renewed interest and advances in using **HFOV in adult ALI/ARDS patients. HFOV is characterized by rapid oscillations** of a diaphragm (at frequencies of 3-10 Hz, ie, 180-600 breaths/minute) driven by a piston pump.

The pressure swings become more attenuated as they move distally from the airways to the alveoli, resulting in a very small V_t. Use of HFOV in inhalation injuries has been an effective treatment. Alsaghir and colleagues demonstrated that prone positioning may improve oxygenation and reduce mortality in patients with ARDS or more severe illnesses. The prone position makes nursing care much more difficult.

VOLUMETRIC DIFFUSIVE RESPIRATION

Volumetric diffusive respiration (VDR), a form of **high-frequency ventilation,** is very effective in cystic fibrosis and smoke inhalation patients due to the copious secretions. VDR requires a high degree of respiratory therapy education and time. VDR acts as a high-frequency percussive ventilator, enabling the ability to clear copious secretions.

SEDATION AND OTHER RELATED MV ISSUES

The major goal of sedation in MV is to control anxiety and provide better coordination between the patients' own breathing efforts and the MV. Propofol (recently made famous by the death of singer Michael Jackson) is a frequently used agent for this purpose. Propofol is a short-acting, *intravenously* administered *hypnotic* agent. Its uses include induction and maintenance of *general anesthesia*, sedation for *mechanically ventilated* adults, and *sedation for procedures*. It is an extremely short-acting agent, which often causes vasodilation with hypotension; the hypotension usually responds to increased fluids or discontinuation of the drug. In critically ill patients, propofol is superior to *lorazepam* both in effectiveness and overall cost. A favorite agent of neurologists and neurosurgeons, it decreases intracranial pressure and is rapid cleared enables quick evaluation of the patient's mental status merely by discontinuing infusion. It has no analgesic properties.

A **propofol syndrome** has been described about 1% of patients, consisting of **rhabdomyolysis and metabolic acidosis.** Propofol produces sedation without causing respiratory depression which makes MV easier to deliver. Paralytic agents should be avoided unless absolutely necessary because of its frequent neurological sequelae.

Acid suppression with a proton pump inhibitor (PPI) or H_2 antagonist is recommended to prevent GI bleeding from gastric sources; the main drawback is increased bacterial overgrowth because of the acid suppression, leading to aspiration pneumonia with potentially antibiotic-resistant pathogens. H_2 antagonists may have an advantage over PPI in this instance. The dose and delivery of aerosolized medications such as β_2 agonist and ipratropium bromide should be doubled above the standard dose (2 U dose vials) for MV patients with an ETT. The ETT increases the area of aerosol deposition thus requiring larger volume of medication to reach the airways. Ninety percent of the volume of aerosolized medications remains in the tubing of the aerosol delivery equipment.

CLINICAL CASE CORRELATION

- **See also Case 8 (Airway Management), Case 11 (Asthmatic Management), and Case 12 (Non-invasive Methods of Ventilatory Support).**

COMPREHENSION QUESTIONS

9.1 Low-volume ventilation is needed for a septic patient with ARDS and severe hypoxia on 90% FIO_2. The chest x-ray shows bilateral infiltrates with a normal heart size, a typical x-ray presentation ARDS. The patient weighs 80 kg. What is the correct amount of tidal volume to begin with for this patient on a mechanical ventilator?

A. 750 mL tidal volume

B. 480 mL tidal volume

C. 300 mL tidal volume

D. 550 mL tidal volume

E. 250 mL tidal volume

9.2 You are called to evaluate a mechanically ventilated patient for new onset hypotension. The patient has a blood pressure of 100/60 mm Hg, with a 20 mm Hg of pulsus paradoxicus and increased JVD at 45 degree of HOB elevation. The patient has wheezing throughout both lungs and is breathing at 35 times/minute on mechanical ventilator settings of SIMV 20 breaths/minute, V_t of 800 mL, PS of 10 mm Hg, a PEEP of 10 mm Hg, and FIO_2 of 40%. ABG results on these setting are pH 7.36, $PACO_2$ 45mm Hg, PAO_2 77 mm Hg. Which of the following would you advise to do next to relieve the hypotension?

A. Decrease the PEEP and auto PEEP by decreasing rate and tidal volume.

B. Start vasopressors to reverse hypotensive effect of PEEP.

C. Increase PEEP to improve hemodynamics

D. Change to assist control mode and keep PEEP the same.

E. Do not make any changes.

ANSWERS TO QUESTIONS

9.1 **B.** Previously, it was thought that tidal volumes (V_t) of 10 to 15 mL/kg were required to prevent atelectasis during MV; however, these higher volumes are no longer used. The Surviving Sepsis Guidelines recommend a strategy of low-volume ventilation using a V_t of 6 to 8 mL/kg with a plateau pressure <30 mm Hg H_2O. This method is referred to as low-volume ventilation and is very effective in supporting patients with sepsis and ARDS. The best initial V_t is approximately 480 mL using 6 mL/kg. The arterial pH should be kept at 7.20 or higher. Bicarbonate treatment should only be considered when the pH is below 7.20. This low-volume ventilation method is effective in preventing and treating ARDS. Sedation will be needed for patient comfort with this method.

9.2 **A.** Increased PEEP or auto PEEP increases the intrathoracic pressure (ITP), and decreases venous return to the heart. This reduces right ventricular filling and can decrease cardiac output, leading to hypotension. Attempts should be made to increase expiratory time to decrease auto PEEP. **With severe hypotension due to auto PEEP, disconnecting the patient from the MV and allowing a long expiration will generally correct the hypotension.** Lowering the auto PEEP levels can be achieved by decreasing the respiratory rate, decreasing the tidal volume, and increasing the expiratory time. Giving IV fluids and expanding the intravascular space helps reverse the decreased preload and assists in restoring the blood pressure by restoring intravascular and right ventricular filling volume.

CLINICAL PEARLS

- Low-volume ventilation is important in patients with ARDS to prevent alveolar barotrauma.
- Pressure support ventilation (PSV) helps reduce the need for sedation.
- Acid suppression with proton-pump inhibitors or histamine-2 (H_2) blockers heightens the risk for resistant bacterial pneumonia in hospitalized patients, PPI more than H_2 blockers.
- PSV increases patient comfort and resistance to spontaneous respiration by patient.
- Avoid neuromuscular blockade since this is associated with long-term neurological defects.
- Do not change the plastic circuitry of MV unless needed. Unnecessary changing of tubing increases the rate of infection.
- The use of artificial noses for humidification in MV circuitry reduces the risk of waterborne respiratory infections compared with the use of inline humidifiers.
- Volumetric diffusive percussive respiration (VDR) enables clearance of copious secretions resulting from smoke inhalation and patients with cystic fibrosis.

REFERENCES

Alsaghir Ah, Martin CM. Effect of prone positioning in patients with acute respiratory distress syndrome: a meta-analysis. *Crit Care Med.* 2008;36(2):603-609.

Loscalzo J. *Harrison's Pulmonary and Critical Care Medicine.* New York, NY: McGraw-Hill; 2011.

Malhotra A. Clinical therapeutics, low-tidal-volume ventilation in the acute respiratory distress syndrome. *N Engl J Med.* 2007;357:1113-1120.

Tobin MJ. Advances in mechanical ventilation. *N Engl J Med.* 2001;344:1986-1996.

Toy EC, Simon B, Takenaka K, Liu T, Rosh A. *Case Files Emergency Medicine.* 2nd ed. New York: McGraw-Hill; 2009.

CASE 10

A 27-year-old woman with cystic fibrosis has a new bacterial pneumonia requiring intubation. On ICU day 3, her oxygen saturation is 93% with an FIO_2 of 30% on MV and a pressure support of 10 cm H_2O. She has a spontaneous breathing rate averaging 14 breaths/minute and a positive end expiratory pressure (PEEP) of 2.5 cm H_2O. Weaning parameters (measurements of a patient's spontaneous respiratory efforts) show she is generating an average tidal volume of 400 mL and a negative inspiratory pressure of −35 cm H_2O. An ABG shows a pH of 7.39, $PACO_2$ 37 mm Hg, and PAO_2 of 100 mm Hg. She has been afebrile for the last 48 hours and her white cell count is now within normal limits. On physical examination, she is in no acute distress and answers questions by nodding or writing on a paper pad. Her temperature is 36.9°C (98.4°F), blood pressure 132/66 mm Hg, heart rate 76 beats/minute, and respiration rate 14 breaths/minute. Auscultation of the chest reveals good air movement throughout. Chest radiographs indicate a clearance of a left-sided pulmonary infiltrate present on the admission x-ray.

- ► What is the best next step in this patient's management?
- ► What other steps should be considered?

ANSWERS TO CASE 10:
Respiratory Weaning

Summary: This 27-year-old woman has markedly improved from her pneumonia and respiratory failure. The weaning parameters all point to a successful extubation. MV is no longer needed and should be removed. After conducting a successful spontaneous breathing trial, the patient should be liberated from MV.

- **Best next management step:** A spontaneous breathing trial (SBT) should be performed since the weaning parameters are acceptable. If the SBT is successful, it would lead to extubation or liberation from MV.
- **Other steps:** Prepare the patient for the weaning and extubation process and observe her closely postextubation. Elevate the head of the bed to minimize the risk for aspiration. In the presence of cystic fibrosis, the clearance and control of secretions are essential.

ANALYSIS

Objectives

1. To understand the clinical and the objective parameters that predict a successful liberation from mechanical ventilation.
2. To understand the predictors of weaning failure.
3. To understand a logical approach to weaning.

Considerations

This 27-year-old woman with cystic fibrosis required intubation for respiratory failure and pneumonia. She has been treated for 2 days in the ICU. The patient is generally alert and responsive. Weaning parameters are favorable, with a PAO_2 of 60 or greater, an FIO_2 <60%, and a PEEP <5 mm H_2O present. When the MV patient reaches these criteria, it is safe to proceed to spontaneous breathing trials; if these trials are successful, then the next step is extubation and liberation from MV. Pressure support ventilation (PSV) or continuous positive airway pressure (CPAP) would be the best way to wean this patient.

APPROACH TO:
Respiratory Weaning

INTRODUCTION

Weaning or liberation from invasive or noninvasive mechanical ventilation is the process of freeing the patient from positive pressure mechanical ventilation (see Case 11 for more information on NIV). Because of the significant morbidity and

Table 10–1 • PROPOSED SIX STEPS TO BE CONSIDERED FOR WEANING PROCESS (PER EXPERT CONSENSUS)

1. Treatment of acute respiratory failure	4. A spontaneous breathing trial
2. Clinical judgment that weaning may be possible	5. Extubation
3. Assessment of the readiness to wean	6. Possible reintubation

mortality associated with prolonged mechanical ventilation, it is generally accepted that all mechanically ventilated ICU patients should be assessed on a daily basis for their readiness to wean. This assessment should include the cessation of sedation and a reevaluation of its need. Weaning can be started after the first formal assessment of the patient's respiratory condition indicates that weaning could be successful. Nearly 50% of unexpected self-extubation during the weaning process do not require reintubation. It is important to be aware of the frequency of weaning failures and predictors of such failures.

APPROACH TO WEANING

Liberation from mechanical ventilation is a central component in the care of the critically ill patient. To start weaning a patient from MV, one must begin with a patient who is ready for the process and who has a good possibility of success (Table 10–1).

Underlying disease should be treated since its persistence can contribute to requiring continued MV. Successful weaning depends on many variables including adequate mental status, muscle strength required to maintain spontaneous breathing, and hemodynamic stability. Are the ABG values acceptable? Are electrolyte values normal including Mg^+, K, Ca^{2+}, and PO_4? Adequate nutrition must be maintained, but overfeeding should be avoided, especially with carbohydrates; increased CO_2 production may result and require increased minute ventilation (V_e). Fatty meals are advised, since fat produces more energy than carbohydrates (8 kcal for each gram of fat vs 4 kcal for every gram of carbohydrates) with much less CO_2 production. Some basic weaning goals should be attained: PAO_2 of 60 or more with an FIO_2 <60% and a peep <5 cm H_2O. When the MV patient reaches these criteria, it is safe to proceed to spontaneous breathing trials and if successful, then moving to extubation and liberation from MV.

WEANING PREDICTORS

Weaning is the progressive reduction in the amount of support provided by a mechanical ventilator. The term **weaning** is frequently used to describe the transition from intubation and full mechanical support to spontaneous breathing by the patient with a protected airway. Weaning predictors act as guidelines to identify those patients that qualify for spontaneous breathing trials and liberation from MV with successful extubation. These predictors are based on measurements of the work of breathing, which help determine whether the patient's respiratory system can adjust to spontaneous unassisted respiration.

An NIF > –25 cm H_2O is predictive of successful weaning from MV. This confirms the patient's respiratory muscle strength is suitable and that the patient's own respiratory system is conditioned to breathe without MV support. Stable vital signs with an improving clinical picture **during the weaning process** is critical. Stable vital signs can be used to predict the stability of the arterial blood gases (ABG) reducing the need for repetitive ABG analyses. ABG studies are costly, painful, and not free of possible complications, including distal arterial occlusion or dissection of the artery. Achievement of a spontaneous minute ventilation (V_e) <10 L/min (maintaining oxygenation without excessive work) is an excellent predictor of successful liberation from MV.

WEANING TECHNIQUES

A **successful trial of spontaneous breathing has become the gold standard for weaning.** Every intubated patient on MV should be evaluated daily with a trial of some form of spontaneous breathing. A sedation holiday should also be attempted; if sedation is still required, it can be restarted at half the previous dose. The patient should be on a minimal sedation dose to avoid depression of respiratory functions. Trials of spontaneous weaning can be performed with or without MV assistance. Weaning trials with MV assistance increase the safety of the procedure since respiratory parameters are more precisely monitored and patient deterioration can be diagnosed earlier. So-called traditional T-piece trial with FIO_2% delivery only via plastic tubing without the aid of MV gives a realistic evaluation of the patient's breathing without MV help or the resistance of MV sensor valves. Surveys of respiratory departments have shown that SIMV with or without PS assistance was the most common method of MV weaning. This was closely followed by T-piece trials and by PS weaning. Use of the rapid shallow breathing index RR/V_t of <105 as shown by Yang and Tobin has an excellent predictive value of extubation failure. Different weaning parameters are better predictors in specific diseases.

T-Piece Trials

T-piece trials are conducted in a spontaneously breathing patient via an ETT connected to an FIO_2 source (thus the T) with the open end of the FIO_2 hose open to ambient air. This method is the oldest and still most effective method of ventilator weaning techniques. Sequentially increasing the amount of time the patient spends on the T-piece will enhance the prospect of complete liberation from MV. A single daily spontaneous breathing trial is as efficient and effective as multiple short trials and is less labor intensive. If needed, PEEP can always be added to the circuit by an expiratory valve or possibly be better accomplished with the patient breathing spontaneously on the MV with the desired PEEP level and a CPAP setting of 0 cm H_2O. These measures are not needed if the patient is on PEEP <5 cm H_2O. The FIO_2 source should be humidified, creating a mist at the open end of the T-piece. If this fine aerosol disappears completely during inspiration, the patient's inspiratory flow is overcoming the inspiratory FIO_2 flow and inhaling 21% room air via the open end of the tube. This circumstance causes a lower actual FIO_2 versus the set FIO_2 affecting the ABG values because of a decrease in FIO_2 reflected in the lower PAO_2 (Table 10–2).

Table 10–2 • APPROACH TO FAILURES OF THE SPONTANEOUS BREATHING TEST
If the patient fails a spontaneous breathing test, the clinician should
(1) Address all contributory causes of failure to wean
(2) Do not perform or repeat a spontaneous breathing trial for 24 h
(3) Support the patient with a nonfatiguing mode of ventilation (most commonly PSV)
(4) Consider NIV if appropriate
(5) Consider tracheostomy

Noninvasive Ventilation

Noninvasive ventilation (NIV) is a useful tool in the difficult-to-wean patient. It avoids the complications of intubation and sedation and reduces the total time of invasive mechanical ventilation. The goal of NIV in weaning can be separated into 2 parts: to prevent extubation failure, and to provide a rescue therapy for postextubation respiratory distress. NIV permits early extubation in patients who fail to meet standard extubation criteria.

Pressure Support Ventilation Weaning

Pressure support ventilation (PSV) allows the patient to determine the most comfortable depth, length, flow, and rate of breathing. It is used as a weaning tool by gradually reducing pressure support by 2 to 4 cm H_2O as long as the patient is successfully tolerating these decreases. This results in a progressive reduction in ventilatory support over hours or days. PSV is superior to SIMV in reducing the duration of mechanical ventilation in difficult-to-wean patients. PSV weaning compared to T-piece weaning revealed T-piece weaning to be superior. However, one small prospective trial has recently suggested that PSV weaning is superior to T-piece weaning in patients with chronic obstructive pulmonary disease (COPD).

Intermittent Mandatory Volume Weaning

SIMV is a poor weaning mode (unless associated with PS), and should not be used in isolation as a weaning tool. SIMV with PS weaning involves a progressive reduction of the respiratory rate in steps of 1 to 3 breaths/minute. SIMV may actually contribute to respiratory muscle fatigue, because of the increased work of breathing due to ventilator factors (increased effort to activate the SIMV demand valve, inspiratory, and expiratory dyssynchrony). SIMV with T-piece spontaneous breathing resulted in a longer duration of MV compared to PSV. SIMV had higher rates of weaning failure. SIMV-based weaning strategies resulted in a longer duration of mechanical ventilation (5 days) compared with a PSV-based strategy (4 days) and T-piece ventilation (3 days).

The Endotracheal Tube

The largest endotracheal tube (ETT) that can be safely be inserted should be used (≥8 mm). A larger caliber facilitates the removal of secretions by suction catheter and decreases in airflow resistance. Reducing high plateau pressures to <30 cm H_2O with V_t volumes of 6 to 8 mL/kg will avoid barotrauma. **The mere presence of an ETT in the trachea can induce significant bronchospasm.** This is often noticed in the operative room postintubation. The presence of the ETT may cause bronchospasm or "rock bag" ventilation as it is sometimes described when this occurs during the anesthetic period. The administration of IV Lidocaine prior to intubation may prevent EET-associated bronchospasm. Intravenous corticosteroids may be used even though most volatile anesthetics are excellent bronchodilators. The addition of aerosolized β_2 agonists may also be used and is easily delivered to the patient.

Role of Tracheostomy in Weaning

Tracheostomies can be important in weaning difficult patients. **A tracheostomy is usually far less irritating to the patient than an endotracheal tube, and the reduced need for sedation usually facilitates weaning.** Tracheostomy provides a secure airway, which reduces the work of breathing and minimizes the risk of pneumonia associated with MV (ventilator-associated pneumonia [VAP]). Studies have not determined whether early or late tracheostomy is superior.

MANAGEMENT OF THE DIFFICULT TO WEAN PATIENT

The difficult-to-wean patient is defined as one who has already failed at least 1 spontaneous breathing trial or has required reintubation within 48 hours of extubation. The failure of a spontaneous breathing trial may be accompanied by a significantly increased inspiratory effort with respiratory muscle fatigue. This may induce short-lasting, high-frequency fatigue. Failure of either a spontaneous breathing trial or extubation demands an identification of the exacerbating factors that caused the failure. Adjustments must be made that will increase the success of weaning and provide adequate ventilatory support. The clinician should conduct a careful physical examination and review the patient's diagnostic tests to uncover and treat any reversible contributory factors leading to weaning failure.

The most widely used modes of ventilation are (volume) assist control ventilation (ACV), synchronized intermittent mechanical ventilation (SIMV), and PSV. One classification system divides ICU patients into those simple to wean, those difficult to wean (also called prolonged weaning) groups.

- **Simple-to-wean patients** are those who are successfully extubated on the first attempt. This group consists of patients in the intensive care unit (ICU) (about 69%) which have a low mortality rate (about 5%).

- The **difficult-to-wean or prolonged-weaning patients** (requiring up to 3 attempts or up to 7 days from the onset of weaning efforts) require greater efforts to successfully liberate them from mechanical ventilation.

These difficult-to-wean and prolonged-weaning patients have a mortality rate of 25%. Longer duration of MV is associated with an increased mortality and expense (mechanical ventilation costs more than $2000/d), and it has been estimated that the 6% of patients who require prolonged MV consume 37% of ICU resources.

More severely ill patients usually require longer periods of mechanical ventilation. Overall, 40% to 50% of the time spent on mechanical ventilation occurs after the weaning process has started. Most critically ill patients require a period of rest after intubation. The weaning process should begin very soon after intubation.

WEANING PROTOCOLS

A lack of attention to the screening process to determine the ability of a patient to pass through the weaning process or unnecessary delays in progression through the weaning steps are associated with increased patient morbidity and mortality. The proper use of weaning protocols has reduced ventilator-associated pneumonia, lowered self-extubation rates, lowered tracheostomy rates, and minimized hospital costs. To be effective, these weaning protocols should include an interdisciplinary team approach with nursing and respiratory therapy personnel in association with physicians all of whom are experienced in the use of MV and weaning procedures.

CLINICAL CASE CORRELATION

- **See also Case 8 (Airway Management/Respiratory Failure), Case 9 (Ventilator Management), Case 11 (Asthmatic Management), and Case 12 (Non-invasive Methods of Ventilatory Support).**

COMPREHENSION QUESTIONS

10.1 You are called to continue mechanical ventilator weaning on a 42-year-old man who is now on day 4 post admission. He has been intubated for adult respiratory distress syndrome (ARDS) secondary to smoke inhalation suffered during his work as a fire fighter. The morning arterial blood gas (ABG) values with the patient awake and alert, sitting up in bed are: pH 7.38, PACO_2 39 mm and PAO_2 99 mm on CPAP mode of 5 cm H_2O, +5 of positive end expiratory pressure (PEEP), spontaneous tidal volume (V_t) of 400 mL, fraction of inspired oxygen (FIO_2) of 28%. His spontaneous weaning parameters reveal a negative inspiratory force (NIF) of –30 cm H_2O, respiratory rate (RR) of 20 breaths/minute, V_t 450 mL, FVC 1.5 L. He is afebrile and breathing comfortably on these settings. Which if the following is the next step in weaning this patient from the ventilator?

A. Decrease ventilatory parameters and continue the weaning process.

B. Stop mechanical ventilation, extubate the patient, and start O_2 via nasal cannula.

C. Change to assist control ventilation.

D. Increase pressure support to 10 cm H_2O.

E. Give a 2-hour spontaneous breathing trial.

10.2 A 35-year-old white male has been on a mechanical ventilator for 7 days. He suffers from ascending paralysis. He has an NIF of –5 cm H_2O and cannot tolerate any spontaneous breathing trials for more than a few minutes without distress. He has copious secretions. The best option for mechanical ventilation (MV) is

A. Trial of pressure support (PSV) weaning.

B. Consider tracheostomy and plan on long-term MV and its needs.

C. Change to assist control ventilation.

D. Perform a spontaneous breathing trial.

E. Trial of noninvasive ventilation (NIV).

ANSWERS TO QUESTIONS

10.1 **B.** The patient has obviously recovered his control and ability to ventilate and oxygenate on his own without MV support. The improving respiratory status is seen clinically and fulfills objective measures of weaning parameters. Weaning parameters are positive predictors of successful extubation. In particular, the NIF of –30 cm H_2O and >300 PAO_2/FIO_2 ratio is informatory. The next best step is to liberate the patient from MV by extubation of the patient and to start the patient on O_2 via nasal cannula with a target O_2 saturation of 92% to 95% O_2 via pulse oxymetry (O_{2Sat}). An aerosol treatment with a β_2 agonist and ipratropium bromide is usually given after the extubation since mild aspiration occurs and the manipulation of the ETT itself during extubation induces bronchospasm and cough.

10.2 **B.** The patient has ascending respiratory paralysis, otherwise known as Guillain-Barre syndrome. The severe respiratory muscle weakness will persists for a significant amount of time and will require long-term ventilator care. Since extubation is not likely in the near future, a tracheostomy for long-term care is indicated. The tracheostomy will allow better management of the copious secretions by frequent suctioning and decrease dead space ventilation, simultaneously improving patient comfort. The performance of a tracheostomy is an important tool in the difficult-to-wean patient. A tracheostomy is usually far less irritating to the patient than an endotracheal tube, and helps to decrease the requirement for sedation, enabling weaning strategies that would otherwise not be possible. Tracheostomy also provides a more secure airway, reduces the work of breathing by decreasing dead space, and carries a reduced rate of ventilator-associated pneumonia. Tracheostomy tubes with fenestrations or by presenting the balloon cuff in a down position may also allow the patient to speak. A one-way valve such as the Passy-Muir valve may be used to aid speech. This valve lets air enter during inhalation and closes during expiration, forcing the expired air to pass through the vocal cords thus allowing the patient to speak. This valve can be used with or without the ventilator. Studies have not determined which is a superior strategy, early <7 days or late tracheostomy >7 days.

CLINICAL PEARLS

- Pressure support ventilation (PSV) is the simplest and most effective method of weaning patients from MV.
- Weaning increases the patient's respiratory effort and increases myocardial oxygen (O_2) demand, making it a cardiopulmonary stress test.
- Assessment of the readiness to wean and reductions in sedative infusions should be considered early and frequently in critically ill patients receiving mechanical ventilation.
- After the acute insult has improved or resolved, clinicians should have a low threshold for conducting a spontaneous breathing trial in all critically ill patients.
- A V_d/V_t ratio of >105 is an excellent predictor of weaning success especially when combined with an NIF exceeding −25 cm H_2O and a stable clinical picture.
- Weaning protocols are not a replacement for expert clinical opinion and management.
- Application of NIV after extubation may assist post extubation from mechanical ventilation.

REFERENCES

Brochard L. Pressure support is the preferred weaning method. Paper presented at the 5th International Consensus Conference in Intensive Care Medicine: Weaning from Mechanical Ventilation. 2005 April 28-29.

Loscalzo J. *Harrison's Pulmonary and Critical Care Medicine*. New York, NY: McGraw-Hill; 2011.

Slutsky AS. Mechanical ventilation. American College of Chest Physicians' Consensus Conference. *Chest* 1993;104:1833-1859.

Toy EC, Simon B, Takenaka K, Liu T, Rosh A. *Case Files Emergency Medicine*. 2nd ed. New York: McGraw-Hill; 2009.

CASE 11

A 35-year-old woman with persistent severe asthma is being seen in the ED. On a previous admission, she required mechanical ventilation and was transferred to the intensive care unit (ICU) for treatment of an asthmatic exacerbation. For the past week, she has increased her use of a β_2 agonist as rescue medication by 6 to 8 times normal, and has nighttime exacerbations every evening. On physical examination she is in acute respiratory distress with nasal flaring and a quiet chest with very distant wheezing. An ABG drawn on 30% oxygen shows a pH of 7.35, $PACO_2$ 42 mm Hg, PAO_2 89 mm Hg, and bicarbonate (HCO_3) of 23 mEq/L. Peak expiratory flow rates are all below 40% of the patient's predicted range. Her respiratory rate is 30 breaths/minute, heart rate is 110 beats/minute and regular, and blood pressure is 150/78 mm Hg with a pulsus paradoxicus of 10 mm Hg.

- ▶ What is the most important next step in the management of this patient?
- ▶ What other treatment options should be undertaken concurrently?
- ▶ What predictors are present that point to a high likelihood of intubation?

ANSWERS TO CASE 11: Asthmatic Exacerbation

Summary: A 35-year-old woman who has a severe asthma exacerbation is seen in the ED. She has respiratory failure. The severe respiratory distress is confirmed with an ABG showing an acute respiratory acidosis. A quiet chest on physical examination, overuse of rescue medications, and a history of MV are all warning signs of an acute asthma exacerbation with respiratory failure and the need for rapid-sequence intubation and safe MV.

- **Most important next management step:** Rapid-sequence intubation and mechanical ventilation.
- **Other treatment options:** High dose and frequent use of aerosolized bronchodilators with albuterol and ipratropium bromide. IV corticosteroids and magnesium infusion should be started. Low-volume MV is likely ideal. Sedation for anxiety and improved coordination with MV should be used.
- **Predictors of high likelihood of intubation:** Prior severe asthmatic episode requiring MV, quiet chest, overuse of rescue agents, frequent nighttime exacerbations, and respiratory acidosis.

ANALYSIS

Objectives

1. To understand the pathophysiology of an acute asthma exacerbation.
2. To describe the classical findings and their correlation with an exacerbation of acute asthma.
3. To understand the correct stepwise treatment of an acute exacerbation of asthma.

Considerations

The patient is in status asthmaticus with hypercarbic respiratory failure. She has a history of a severe asthmatic episode requiring endotracheal tube (ETT) and MV. RSI with MV for relief of respiratory insufficiency is indicated. A large-bore (≥8 mm) ETT should be used to facilitate the suctioning of secretions and to decrease resistance to airflow during MV of asthmatic patients. Bronchodilator agents, corticosteroids, and magnesium sulfate should be started immediately. NIV would be useful in more stable patients, and likely not effective in this patient.

APPROACH TO:
Asthmatic Exacerbation

INITIAL PRIORITIES

Providing relief to the failing respiratory system and airway control is foremost here.

> *"[He} presents with a distressing sense of want of breath and a feeling of great oppression in the chest. Soon the respiratory efforts become violent, and all of the accessory muscles are brought into play. In a few minutes the patient is in a paroxysm of the most intense dyspnea."*
>
> **Sir William Osler**

APPROACH TO THE ASTHMATIC PATIENT

ICU admissions for refractory asthma range from 2% to 20%, affected somewhat by adherence to best practice protocols. When protocol therapies are used, ICU admissions fall by 41%; in contrast, when a new group of physicians assumes responsibilities for the ED, admissions generally increase. Aggressive bronchodilation with inhaled short-acting β_2-adrenergic agonists (SABA) such as albuterol and recently the addition of ipratropium bromide either in high-volume aerosolized form or via frequent aerosol treatments are indicated. IV corticosteroids for the relief of inflammation and bronchodilation are also used. Steroids increase the number of β_2 receptor sites available, thereby enhancing the effectiveness of β_2 agonists and avoiding tachyphylaxis to these agents. Aerosol treatments in intubated patients should be with double the amount normally recommended; this overcomes the increased deposition in the ETT. Sedation with IV propofol adds patient comfort and reduces the pressure needed to effectively mechanically ventilate. Propofol causes relaxation of the respiratory muscles, increasing the compliance of the chest wall; it also decreases cardiac output and causes vasodilation, which can lower the BP. This requires increased fluid administration. The use of safe pressures for MV may require an acceptance of a passive hypercapnia. Sedation helps the patient tolerate the feeling of the elevated $PACO_2$. Intravenous magnesium sulfate may also help respiratory muscle strength. Careful attention to MV and ventilating the patient with the safest airways pressures are needed to avoid barotrauma and pneumothorax. Low-volume MV with a tidal volume (V_t) of 6 to 8 mL/kg of ideal body weight is needed to avoid unsafe high pressures. The pH should be maintained above 7.20 regardless of the $PACO_2$ level as long as there is no hypoxia.

Overall, the national asthma prevalence rate is 10%, and has risen by 61% in the last 20 years. Patients are predisposed to a severe exacerbation from many different sources: allergen, exercise, infection (both viral and bacterial), cold air, emotional stress, gastroesophageal reflux (GERD), sinusitis, and post nasal drip. The underlying cause of asthma still remains unknown. Asthma accounts for about 2 million ED visits, 500,000 admissions, and 5000 deaths per year in the United States and is the third leading cause of preventable admission. Asthma is responsible for 10 million lost school days each year at a cost of >$12 billion/y.

The mortality from asthma has not decreased over the last 20 years even with advancements in the treatment. An inflammatory process leads to airway obstruction, increased mucus production, and smooth muscle hypertrophy; these changes lead to airway narrowing and airflow obstruction during the expiratory phase. If uncontrolled, airway remodeling and irreversible airway obstruction develops.

The early and late phases of an allergic response contribute to airway inflammation and increased mucus production. The **early response**, occurring within 1 hour of allergen exposure, is marked by histamines and other mediators released and allergic symptoms such as sneezing, itchy eyes, and runny nose, and respiratory symptoms such as wheezing, coughing, and shortness of breath. The **late-phase response**, occurring 3 to 10 hours after exposure, can last for as long as 24 hours, and prolongs the asthma attack and results in more severe congestion and inflammation.

DIAGNOSIS

Patients presenting to the ED with asthma should be evaluated and triaged quickly to assess the severity and the need for urgent intervention, but assessment should not delay treatment. Clinicians should search for signs of life-threatening asthma and identify high-risk patients (Table 11–1). Any of these conditions usually necessitate admission. Attention should be paid to factors that are associated with an increased risk of death from asthma, such as previous intubation or admission to an ICU, 2 or more hospitalizations for asthma during the past year, low socioeconomic status, and various coexisting illnesses.

MANAGEMENT

All patients should be treated with oxygen to achieve an arterial O_{2Sat} exceeding 90%, with inhaled SABAs, and systemic corticosteroids. High-dose ipratropium bromide given in combination with SABAs has been shown to **increase** bronchodilation.

Oxygen, Compressed Air, and Heliox

Oxygen should be administered. Patients with chronic severe asthma and chronic hypercarbia should be carefully monitored, since excessive oxygen may lead to

Table 11–1 • HIGH-RISK FACTORS IN ASTHMATIC EXACERBATION
• Altered mental status (AMS)
• Paradoxical chest or abdominal movement
• Absence of wheezing or quiet chest
• Previous intubations or previous admission to the intensive care unit (ICU)
• Overuse of rescue agents
• Frequent nighttime awakenings and exacerbations
• High frequency of emergency department (ED) visits
• Comorbid conditions such as congestive heart failure (CHF), chronic obstructive pulmonary disease (COPD), coronary artery disease (CAD)
• A second visit to the ED on the same day

increasing hypercarbia due to hypoventilation. The **elbow of the oxyhemoglobin dissociation curve lies at 90% saturation, equivalent to a P_{AO_2} of 60 mm Hg.** Small decreases below this point leads to dramatic fall in oxygen delivery. **PEEP, which is already increased intrinsically because of the reduced expiratory time, should be avoided.** The use of 100% inspired oxygen (F_{IO_2}) is not uncommon. Oxygen can be toxic and is a potent oxidizing agent when used at high concentrations over prolonged periods of time. Heliox, which is a mixture of helium and oxygen with a density about one-third that of air, reduces airflow resistance in the bronchial tree where turbulent flow predominates. **Heliox reduces airway flow resistance,** eases the work of breathing, and improves the delivery of aerosolized medications. A heliox mixture can be used in severe cases. Since helium occupies some of the inspired volume, the higher the percent of helium used, the lower the maximum F_{IO_2} that can be achieved. The roles of IV magnesium sulfate and heliox are controversial. The major benefit in their use may be avoiding the need for intubation.

Adrenergic Agents

SABAs should be administered immediately to a patient with an asthmatic exacerbation. The administration of SABAs can be repeated up to 3 times every 20 minutes via aerosols or by high-volume continuous nebulizer treatment. Rescue inhaler use of a SABA agent such as albuterol is the drug of choice. Levalbuterol, the R-isomer of albuterol, is effective at half the dose of albuterol, but trials have not consistently shown an advantage over racemic albuterol. Continuous high-dose inhalation of SABAs for acute rescue bronchodilation with the addition of ipratropium bromide adds a second but different short-acting bronchodilator. Should the patient need intubation, doubling the normal recommended dose of inhaled albuterol and ipratropium is advised, because of the increased deposition of these drugs in the ETT. Oral or parenteral administration of β_2-adrenergic agonists is not recommended, and is associated with an increased frequency of side effects. In severe cases, parenteral use of a β_2 agonist such as epinephrine (1/1000 solution) SC can be used with as many as 3 doses sq 20 minutes apart. This is generally reserved for younger patients with severe anaphylaxis with upper airway obstruction. Brethine in SC form or epinephrine IV may have a better side effect profile in these cases.

Anticholinergic Agents

When added to an inhaled β_2-adrenergic agonist, **ipratropium bromide** improved symptoms and lung function equivalent to the addition of salmeterol, a long-acting inhaled β_2-adrenergic agonist (LABA). In poorly controlled asthmatics, the addition of tiotropium in once-a-day metered dose inhaler (MDI) form was superior to the doubling of the dose of an inhaled glucocorticoid and was equivalent to the addition of inhaled salmeterol, an LABA. Ipratropium or tiotropium added to an SABA caused a greater and longer lasting bronchodilator effect. The use of ipratropium together with an SABA in severe airflow obstruction, compared with an SABA alone, reduced the rate of hospitalization by 25%. Benefit of continuing ipratropium after hospitalization was seen in smokers or patients with a chronic bronchitis or COPD.

Glucocorticoids

Systemic corticosteroids are a **cornerstone** to successful treatment of most individuals with asthmatic exacerbations. Their use is associated with a faster improvement in lung function, fewer hospitalizations, and a lower rate of relapse after ED discharge. Although the optimal dose of corticosteroids is unknown, clinical trials have shown no added efficacy in doses of prednisolone exceeding 100 mg/d. The most recent guidelines recommend the use of 40 to 80 mg of prednisolone each day in 1 or 2 divided doses.

Inhaled Corticosteroids, Hydration

Evidence does not support the use of inhaled corticosteroids (ICS) for acute exacerbations of asthma. **Aggressive hydration or mucolytic agents are not recommended in asthmatic exacerbations.** Autopsy of asthmatics show impacted mucous in the airways. Elevation of the head of the bed (HOB) at 45 degree is important to prevent aspiration.

Leukotriene Antagonists

The efficacy of leukotriene antagonists (LTAs) in the acute setting is unclear. They are excellent agents with a favorable safe side effect profile in moderate and mild cases of asthma. A 20% improvement in PFTs and PEFR which is the same response expected due to the normal diurnal rhythm, may be accentuated in asthmatics.

Magnesium

Magnesium (Mg^+) plays a role in neuromuscular function, and is more effective in relieving **severe** asthmatic exacerbations but less so in mild to moderate instances. **Magnesium decreases muscle constriction via competition with calcium and prevents acetylcholine release, thereby decreasing cyclic GMP.** Histamine release is also reduced. Magnesium is an important cofactor in many enzymatic reactions and there is evidence that IV magnesium can induce bronchodilation and reduce the neutrophilic burst of the inflammatory response. The effects of IV magnesium are rapid, within 5 to 10 minutes but the duration of action is also short. It has an excellent therapeutic-to-toxicity ratio at dosages of 2 to 4 g per hour as a continuous IV drip, and is widely used in asthmatics refractory to standard treatment. In **children, intravenous magnesium sulfate has been shown to significantly improve lung function and reduce rates of hospital admission**. A beneficial effect of nebulized magnesium sulfate is less substantiated.

Methylxathines and Antibiotics

Methylxanthines, once a standard treatment for asthma in the ED, are now rarely used because of their adverse effects (narrow therapeutic-to-toxic ratio) and lack of proven efficacy. These agents (theophylline, aminophylline) are no longer recommended for routine use. Theophylline is still used in the most severe cases where any improvement is welcome. The main side effects of methylxanthines include tachycardia, cardiac arrhythmias, and nausea and vomiting. Serum levels should be targeted to about 8 μg/dL since this level is associated with maximum bronchodilator effect and minimum side effects.

Antimicrobial Agents

Antibiotics should not be used routinely, but rather reserved for patients in whom a bacterial infection (eg, pneumonia or sinusitis) seems likely. The majority of asthmatic exacerbations are caused by viral infections, which can lead to a secondary bacterial superinfection. The antibiotic chosen should be directed toward the most likely pathogens (pneumococcus, *Haemophilus influenzae*, or mycoplasma).

Volatile Anesthetics

Volatile anesthetics are potent bronchodilators. Conventional tests of airway resistance demonstrate little difference between halothane, isoflurane, or enflurane (Ethrane). Halothane appeared to be a more potent bronchodilator than isoflurane. ETI by itself can induce severe bronchospasm. Volatile anesthetics are useful in treating severe status asthmaticus when the patient is unresponsive to conventional treatments. Isoflurane may be the most appropriate choice of volatile anesthetics due to its minimal depressive influence on cardiovascular and arrhythmogenic potential. Increased cerebral flow, cerebral edema, and increased intracranial pressure may be associated with the use of volatile agents in hypercapnic patients who may have suffered a degree of hypoxic brain injury.

BiPAP, CPAP, and Positive Pressure Ventilation

Please refer to Chapter 12 on noninvasive ventilation.

Intubation and Mechanical Ventilation

The use of invasive ventilatory support can be life saving in patients with an asthmatic exacerbation. **About 30% (range 2%-70%) of such individuals admitted to the ICU require intubation.** The decision for MV is based on clinical judgment. **Progressive hypercapnia, deterioration of mental status, exhaustion, and impending cardiopulmonary arrest** strongly suggest the need for ventilatory support. Authorities agree that intubation should be considered before these signs develop. A physician who has experience with intubation and airway management should ideally be managing the MV. The high pressures encountered by MV should be attained with low tidal volumes of 6 to 8 mL/kg of ideal body weight and started in the assist control mode at a low rate of 8 to 10 breaths/minute to avoid high plateau pressures and auto–positive end expiratory pressure (auto-PEEP). Plateau pressures should be kept <30 cm H_2O when possible to avoid barotrauma. Passive hypercapnia with a pH of 7.20 or greater may be needed to attain safe ventilation pressures. Sedation with short-acting agents like propofol will assist the patient in tolerating this treatment. Bicarbonate therapy should be reserved for patients with arterial pHs lower than 7.20. Permissive hypercapnia is not uniformly effective, and consultation with or comanagement by physicians who have expertise in ventilator management is appropriate to avoid risks.

Quick access to chest tube placement in the case of pneumothorax should be available. Strategies to reduce auto-PEEP often result in hypoventilation. The ensuing hypercapnia, termed *permissive hypercapnia*, is well tolerated as long as it develops slowly and the carbon dioxide tension remains at 90 mm Hg or less. When necessary, the pH can be managed pharmacologically. Daily ABGs and chest x-rays should be performed. Sedation may be needed to keep the patient comfortable and breathing in synchrony with the MV. This can usually be achieved with benzodiazepines combined with opioids or propofol. Ketamine is an attractive agent because of its bronchodilating properties; however, its CNS effects, tachycardia, and hypertension limit its use. Switching to CPAP with PSV when possible will help the patient tolerate MV via better coordination with the MV. Patients should be kept at an elevation of the head of the bed of 45 degrees to avoid aspiration. Auto-PEEP is a common problem in patients receiving full or partial ventilatory support, especially those needing high pressures for ventilation or having short expiratory times.

Physicians should be alert for air trapping and take measures to reduce it, as it can have serious consequences. The clinician needs to fully understand the physiology of auto-PEEP so as to choose the appropriate ventilator settings. Some of these maneuvers should include arranging the longest expiratory time possible and avoiding high respiratory rates and tidal volumes. The recommended settings for initial ventilation are as follows: tidal volume of 6 to 8 mL/kg, respiratory rate of 11 to 14 breaths/minute, flow rate of 100 L/min, and PEEP of 5. Allow the maximum possible time for exhalation by combining small tidal volumes with slow respiratory rates and short inspiratory times. Static end-inspiratory pressures (plateau pressures) levels of 30 cm H_2O or greater correlate with hyperinflation and auto-PEEP. Auto-PEEP rises directly with minute ventilation. The lungs and chest walls become less elastic and work of breathing rises. Venous return, BP, and cardiac output fall. Paralyzing agents are associated with myopathy, which prolongs hospitalization by 1 day, and intubation increases this time to 4.5 days. Fatalities due to asthma in the ICU averaged 2.7%. In intubated patients, the rate rises to 8.1%. Deaths from acute exacerbations of asthma in general are reported in <0.5% of patients. Pulmonary lavage via flexible bronchoscope is used to remove mucous plugs frequently found in patients with severe asthma. This procedure carries some risk.

ADMISSION/DISCHARGE CRITERIA

The decision to admit or discharge a patient should be made within 4 hours after presentation to the ED. **Patients may be discharged if the FEV_1 or PEF after treatment is 70% or more of the personal best or predicted value.** The initiation of therapy with ICS at the time of discharge reduces the risk of relapse. Discharging a patient who is on oral steroids and tapering the dosage schedule is needed only if steroids were used at high doses and for periods longer than 2 weeks. The patient should be free of symptoms at bedtime with a minimal need for rescue medication during the day. Patients should be educated about medications, inhaler technique, and reduce exposure to triggers of allergic reactions; they should have an asthma action plan and receive instructions for monitoring their symptoms and implementing their plan at home. A follow-up appointment should be scheduled with the treating physician 1 week after discharge.

To prevent readmission, discharge treatment should include rescue use of β_2 agonist as needed, maintenance use of an ICS and an LABA combination, and LTA use such as monteleukast at bedtime. Additionally, if the patient has a history of smoking or chronic bronchitis, ipratropium bromide or oral steroids, or azithromycin (Zithromax) should be considered when an impending acute exacerbation occurs. Instruction of the appropriate use of MDI and home aerosol machines should be provided. Immunization with the influenza and pneumococcal vaccines should be given.

CONCLUSION

Severe asthmatic exacerbations remain an enormous challenge. Physicians have proven to be poor judges of the severity of an asthma attack, and it is essential to use objective criteria when triaging a patient to an unmonitored bed or an ICU bed. SABAs and early administration of systemic corticosteroids are the mainstays of treatment now with the additional benefit of an anticholinergic agent. When ventilatory support is needed, noninvasive ventilation can be attempted but not delay intubation and MV. Status asthmaticus carries significant complications, including death.

CLINICAL CASE CORRELATION

- **See also Case 9 (Ventilator Management), Case 10 (Respiratory Weaning), and Case 12 (Noninvasive Methods of Ventilatory Support).**

COMPREHENSION QUESTIONS

11.1 A 45-year-old man who is intubated because of a severe asthma exacerbation starts to show a significant decrease in BP, high RR, decreased expiratory time, and increased airway pressure on the MV. The O_2 saturation reads 95% on the current settings. What should be performed to rule out auto-PEEP as a cause of deterioration?

A. Perform a stat arterial blood gas on present ventilator settings.

B. Disconnect the patient from the ventilator and see if there is rapid improvement.

C. Perform a stat chest radiograph.

D. Start the use of heliox mixture.

E. Insert a chest tube for probable pneumothorax.

11.2 A 22-year-old woman presents with a severe asthmatic exacerbation and respiratory distress. Which of the following would be the most important first step in her treatment?

A. A combination of ICS and long-acting inhaled β_2-adrenergic agonists (LABA)

B. Intravenous (IV) corticosteroids

C. Heliox mixture

D. Magnesium infusion

E. Inhaled SABA therapy

ANSWERS TO QUESTIONS

11.1 **B.** Auto-PEEP occurs more frequently that previously thought. Decreased expiratory time results in air-trapping and increased intrathoracic pressure. Progressive vascular collapse ensues, decreasing preload resulting in hypotension with tachycardia. Auto-PEEP and dynamic hyperinflation cause significant discomfort and precipitate patient–ventilator asynchrony. Auto-PEEP increases the work of breathing, lowers gas exchange, and decreases cardiac output, which causes hypotension. Disconnecting the patient from the MV immediately alleviates the high intrathoracic pressure; a dramatic improvement in BP is strong confirmation that auto-PEEP was the cause of the hypotension.

11.2 **E.** Inhaled SABAs should be immediately administered when an asthmatic patient presents with an exacerbation. SABAs can be repeated every 20 minutes or used as a high-volume continuous nebulizer treatment. SABAs such as albuterol is the first drug of choice for relief of the bronchoconstriction. Levalbuterol, the R-enantiomer of albuterol, is effective at half the dose of albuterol; trials have not consistently shown a clinical advantage of levalbuterol over racemic albuterol. Continuous high-dose inhalation of SABAs and ipratropium bromide are an excellent treatment combination as acute rescue bronchodilators.

CLINICAL PEARLS

- ► An ETT should be greater than or equal to 8 mm to allow for suctioning and to decrease resistance during the MV of asthmatics.
- ► V_t of 6 to 8 mL/kg of ideal body weight should be used when MV to avoid barotrauma.
- ► Heliox and general anesthesia are beneficial in patients unresponsive to initial treatments.
- ► A quiet chest in an asthmatic exacerbation is a bad prognostic sign with decreased ventilation.
- ► Previous intubation, overuse of rescue medications, frequent nighttime awakenings are all high-risk signs of asthmatic exacerbation, need for admission, and aggressive treatment.
- ► Continuous high-dose inhalation of SABAs and ipratropium bromide is of great value for bronchodilation and in the acute treatment regimen.
- ► Intravenous magnesium and heliox can be used as adjunctive therapy.
- ► Complications from positive-pressure ventilation are common in asthmatic patients.

REFERENCES

Bordow RA, Ries AL, Morris TA. *Manual of Clinical Problems in Pulmonary Medicine*. 6th ed. Philadelphia, PA: Lippincott Williams and Wilkins; 2005.

Deutschman CS, Neligan PJ. *Evidence Based Practice of Critical Care*. Philadelphia: Saunders; 2010.

Lazarus SC. Emergency treatment of asthma. *N Engl J Med*. 2010;363:755-764.

Toy EC, Simon B, Takenaka K, Liu T, Rosh A. *Case Files Emergency Medicine*. 2nd ed. McGraw-Hill Medical, 2009.

CASE 12

A 75-year-old man is admitted to the ICU for exacerbation of chronic obstructive pulmonary disease (COPD) and congestive heart failure (CHF). The patient experienced retrosternal chest pain lasting 4 minutes, which was relieved by 1 sublingual nitroglycerin tablet 1/150 mg. On initial physical examination, the respiratory rate is 35 breaths/minute, heart rate 123 beats/minute with a regular rhythm, and blood pressure 189/98 mm Hg. Rales and scattered wheezing are heard in the bilateral lung bases. There is a fixed split second heart sound (S_2) and a third heart sound (S_3) gallop present. The lower extremities show 2+ pitting edema. A chest x-ray (CXR) reveals a CHF pattern and cardiomegaly as well as hyperinflation and COPD changes, without acute infiltrates. Arterial blood gas (ABG) shows a pH of 7.45, P_{ACO_2} of 35 mm Hg, and P_{AO_2} of 100 mm Hg on 100% F_{IO_2}. The β natriuretic peptide (BNP) level is 1000 pg/mL (normal <100) and troponin I cardiac enzyme level is 5 ng/mL (normal <0.5).

- ▶ What is the next best step in managing this patient's respiratory status?
- ▶ What other treatment options should also be considered concurrently?

ANSWERS TO CASE 12:
Noninvasive Methods of Ventilator Support

Summary: This 75-year-old man is in obvious respiratory distress from pulmonary edema after an acute myocardial infarction.

- **Next step in management:** This patient is in need of ventilatory support, and bi-level positive airway (BiPAP) is an ideal choice since the patient has COPD, acute cardiogenic pulmonary edema (ACPE), and CHF. BiPAP can be started at 10 cm H_2O of inspiratory positive airway pressure (IPAP) and 5 cm H_2O of expiratory positive airway pressure (EPAP)/PEEP with 100% FIO_2.
- **Other considerations:** Other interventions should be directed at improving cardiac perfusion and improving cardiac output: intravenous angiotensin-converting enzyme inhibitors (ACE), IV nitrate therapy for coronary vasodilation relief of chest pain and as preload-reducing agent all improve CO. Diuresis with loop diuretics like furosemide, inhaled β_2 agonists, and ipratropium bromide plus IV corticosteroids are also indicated.

ANALYSIS

Objectives

1. To be familiar with noninvasive methods of ventilatory support (NIV).
2. To learn the indications for the use of noninvasive methods of ventilatory support.
3. To understand and know the settings for noninvasive methods of ventilatory support.
4. To understand how to wean the patient from noninvasive methods of ventilatory support.

Considerations

This is a 75-year-old patient with COPD and acute pulmonary edema due to myocardial infarction. The best approach to this awake and cooperative patient is to initially use NIV to relieve the respiratory failure caused by the pulmonary edema. Respiratory failure increases the work of breathing; accordingly, the respiratory-related cardiac output needs is increased from 1% to >20% of the total cardiac output. If not treated quickly, RSI and MV may be required. NIV is indicated in this patient to alleviate the increased work of breathing; give O_2 and bronchodilators. If improvement is not rapidly seen after NIV use, intubation and mechanical ventilation should not be delayed. BiPAP NIV serves to decrease the work of breathing, decrease anxiety, and improve the status of the pulmonary edema by decreasing cardiac and pulmonary preload and venous return to the right ventricle. NIV can avoid the need for invasive rapid-sequence intubation. NIV decreases both preload and afterload, thereby improving cardiac output.

APPROACH TO: Noninvasive Ventilatory Support

INTRODUCTION

NIV is an effective treatment for 2 main diseases: (1) exacerbations of COPD and (2) exacerbations of CHF. Successful use of NIV avoids the higher risk of ETI and MV. Positive pressure increases intrathoracic pressure and decreases venous return, causing a decreasing preload and acting as immediate treatment of the CHF. The application of pressure support ventilation (PSV) in an NIV delivers relief from respiratory distress by improving ventilation and oxygenation. Oxygenation occurs by diffusion while the exchange of CO_2 requires changes in ventilation. **NIV use may also reduce mortality in these diseases.** BiPAP is the most common mode of NIV. It delivers a preset amount of IPAP and EPAP. The difference between the IPAP and EPAP is the actual PSV provided to the patient.

INITIAL INTERVENTIONS

Supplemental oxygen is used to deliver the desired FIO_2 with PSV via a tight-fitting facemask. This has become the predominant method of providing NIV. Successful NIV support leads to a decrease in respiratory rate (RR), increase in tidal volume (V_t), and decrease in dyspnea. Other improved measures include decreased diaphragmatic electromyography (EMG), transdiaphragmatic pressures, hypercapnia, and work of breathing. **NIV is achieved through a variety of interfaces such as mouthpieces, nasal masks, facemasks, even a helmet mask, with the facemask being the most common.** These aids are used with a variety of NIV modes such as volume ventilation (VV), pressure support (PS), BiPAP, proportional assist ventilation (PAV), continuous positive airway pressure (CPAP) either with ventilators dedicated to NIV or standard mechanical ventilators fitted to these masks.

NIV support has markedly increased over the past 2 decades, and has become an integral tool in the management of both acute and chronic respiratory failure in the acute care, critical care, and chronic care settings. NIV has been used as a replacement for invasive ventilation.

INDICATIONS FOR NIV

Selection of patients for NIV must be considered carefully. **Respiratory failure due to acute cardiogenic pulmonary edema (ACPE) CHF** and COPD are the principal indications, since respiratory failure in these settings is rapidly reversible. NIV is an ideal adjunct in the management of the respiratory distress in these conditions.

Patient Inclusion Criteria

- Spontaneously breathing cooperative patient
- Dyspnea is moderate to severe, but short of respiratory failure
- Tachypnea (>24 breaths/minute)

- Increased work of breathing (accessory muscle use, pursed-lips breathing)
- Hypercapnic respiratory acidosis (pH range 7.10-7.35) ($PACO_2$ >42 mm Hg)
- Hypoxemia (PAO_2/FIO_2 <200 mm Hg, PAO_2 <60 mm Hg on room air)

The 2 most suitable clinical conditions for NIV are chronic obstructive pulmonary disease and cardiogenic pulmonary edema. Some other conditions that also respond to noninvasive ventilation are noted in Table 12–1. **Patient exclusion criteria are principally** mild disease or very severe distress.

Application of Noninvasive Ventilation

The experience and expertise of health-care providers, specifically nursing and respiratory therapy staff, cannot be underestimated. NIV implementation is dependent on the staff learning curve and the time demands of nursing and respiratory therapy (Table 12–2). Another important consideration is the potential for delay in definitive therapy.

Patient Interfaces and Mask Devices

NIV differs from invasive ventilation by nature of the interface between the patient and the ventilator. Invasive ventilatory support is provided via either an ETT or tracheostomy tube. NIV support uses a variety of interfaces, and these have continued

Table 12–1 • INDICATIONS FOR NIV

After discontinuation of mechanical ventilation
Pneumonias
Community-acquired pneumonia (CAP)
Mild *Pneumocystis jiroveci* pneumonia
Mild bacterial pneumonia
Cystic fibrosis
Asthmatic exacerbation
Acute respiratory distress syndrome (mild)
Immunocompromised state with respiratory distress
Do-not-intubate status
Neuromuscular respiratory failure
Postoperative respiratory distress and respiratory failure
Decompensated obstructive sleep apnea or cor pulmonale

Table 12–2 • LOCATION OF APPLICATION OF NIV

ICU	Telemetry Units	Intermittent/ Nocturnal Support	Ward Setting (no if Intubation Is Consideration)	Emergency Department
Step-down unit (lower severity of illness)	Moderately severe COPD (pH >7.30)	Suitable in specialized units	Same considerations as step-down unit	Local expertise may mirror ICU or step-down unit

Table 12–3 • ADVANTAGES AND DISADVANTAGES OF OROFACIAL MASKS

Advantages	Disadvantages
Best suited for less cooperative patients	Claustrophobic
Better in patients with a higher severity of illness	Hinder speaking and coughing
Better in edentulous patients, mouth or pursed-lips breathing	Risk of aspiration with emesis
Generally more effective ventilation	

to evolve with modifications based on patient comfort and efficacy. **Nasal masks and orofacial masks** were the earliest interfaces, followed by the subsequent development and use of **full-face masks, mouthpieces, and nasal pillows.** Nasal masks and orofacial masks are still the most commonly used devices. Orofacial masks are used almost twice as frequently as nasal masks.

Proper fitting of the mask is a key component to successful NIV. The mask should be held in place without straps first by the therapist to familiarize the patient with the mask and the ventilator. Typically, the smallest mask providing a proper fit is the most effective. Straps hold the mask in place. Leaking masks are the biggest problem in the use of all masks. Care must be taken to minimize excess pressure on the face or nose, which would otherwise create pressure ulcers. Excess pressure increases the risk of pressure necrosis and skin breakdown. Any cuff used in these interfaces should be kept below 25 mm Hg to prevent tissue necrosis. The main considerations regarding the choice of an orofacial mask or nasal mask are outlined in Tables 12–3 and 12–4.

Ventilators Used in NIV Support

Ventilator options providing NIV have continued to increase. The specialty ventilators have fewer options and range, but are more leak tolerant. Many critical care ventilators currently in use also have an NIV option, either as part of the original device or available as an upgrade option. Selection of the ideal device is dependent on a number of factors, including familiarity of the staff with the equipment chosen and the availability of alternative options. Many hospitals continue to provide noninvasive support with the specialty ventilator.

Modes of Noninvasive Ventilation

Most patients treated with NIV receive PSV, with CPAP, which is the most basic level of support. BiPAP is the most common mode of support and requires provision

Table 12–4 • ADVANTAGES AND DISADVANTAGES OF NASAL MASKS

Advantages	Disadvantages
Generally better tolerated, best for more cooperative, non-claustrophobic	More leaks possible
Patients with lower severity of illness, less aspiration risk with emesis	Effectiveness limited in nasal deformities or blocked nasal passages
Allows speaking, drinking, coughing, and secretion clearance	Effectiveness limited in claustrophobic patients

and control in the amount of both IPAP and EPAP. The difference between IPAP and EPAP is the amount of pressure support provided to the patient by the ventilator. EPAP is equivalent to positive end-expiratory pressure (PEEP). While volume ventilators can be used to provide NIV support, the previously described dedicated models are the best. Less sedation is needed because of increased patient comfort with the use of NIV.

Initial Ventilator Settings and Adjustments

The primary goals of NIV are: (1) adequate ventilation and oxygenation, (2) correction of respiratory failure, and (3) an acceptable level of patient tolerance and comfort. Adjustments are often necessary to achieve these endpoints. The initial settings should focus on achieving adequate tidal volumes, usually in the range of 5 to 7 mL/kg. Additional support is provided to reduce the respiratory rate to be <25 breaths/minute. FIO_2 is adjusted to achieve adequate oxygenation with a pulse oximetry level of 90% to 92%. Serial ABG measurements are essential to monitor the response to therapy and guide further adjustments.

Initial IPAP/EPAP Settings

Start at 10 cm H_2O IPAP/5 cm H_2O EPAP, pressures <8 cm H_2O IPAP/4 cm H_2O EPAP are not advised as this may be inadequate, make adjustments to achieve tidal volume of 5 to 7 mL/kg (IPAP and/or EPAP).

Subsequent Adjustments Based on Arterial Blood Gas Values

- Increase IPAP by 2 cm H_2O if persistent hypercapnia exists.
- Increase IPAP and EPAP by 2 cm H_2O if persistent hypoxemia exists.
- IPAP limited to 20 to 25 cm H_2O (avoids gastric distension, improves patient comfort).
- Maximal EPAP should be limited to 10 to 15 cm H_2O.
- Begin FIO_2 of 100% and adjust to the lowest level with an acceptable pulse oximetry value.
- Back up the respiratory rate to 12 to 16 breaths/minute.

Predictors of success include a good response to a trial of NIV for 1 to 2 hours with a decrease in $PACO_2$ >8 mm Hg from baseline and an improvement in pH >0.06 units. Predictors of failure include an increased severity of illness and acidosis (pH <7.25) especially if due to hypercapnia ($PACO_2$ >80). Certain patients may benefit from a trial of NIV, limiting the duration of trials is important to avoid delays in definitive therapy. NIV trials may be as short as a few minutes in patients with immediate failure and probably should not exceed 2 hours if patients fail to improve. Follow intubation criteria when NIV fails. It is important to use the following guidelines to assist in the decision of when to intubate a patient.

COMPLICATIONS OF NIV

Complications common to both NIV and invasive ventilation occur less frequently in patients undergoing NIV. When compared to CPAP, BiPAP has less morbidity, lower mortality, fewer adverse events, and lower medical utilization in adults with COPD and acute respiratory failure. NIV is also effective in the perioperative and posttransplantation settings. **Facial and nasal pressure sores and air leaks** are the main complications of NIV. This pressure can be minimized by intermittent NIV application at scheduled breaks of 30 to 90 minutes. Rebalancing of strap tension to minimize mask leaks without excessive mask pressures is also helpful. Early wound care is important. Gastric distension can be avoided by limiting peak inspiratory pressures to <25 cm of H_2O. Nasogastric tubes can be placed but can increase leaks from the mask. The use of nasogastric tubes also bypasses the lower esophageal sphincter and permits reflux to occur with more ease. Aspiration of gastric contents especially with emesis during NIV can also occur. NIV should be avoided in patients with ongoing emesis or hematemesis.

Barotrauma complicates both NIV and invasive ventilation, but occurs less frequently with NIV. Hypotension related to increased positive intrathoracic pressure can be reversed with increased intravenous fluids. Sedatives were used in <15% of NIV patients. It is used extensively in Europe (>80% of ICU patients). Current NIV practice guidelines suggest an increase in the usage of NIV because of the increased use of protocol, which avoids the costs of endotracheal intubation and mechanical ventilation, provides shorter ICU and hospital stays, and eliminates costs associated with infectious complications. Episodes of ventilator-associated pneumonia are reduced by half or more when NIV is used.

CONCLUSIONS

COPD is the most suitable condition for NIV. It is most effective in patients with moderate to severe disease. Those with hypercapneic respiratory acidosis are generally the best responders (pH 7.20-7.30). CPAP and BiPAP modalities are effective, with CPAP possibly being more effective. The greatest benefits are realized in the relief of symptoms and dyspnea. A decrease in intubation and mortality rates is not a universal experience. NIV is effective as a bridge support to freely breathing patients after early extubation. Patients with underlying COPD are most likely to benefit from this modality after early extubation. **NIV has not shown benefit in patients with community-acquired pneumonia (CAP).** Secretions may be a limiting factor to the use of NIV.

NIV is effective in patients with muscular dystrophy, kyphoscoliosis, and post-polio syndrome, as well as in cases of obesity-hypoventilation or obstructive sleep apnea (OSA). In OSA, NIV corrects hypercapnia, facilitates diuresis, and provides an opportunity for restorative sleep. NIV should be used carefully in cases of partial upper airway obstruction, but an even greater caution should be used if a potential for complete obstruction exists. NIV is also used during invasive procedures such as bronchoscopy, percutaneous gastrostomy.

CLINICAL CASE CORRELATION

- **See also Case 8 (Airway Management/Respiratory Failure), Case 9 (Ventilator Management), Case 10 (Respiratory Weaning), and Case 11 (Asthmatic Exacerbation).**

COMPREHENSION QUESTIONS

12.1 NIV is started on a 72-year-old man who presents to the emergency department with a non-ST-segment elevation myocardial infarction and acute onset of pulmonary edema. He has a medical history of chronic obstructive pulmonary disease with a 40 pack per year history of cigarette smoking. He complains of air hunger and is breathing at 30 breaths/minute with pursed lip breathing and accessory muscle use. His heart rate is 120 beats/minute and regular. His blood pressure is 140/80 mm Hg and he has a temperature of 98°F. His oxygen saturation is 90% while breathing on 1 L of oxygen via nasal cannula. He is awake and cooperative and free of chest pain on a nitroglycerin drip. What initial treatment with noninvasive ventilation would be best for this patient?

A. BiPAP at a pressure of 10 cm H_2O IPAP and 5 cm H_2O of EPAP

B. Intermittent positive pressure breathing

C. CPAP at 5 cm H_2O

D. Nasal CPAP

E. CPAP at 35 cm H_2O

12.2 A 35-year-old woman has been receiving BiPAP for 2 days because of CAP and an exacerbation of asthma with moderate respiratory distress. On day 3 she is now afebrile, alert, and cooperative; secretions are well controlled, the respiratory rate is 10 breaths/minute, wheezing cannot be heard, and breath sounds are normal. There is no use of accessory muscles while breathing. The O_2 saturation reads 95% on the current settings of 8 cm H_2O IPAP and 4 cm H_2O EPAP with an FIO_2 of 30%. These settings have been decreased from the admission values of 10 cm H_2O IPAP and 5 cm H_2O EPAP with an FIO_2 of 50%. What should be the next best step in the use of BiPAP in this patient?

A. Continue present BiPAP settings.

B. Stop BiPAP and observe the patient closely.

C. Further decrease the IPAP and EPAP.

D. Switch to CPAP.

E. Apply BiPAP use for nighttime use only.

ANSWERS TO QUESTIONS

12.1 **A.** When a patient has respiratory distress especially if caused by COPD or cardiogenic pulmonary edema (CPE) the application of NIV is the treatment of choice. Delivery of NIV would be best accomplished by the use of BiPAP at minimum starting level of 10 cm H_2O of IPAP, and 5 cm H_2O of EPAP with an appropriate oxygen concentration (FIO_2) for acceptable ABG. This provides a PEEP of 5 cm H_2O or the same as the EPAP and a net pressure support of 5 cm H_2O, the difference between IPAP and EPAP. The maximum numbers that are usually effective are 15 IPAP, 8 EPAP, and minimum numbers of support during weaning off BiPAP 8 IPAP and 4 EPAP.

12.2 **B.** An improving clinical picture with the use of NIV should lead to a trial discontinuation of the NIV. The improvement and stability of the patient's condition would suggest the discontinuation of the NIV and a continued clinical evaluation of the patient. The blood gases are acceptable with BiPAP settings at the minimum recommended pressures of 8 IPAP and 4 EPAP. Follow the patient closely after extubation but with continuous ECG/O_2 saturation monitoring. Use ABGs as needed. Being on the minimum BiPAP settings is equivalent to a spontaneous breathing trial and a successful respiratory stress test. Do not prolong these trials since in some cases they may lead to fatigue and failure. Liberate the patient from NIV once the patient shows she can breathe on her own.

CLINICAL PEARLS

- NIV is best used for patients with moderate exacerbations of chronic obstructive pulmonary disease and/or cardiogenic pulmonary edema.
- Nasal masks and orofacial masks are the most commonly used NIV interfaces, with orofacial masks more commonly used in the acute setting.
- BiPAP is the most commonly used NIV.
- NIV works best in patients in **moderate** distress, is less useful in severe or mild conditions, and should be avoided in patients with decreased mental status.
- The complications of NIV are similar to but occur less often than associated with invasive (intubated) mechanical ventilation.
- Rates of intubation and mechanical ventilation have decreased with the increased use of NIV.

REFERENCES

Bordow RA, Ries AL, Morris TA. *Manual of Clinical Problems in Pulmonary Medicine*. Philadephia: Lippincott Williams and Wilkins, 6th ed., 2005.

Rabe KF, Hurd S, Anzueto A, et al. Global strategy for the diagnosis, management, and prevention of chronic obstructive pulmonary disease: GOLD executive summary. *Am J Respir Crit Care Med*. 2007;176(6):532-555.

Tobin MJ, ed. *Principles and Practice of Mechanical Ventilation*. 2nd ed. New York, NY: McGraw-Hill; 2006:1442; ISBN: 978-0-07-144767-6.

Toy EC, Simon B, Takenaka L, Liu T, Rosh A. *Case Files Emergency Medicine*. 2nd ed. McGraw-Hill Medical, 2009.

CASE 13

A 43-year-old woman was struck by an automobile while crossing the street. She sustained bi-frontal cerebral contusions, a right tibial plateau fracture, left-sided rib fractures, and a grade 2 splenic laceration. Her brain, chest, and abdominal injuries are being managed nonoperatively. On hospital day 4, the patient develops respiratory distress and is transferred to the ICU. On examination, her blood pressure is 130/80 mm Hg, pulse rate is 110 beats/minute, respirations are 32 breaths/minute, and Glasgow coma scale (GCS) is 15. Her chest radiograph is normal. You are called to evaluate and manage the patient.

- What is the most likely diagnosis and risk factors for the patient's respiratory condition?
- What are the priorities in this patient's management?
- What is the differential diagnosis of the patient's respiratory condition?

ANSWERS TO CASE 13:

DVT/Pulmonary Embolism

Summary: A 43-year-old woman with multiple injuries following blunt trauma develops acute respiratory distress requiring transfer to the ICU on hospital day 4.

- **Likely diagnosis and risk factors: Pulmonary embolism (PE).** Risk factors for venous thromboembolic diseases include **stasis** (bed rest, immobilization), **hypercoaguability** (trauma, estrogen), and **endothelial injury** (trauma). Factors that are associated with increased risk of PE after trauma include age ≥40, pelvic fracture, lower extremity fracture, shock, spinal cord injury, and brain injury. Variables associated with very high risk for PE are major operative procedure, venous injury, >3 ventilator days, and having 2 or more high-risk factors.
- **Priorities in management:** The initial priority is to determine adequacy of oxygenation and ventilation. In this case, we must determine her ability to maintain airway patency; she should be placed on high-flow oxygen. The patient's mental status, level of pain, oxygenation, and acid/base status must also be taken into account as we determine whether intubation and/or mechanical ventilation is needed. Given her recent history of major multisystem trauma, she is at high risk for venous thromboembolic complications. A contrast-enhanced helical CT scan and PE protocol should be obtained to confirm or exclude the diagnosis. Documenting the presence of a deep venous thrombosis (DVT)/PE would be important prior to starting anticoagulation, given the bleeding risks associated with her brain and splenic injuries. In a patient with a low risk of bleeding and/or if a long delay is expected before CT scan evaluation can be obtained, immediate anticoagulation therapy is appropriate when a PE is suspected.
- **Differential diagnosis:** Other possible causes of the respiratory distress include pneumonia, mucus plugging, pneumothorax, acute lung injury, fluid overload, PE, and cardiac ischemia.

ANALYSIS

Objectives

1. To learn the risk factors and preventive strategies for DVT/PE in the critical care setting.
2. To learn the diagnostic strategies for patients with suspected DVT/PE.
3. To learn the treatment strategies for patient with PE.

Considerations

This woman who is a victim with multiple trauma including closed head injury, chest injury, splenic injury, and orthopedic injuries develops acute respiratory distress on hospital day 4. Immediately following the stabilization of the respiratory status, we need to determine the cause responsible for her sudden clinical deterioration.

A chest x-ray, EKG, and serum troponin levels are helpful to identify causes such as primary cardiac process, acute lung injury, and pulmonary infections. A CT angiography of the chest would help determine if pulmonary embolic disease is the cause of her problem. Systemic anticoagulation would be indicated if PE is identified.

APPROACH TO: Venous Thromboembolism

DEEP VENOUS THROMBOSIS

Deep venous thrombosis refers to clot formation in the deep veins of the body located predominantly in the lower extremities and pelvis. A **deep vein** is defined as any vein paired with a named artery. The majority of deep venous thrombosis occurs when clots form in the valve cusps of the calf. Once developed, 20% of distal lower extremity (tibial level) DVTs will propagate proximally, resulting in the potential for PE. Rudolph Virchow, a 19th century German physician, first described the triad of circulatory stasis, hypercoaguability, and endothelial injury as factors that contribute to venous thromboembolic diseases. **Circulatory stasis** refers to stagnation of normal blood flow in the veins. Stagnation of blood allows time for the cross-linking of fibrin polymers and clot formation. Conditions associated with stasis are bed rest, travel (eg, long airline flight), immobility (eg, casting a lower extremity in extension), limb paralysis, spinal cord injury, and obesity.

Under usual circumstances, the coagulation/fibrinolytic systems maintain a delicate balance between thrombogenesis and thrombolysis. A **hypercoaguable state** implies an imbalance in coagulation homeostasis usually associated with a derangement of a protein or protein receptor involved in the clotting cascade. Clinical examples of hypercoagulable states include malignancy, trauma, pregnancy, inflammatory conditions, and thrombocythemia.

Deficiency of protein S, protein C, and antithrombin III are host conditions producing hypercoagulable states. Protein S and C deficiency leads to an overabundance of Factors Va and VIIIa, causing thrombosis. Antithrombin III deficiency results in the activation of factors XIIa, XIa, and IXa leading to thrombosis. Factor V Leiden mutation renders factor V resistant to protein C, and this mutation is the most common genetic cause of hypercoagulability and occurs in 5% to 8% of the population; heterozygotes with factor V Leiden mutation carry a 7-fold increased risk of thrombosis, and homozygotes have an 80-fold increased risk in comparison to the general population.

Endothelial injury may occur as the result of surgery or injury, which then activates the extrinsic pathway of the coagulation cascade. Activation of the extrinsic pathway leads to the activation of factor VIIa, and tissue factor/factor VIIa/calcium complex then activates factor Xa and joins the common pathway of the coagulation cascade.

DVT/PE Prevention (Thromboprophylaxis) Strategies

Prevention strategies should be implemented for all hospitalized patients, especially those with **moderate** and **high** risk. Low-risk patients are minor surgery patients and medical patients who are fully mobile, and these individuals are generally not encountered in the ICU setting. Moderate-risk patients include most general surgery, open gynecological surgery, and urological surgery patients, as well as medical patients who are sick or bedridden. High-risk patients include those following hip or knee arthroplasty, hip fracture surgery, major trauma, and spinal cord injury. With this risk-stratification scheme, **the estimated DVT risk without prophylaxis is <10% for low-risk patients, 10% to 40% for moderate-risk patients, and 40% to 80% for high-risk patients.** The recommended prophylaxis strategy for low-risk group is simply early and aggressive ambulation. The recommendation for the moderate-risk group include low molecular weight heparin (LMWH), low-dose unfractionated heparin (LDUH), or fondaparinux; however, if the patient has a high bleeding risk, then mechanical thromboprophylaxis should be implemented instead. For high-risk patient, prophylaxis with LMWH, fondoparinux, or oral vitamin K antagonist (INR 2-3) is recommended, and for high-risk patients with a high bleeding risk, mechanical thromboprophylaxis is recommended.

Diagnosis of DVT

The diagnosis of DVT can be made by a combination of clinical, laboratory, and imaging data. Imaging studies provide the most sensitive and specific diagnostic information. The **Wells score** consists of a list of clinical criteria with a single point awarded per criteria (Table 13–1) and calculates the clinical probability of the diagnosis of DVT in hospitalized patients.

- **Wells scores ≥3 is associated with a high probability of DVT.**
- **Scores from 1 to 2 are associated with a moderate probability.**
- **Scores of 0 represent a low probability of DVT.**

The Wells score has correlated with imaging confirmation of DVT in 76%, 21%, and 10% of patients in the high-, medium-, and low-probability groups, respectively. **The Homans sign, or pain in the calf with ankle flexion, is not reliable for DVT diagnosis,** as it is only present in one-third of DVT cases.

The fibrin degradation product D-dimer can be elevated with DVT. The most common method of D-dimer quantification is the ELISA test. D-dimer screening

Table 13–1 • WELLS SCORE CRITERIA FOR PREDICTION OF DVT
1 point per criteria. Scores ≥3 have a high probability of DVT, scores 1 to 2 have a moderate probability of DVT, and scores of 0 have a low probability of DVT.
Malignancy
Bed rest for >3 days
Pain along the course of a deep vein
Paralysis
Swelling of the entire leg
Calf circumference > 3 cm compared with the asymptomatic leg
Pitting edema in the affected leg
Collateral superficial veins—not varicose veins

is useful for the evaluation of asymptomatic medical patients and outpatients. In the **ICU patient population, D-dimer elevations can occur as a result of medical interventions, thus making it an unreliable test in this population.**

The diagnosis of DVT is generally confirmed with imaging studies. **Duplex ultrasound** is a noninvasive, reproducible examination that can demonstrate the flow characteristics and compressibility of the popliteal and femoral veins. It should be the first imaging study ordered. Ultrasound of the popliteal and femoral veins has a sensitivity and specificity for proximal DVT of 100% and 99%, respectively. **Duplex ultrasound is less sensitive and specific (70% and 60%, respectively) for DVT of the calf.** Two negative ultrasounds performed 1 week apart essentially excludes the diagnosis of DVT.

Treatment of DVT

Systemic anticoagulation is the standard treatment of DVT. Anticoagulation options include subcutaneous low molecular weight heparin (SC LMWH), intravenous unfractionated heparin (IV UFH), monitored subcutaneous unfractionated heparin (SC UFH), fixed-dose SC UFH, or subcutaneous fondaparinux. When possible, an oral vitamin K antagonist (warfarin) should be initiated concurrently with heparin or LMWH. When administering IV UFH, a bolus of 80 U/kg should be given, followed by a continuous infusion of 18 U/kg/h titrated to a target PTT >1.5 times normal. In adults, 150 to 200 U/kg of SC LMWH once a day is as effective as 100 U/kg of SC LMWH twice a day and continuous IV UFH titrated to a PTT >1.5 times normal. Daily LMWH has the advantage of a stable dose–response curve thus obviating the need for frequent laboratory monitoring. **In comparison to a heparin drip, LMWH has the advantages of being associated with a lower risk of heparin-induced thrombocytopenia (HIT)** and lower cost.

To prevent recurrence, patients with DVT and DVT/PE require an extended period of anticoagulation with either LMWH or warfarin. The duration of anticoagulation therapy depends on the circumstances of clot formation. DVT that occurs after a reversible inciting event (eg, surgery, trauma, pregnancy) requires a minimum of 3 months treatment. Unprovoked DVT formation in patients with no risk factors for bleeding requires a minimum of 3 months treatment and the possibility of indefinite treatment should be entertained. Isolated distal DVT formation may be treated with 3 months of anticoagulation therapy.

Systemic fibrinolysis is not recommended for DVT treatment. Compared to heparin therapy, systemic fibrinolytic therapy results in increased thrombolysis, lower risk of postphlebitic syndrome; however, this treatment is associated with **significantly increased risk of bleeding complications**. There is no significant difference in the risk of death or DVT recurrence between systemic fibrinolysis and continuous heparin infusion. Catheter-directed fibrinolysis has had moderate success when used to treat DVT, with total clot dissolution in 31% and partial dissolution in 52% of the treated patients. Catheter-based treatment with fibrinolytics has evolved and may be combined with percutaneous mechanical thrombectomy. Several case series have reported this combination therapy as being 82% to 100% successful and catheter-directed thrombolysis is associated with 1% incidence of PE and no increase in deaths or strokes. Catheter site bleeding is a potential complication

Table 13–2 • INDICATIONS FOR VENA CAVA FILTER

Evidence of PE or iliofemoral DVT in a patient with: a contraindication to anticoagulation, or a complication from anticoagulation, or a failure of anticoagulation
Massive PE with evidence of ongoing DVT
Free-floating iliofemoral or IVC thrombus
DVT in the setting of severe cardiopulmonary disease
Poor compliance with anticoagulation

requiring blood transfusions in 4% to 14% of the treated patients. Percutaneous mechanical thrombectomy appears safe, but there is insufficient evidence to support routine use at the present time.

Vena Cava Filters

The indications for inferior vena cava (IVC) filter are summarized in Table 13–2. Although rarely applied, the relative indications for IVC filters are: (1) prophylactic IVC filter placement for trauma patients, and (2) very high-risk patients, for example, immobilized hypercoagulable patients.

The PREPIC study is the only randomized controlled trial to evaluate the efficacy of IVC filter placement for the prevention of PE in patients with proximal DVT. The study found that PE occurred in 1.1% of patients with an IVC filter and 4.8% of patients without an IVC filter in place. At 2 years, recurrent DVT was found in 20.8% of the IVC filter patients compared with 11.6% of the patients without a filter. At 8-year follow-up, symptomatic PE was found in 6.2% of the IVC filter patients and 15.1% of patients without a filter. The incidence of post-thrombotic syndrome and death were the same in both groups. **The study concluded that IVC filters are only beneficial in high-risk patients and that widespread use of filters is not recommended.**

Thromboembolism After Trauma

Factors associated with a high risk of PE after trauma include age ≥40 years, pelvic fracture, lower extremity fracture, shock, spinal cord injury, and head trauma. High-risk variables associated with major operations include venous injury, >3 days on the ventilator, and having 2 or more high-risk factors. The highest risk trauma patients are those with a spinal cord injury, with reported DVT rates of 80% and PE rates of 5%. **PE is the most common cause of death in spinal cord injury patients.**

The authors of a National Trauma Data Bank study have proposed a thromboprophylaxis strategy for trauma patients at risk for DVT/PE. Patients at high-risk for DVT/PE and without contraindications for heparin should receive prophylactic doses of LMWH. Those patients with a contraindication for heparin should have mechanical compression stockings in place at all times. Those patients at very high risk for DVT/PE without contraindications for heparin should be treated with a prophylactic dose of LMWH combined with mechanical compression. If the very high-risk patient has a contraindication for heparin, mechanical compression stockings should be worn and either serial color-flow Doppler studies to monitor for DVT or a temporary IVC filter should be considered.

PULMONARY EMBOLISM

Most PEs occur when a thrombus breaks free from the endothelial wall, traveling through the right heart, and lodging in the pulmonary artery. PE causes ventilation/perfusion mismatching, increased pulmonary vascular resistance, and cytokine-mediated pulmonary vasoconstriction. Symptoms depend on the degree of pulmonary arterial obstruction, severity of the inflammatory response, and the patient's physiological reserve. Most patients have dyspnea (79% of patients in PIOPED II study), while some patients have hypoxemia and an increased A-a gradient. At times, extravasation of blood into the alveoli can produce pleuritic chest pain, cough, or hemoptysis.

Large PEs can present as acute right heart failure and cardiac arrest. Patients with larger PEs can demonstrate right heart strain. **T-wave inversions in lead V_1 and V_2 may be present on EKG and are 99% specific for PE**. Echocardiography is a useful adjunct in the diagnosis of PE, with sensitivity and specificity reported at 51% and 87%, respectively. Echocardiography has a 97% sensitivity and 98% specificity in patient with passive PEs. CT angiography (CTA) is the diagnostic image of choice, with 82% to 100% sensitivity and 89% to 98% specificity. The sensitivity and specificity of CTA are affected by the pretest probability of disease; thus, in the high-risk patients, the negative predictive value of CTA is only 60%. For the high-risk patients, the combination of a CTA and CTV (CT venography of the upper thigh and pelvis) helps improve the negative predictive value to 82%.

Empiric anticoagulation should be considered in high-risk patients without significant bleeding risks. Treatment with either unfractionated heparin or LMWH is acceptable, and treatment principles for PE are similar to those for the treatment of DVT. Hemodynamically unstable patients with large central PEs can be considered for catheter-directed therapy such as catheter-directed thrombolytic therapy or catheter-directed mechanical clot disruption therapy.

CLINICAL CASE CORRELATION

- **See also Case 8 (Airway Management/Respiratory Failure), Case 9 (Ventilator Management), Case 10 (Respiratory Weaning), Case 11 (Asthmatic Exacerbation), and Case 12 (Noninvasive Methods of Ventilator Support).**

COMPREHENSION QUESTIONS

13.1 A 24-year-old woman is brought in by ambulance to the emergency department as a Level I trauma after crashing into a tree at 75 mph. The paramedics found the patient ejected from the automobile, semiconscious with an open left femur fracture. The patient's initial systolic blood pressure in the ER was 80 mm Hg. After a blood transfusion, the patient's mental status improved and her blood pressure increased to 96/40 mm Hg. Upon reviewing the pelvic film, you notice a diastasis of the right sacroiliac joint and pubic symphysis. The patient gives no history of medical conditions. She is currently taking oral contraceptive pills. All of the following are risk factors for venous thromboembolism in this patient *except*:

A. Age
B. Lower extremity fracture
C. Hypotension
D. Pelvic fractures
E. Oral contraceptive pills

13.2 After placement of a pelvic binder and rapid splinting of the left femur fracture, the patient in Question 13.1 went to the CT scanner and was found to have a 4-cm cerebral contusion in the right frontal lobe, 3 right-sided rib fractures, a grade II splenic laceration, and an extra-peritoneal pelvic hematoma with no active extravasation. All of the following thrombosis prophylaxis measures are indicated *except*:

A. Using bilateral sequential compression devices
B. Immediately starting prophylactic SC UFH upon arrival in the ICU
C. Using graduated compression stockings
D. Starting SC UFH after 48 hours in the ICU if there is no enlargement of the cerebral contusion
E. Administering low-dose Coumadin

13.3 The patient in question 13.1 is taken to the ICU for continuous monitoring and hourly neurological examinations. The patient develops some pain and swelling of the right thigh. What is the best test to screen for DVT?

A. D-dimers level
B. Platelets
C. CT venography
D. Ultrasound examination
E. Coagulation profile

13.4 By hospital day 4 the patient has been started on LMWH, her pelvis and femur fractures stabilized with external fixation devices, and she has been hemodynamically stable. She has now developed swelling and pain in her right thigh and calf. What is the best diagnostic approach for her at this time?

A. CT angiography
B. CT venography
C. Duplex ultrasonography
D. Echocardiography
E. Venography

13.5 In the absence of contraindications for anticoagulation, the most appropriate therapy for femoral DVT with associated PE is:

A. Inferior vena caval filter
B. SC UFH upon arrival in the ICU
C. SC LMWH 150 to 200 U/d followed by transition to warfarin
D. Unmonitored IV UFH drip followed by transition to warfarin
E. Aspirin 325 mg PO daily

ANSWERS TO QUESTIONS

13.1 **A.** The patient is at very high risk for DVT/PE because she has 2 or more high-risk factors for DVT/PE. Her risk factors are pelvic fractures, a lower extremity fracture, and shock. Oral contraceptive pills contribute to and increase estrogen state, which is also a risk factor for DVT/PE. Her age in this case is not a contributing risk factor, because only age >45 is generally considered a risk factor.

13.2 **B.** The patient is at very high risk for a DVT/PE given her long bone fracture, pelvic fractures, and hypotension; however, she has multiple contraindications to systemic anticoagulation therapy at this time, and these are intracerebral hemorrhage and splenic injury. In the initial 48 hours, the patient should have graduated compression stockings and sequential compression devices on both lower extremities. The patient should *not* be started on SC UFH immediately due to the risk of bleeding. If the patient's head injury and splenic injury remain stable, she should be started on prophylactic dosing of SC UFH after 48 hours. Low-dose Coumadin is not indicated as prophylaxis in the trauma patient population.

13.3 **D.** The bedside ultrasound is the standard for screening for DVT. A CT venography is not an appropriate screening examination for DVT. A platelet count and coagulation profile do not diagnose the presence of DVT. The patient will have elevated D-dimer levels due to continuous clot formation and degradation occurring in the trauma patient. Although screening duplex examinations are done at a number of trauma centers, the 2008 American College of Chest Physicians Evidence-Based Clinical Practice Guidelines specifically recommend against screening studies for asymptomatic patients.

13.4 **C.** The concern at this time should be DVT involving the proximal veins. This can be diagnosed by CT venography, venography, or duplex sonography. Venography has the disadvantage of being invasive and requiring the administration of intravenous contrast. The CT venography is a study that requires contrast administration; therefore the duplex is the preferred diagnostic study for DVT diagnosis. CT angiography is useful only if the patient has a PE. Echocardiography would not be useful for DVT diagnosis.

13.5 **C.** The patient should be started on a full anticoagulation regimen starting with an LMWH, monitored IV UFH, fixed-dose SC UFH, or SC fondaparinux. The LMWH is dosed at 150 to 200 U/kg/d or 100 U/kg/twice daily. To initiate a heparin drip, give an 80 U/kg bolus and titrate the PTT to 1.5 times normal starting with 18 U/kg/h. Regardless of which anticoagulation regimen is started, warfarin should be started simultaneously and titrated to an INR of between 2.5 and 3.0. IVC filter would only have a role if the patient develops PE while on appropriate DVT treatment or if anticoagulation is contraindicated.

CLINICAL PEARLS

- DVT prophylaxis is variable depending on the patients' risks for thromboembolism development.
- The combination of CTA and CTV has greater negative predictive value than CTA alone for pulmonary embolism in high-risk patients.
- Dyspnea is the most common presenting symptom in patients with PE.

REFERENCES

Karthikesalingam A, Young EI, Hinchiliffe RJ, et al. A systematic review of percutaneous mechanical thrombectomy in the treatment of deep venous thrombosis. *Euro J Vasc Endovasc Surg*. 2011;41(4): 554-565.

Kearon C, Kahn SR, Agnelli G, Goldhaber S, Raskob GE, Comerota AJ. Antithrombotic therapy for venous thromboembolic disease: American College of Chest Physicians Evidence-Based Clinical Practice Guidelines (8th ed). *Chest*. 2008;133(6 suppl):454S-545S.

Knudson,MM, Ikossi DG, Khaw L, et al. Thromboembolism after trauma: an analysis of 1602 episodes from the American College of Surgeons National Trauma Data Bank. *Annals of Surgery*. 2004;240(3): 490-496; discussion 496-498.

Lensing AW, Prandoni P, Brandjes D, et al. Detection of deep-vein thrombosis by real-time B-mode ultrasonography. *N Engl J Med*. 1989;320(6):342-345.

Wells PS, Hirsh J, Anderson DR, et al. Application of a diagnostic clinical model for the management of hospitalized patients with suspected deep-vein thrombosis. *Thrombosis Haemostasis*. 1999;81(4): 493-497.

CASE 14

A 55-year-old woman presented 2 hours previously with the sudden onset of chest pain, and shortness of breath (SOB) out of proportion to the severity of her chest pain. The ECG shows a heart rate of 55 beats/minute and ST segment elevations of 3 mm on leads II, III, and aVF. She has no contraindications for anticoagulation therapy. Troponin levels are elevated and blood pressure is 130/70 mm Hg. She has required a nitroglycerin drip at 5 μg/kg/min keeping her free of chest pain, but ECG changes persist though now only a 1-mm elevation of the ST segment is seen. Mild JVD is diagnosed on physical examination. The lungs have minimal rales at both lung bases. The patient is breathing at 25 breaths/minute without labor. She smokes 1 pack per day (PPD) and admits to having had a diagnosis of COPD by her physician. The S_1 and S_2 heart sounds are normal without murmurs, and there are no S_3 and S_4 sounds heard. There is no lower extremity edema. The patient was given 325 mg of aspirin (ASA) on arrival in the ED.

- What is the most likely diagnosis?
- What immediate therapeutic steps are indicated?
- What are the different treatment options for her condition?

ANSWERS TO CASE 14:
Acute Coronary Syndrome

Summary: The patient presents with an acute ST elevation myocardial infarction (STEMI). She has no contraindications to anticoagulation. She has already received 325 mg of ASA.

- **Most likely diagnosis:** Inferior wall ST segment elevation MI (STEMI).
- **Immediate steps in treatment:** Administer ASA, anticoagulation, pain control, β-blockade, prepare patient for percutaneous coronary intervention (PCI) and notify the cardiology and catheterization team.
- **Treatment options:** Individualized depending upon whether the MI is an STEMI or a non-STEMI, with PCI being the preferred treatment and thrombolytic therapy (TPA) being an option when PCI is not possible. In rare cases, bypass surgery may be indicated.

ANALYSIS

Objectives

1. To understand the difference in acute coronary syndromes (ACS).
2. To understand the difference in treatment of STEMI and non-STEMI.
3. To understand the different treatment options for ACS.

Considerations

This is a 55-year-old woman with ACS, STEMI as evidenced by the EKG changes, and elevated cardiac troponin levels. The EKG ST segment elevation in the inferior leads and the bradycardia speak for an inferior wall MI. Because the SA node as well as the inferior portion of the heart is usually supplied by the right coronary artery, inferior wall cardiac injury and sinus bradycardia are often seen together. The saying is, "Time is myocardium," and within several hours of diagnosis of ACS, the patient should have intervention, which can include TPA or PCA. PCI, placement of a stent in the affected coronary artery, is associated with a lower 30-day mortality rate compared with TPA.

APPROACH TO:
Acute Coronary Syndrome

INTRODUCTION

ACS refers to acute myocardial ischemia. It encompasses unstable angina, non-STEMI, and STEMI. Troponin elevations are common in ICU patients although not always due to myocardial ischemia or MI, elevations are associated with poor patient outcome. Loss of a viable myocardium is diagnosed when the troponins exceed the 99th percentile with at least one of the following:

- Ischemic ST- and T-wave changes
- New left bundle branch block (LBBB)
- New Q waves
- Percutaneous coronary intervention

Cardiac enzymes may be elevated due mechanical injury, which may occur in the setting of CABG or from sepsis, chest trauma, or cardioversion. STEMI has a clinical presentation consistent with acute MI and ECG changes with evidence of ST-segment elevation. Unstable angina and non-STEMI are related and differ only in the severity of the ischemia. Non-STEMI is associated with elevated biomarkers of myocardial injury while unstable angina is not. The therapy is identical for both unstable angina and non-STEMI. ACS is characterized by atherosclerotic plaque rupture, formation of a platelet and fibrin thrombi, and local release of vasoactive substances. Unstable angina and non-STEMI are caused by thrombi that are not entirely occlusive. A form of unstable angina and non-STEMI can include vasospasm of an epicardial coronary artery (Prinzmetal angina) and secondary angina (eg, hypoxemia, anemia, tachycardia, or thyrotoxicosis). Vasospastic angina can also be seen in Raynaud disease and scleroderma. The most common cause of STEMI is a totally occlusive thrombus.

PREVENTION

Asymptomatic adults ≥30 years old should be periodically screened for dyslipidemia, hypertension, and diabetes. Patients who smoke should stop, since this is the most significant modifiable cardiovascular risk factor. ASA reduces the risk of cardiovascular events by inhibiting platelet activation. Moderate strenuous exercise is indicated and raises protective HDL levels as well as low alcohol intake. A high-fiber diet rich in fresh fruits and vegetables, low in cholesterol, saturated fats, and refined sugars should be instituted. Hormone replacement therapy in postmenopausal women may increase the incidence of nonfatal MI.

Screening of Asymptomatic Individuals

Routine screening for CAD in asymptomatic persons without cardiovascular risk factors is not recommended. Exercise testing is limited by the low prevalence of CAD in asymptomatic adults. The presence of calcification in coronary arteries, detected by electron-beam CT scanning, is predictive of nonfatal MI. In 2007, the use of electron-beam CT-identified patients with an estimated 10% to 20% risk of a coronary event over the following 10 years.

DIAGNOSIS

Analysis of an ECG is essential for patients with suspected cardiac ischemia or infarction. ECG findings such as the evolution of ST-segment abnormalities and Q waves can provide essential information regarding the duration, size, and location of injury. When inferior MI is suspected, a right-sided ECG should be recorded to evaluate right ventricular infarction. Typical angina, characterized by substernal discomfort, exertional onset, and prompt relief with nitroglycerin or rest, is associated with a 94% probability of CAD. The failure to diagnose acute MI may be because the patient has either "noncardiac" or "atypical" symptoms of dyspnea, fatigue, nausea, abdominal discomfort, or syncope. Any of these symptoms should prompt a consideration of ACS.

Up to 25% of women, diabetics, and the elderly with ACS have atypical symptoms. Chest pain that is pleuritic, sharp, stabbing, or positional significantly increases the chance of pulmonary disease and not ACS. Physical findings alone cannot exclude the diagnosis of ACS. A new murmur may suggest valvular incompetence caused by papillary muscle dysfunction or rupture which requires immediate attention and possibly an intra-aortic balloon pump (IABP) and/or open heart surgery. A **new S_4 gallop can represent decreased diastolic compliance.** Heart failure may be present if ischemia results in left ventricular diastolic, systolic dysfunction or valvular incompetence and is a high-risk feature for death. **Physical examination features most predictive of MI are: (1) elevated central venous pressure, (2) hypotension, (3) bibasilar crackles, and (4) an S_3 heart sound.**

An electrocardiogram (ECG) should be performed immediately in patients suspected of ACS. **New ST-segment elevation and Q waves** are the most powerful predictors for MI. Half of the time, the initial ECG may be nondiagnostic, and serial ECGs are essential. The diagnostic yield of the ECG is improved if a tracing can be recorded during an episode of chest discomfort. STEMI is characterized by chest pain and ST elevations >1 mm in 2 or more contiguous leads, new left bundle-branch block, or evidence of true posterior infarction on electrocardiography. Non-STEMI is defined by elevated cardiac biomarkers and an absence of ST-segment elevation. A persistently normal ECG decreases the probability of MI.

Transthoracic Echocardiogram

Transthoracic echocardiography (TE) in patients with myocardial ischemia provides valuable diagnostic and prognostic information and detects complications. **TE is recommended when acute ischemia is not detected despite a high suspicion.** The presence of left ventricular (LV) dysfunction or mitral regurgitation after MI is an adverse prognostic finding. After MI, TE can detect complications such as residual ischemia, ventricular septal defects, papillary muscle rupture or dysfunction, free wall rupture, regurgitant lesions, LV thrombus, or tamponade. Radionuclide ventriculography, myocardial perfusion scintography (MPS), and magnetic resonance imaging (MRI) are techniques that assess the viability of myocardial tissue and characterize the extent of tissue injury.

During MI, the cardiac myocytes lose membrane integrity and leak proteins (eg, creatine kinase, myoglobin, cardiac troponin), see Figure 14–1. By serially measuring the presence and concentration of these cardiac marker proteins, evidence of myocardial damage that has occurred within the past 24 hours can be detected. Repetition of these determinations is advised 6 and 12 hours after the onset of symptoms. In patients with acute ST elevations, further management should not be delayed awaiting biomarker data. An echocardiogram detecting abnormality in regional wall

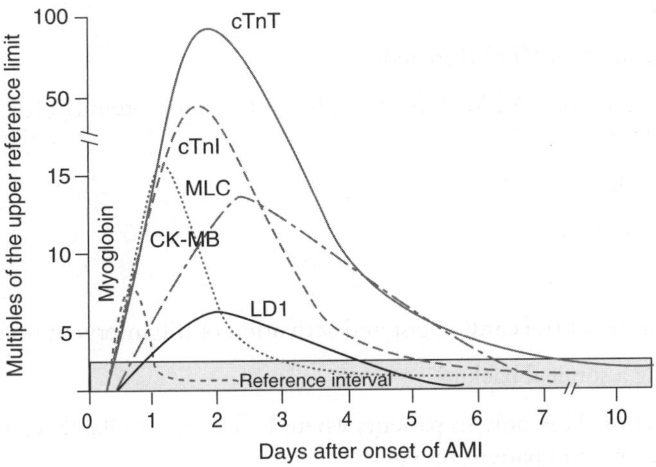

Figure 14–1. Serum markers after acute myocardial infarction. CK-MB, MB fraction of creatine kinase; cTnI, cardiac troponin I; cTnT, cardiac troponin T; LD1, lactate dehydrogenase isoenzyme 1; MLC, myosin light chain. (Reproduced, with permission, from Tintinalli JE, Stapczynski S, Cline DM, et al. *Tintinalli's Emergency Medicine*. 7th ed. New York, NY: McGraw-Hill Education; 2011. Figure 52-1.)

motion may be helpful, especially in cases of nondiagnostic electrocardiogram when non-STEMI or unstable angina is suspected. Echocardiography can show the progressive course from hypokinesis to akinesis during ischemia, and identify impaired myocardial relaxation during diastole.

An echocardiogram that demonstrates normal wall motion excludes the possibility of extensive myocardial damage but does not rule out non-STEMI. The differential diagnosis of acute chest pain is broad. Echocardiography can be used to identify nonischemic conditions that cause chest pain, such as myocarditis, aortic stenosis, aortic dissection, pulmonary embolism, and mechanical complications of acute infarction, such as papillary muscle dysfunction or rupture and ventricular septal defect. PCA provides detailed information about the coronary anatomy and facilitates invasive management of occluded coronary arteries. It is most often considered in the setting of ACS in patients with STEMI or new LBBB in whom immediate angioplasty is an option. Other such settings include, unstable angina, non-STEMI. and high-risk features as hypotension, CHF, mitral regurgitation, and repeated episodes of ACS despite optimal therapy.

Mechanical complications occur in 0.1% of post-MI patients between days 2 and 7. These complications include **ventricular septal defect, papillary muscle rupture leading to acute mitral valve regurgitation, and left ventricular free wall rupture**, which will lead to **cardiac tamponade.** Ventricular septal defect and rupture of papillary muscle usually lead to a new, loud systolic murmur and acute pulmonary edema or hypotension. Diagnosis is critical because the 24-hour survival rate is approximately 25% with medical therapy alone but increases to 50% with emergency surgical intervention. Pericardial tamponade from free wall rupture usually leads to sudden hypotension, pulse-less electrical activity on electrocardiography, and death.

THERAPY

The management for STEMI includes

1. Anticoagulation (ASA, clopidogrel, heparin, glycoprotein IIb/IIIGa inhibitor) and LMWH
2. β-Blockade
3. ACE inhibitors
4. Statins
5. Notification of the cardiologist and activation of the interventional lab
6. Enlisting a surgical backup
7. Considering TPA only in patients where PCI is not available, cannot be done on time, or upon patient refusal

Effective analgesia early in the course of ACS is an important therapeutic intervention. Morphine sulfate reduces sympathetic tone through a centrally mediated anxiolytic affect, and also reduces myocardial oxygen demand by reducing preload and by a reduction in vagally mediated heart rate. The **vasodilating action of nitroglycerin results in combined preload and afterload reduction, decreased cardiac work, and lowered myocardial oxygen requirements.** Nitrates may reduce infarct size, improve regional myocardial function, prevent left ventricular remodeling, and provide a small reduction in mortality rates. In the ICU nitrates are administered IV. Endpoints are the control of symptoms or a decrease in mean arterial blood pressure (MAP) by 10%, and an MAP goal of ≥60 mm Hg.

Mean arterial blood pressure (MAP) = [(2 × diastolic) + systolic]/3)

Antithrombotic Therapy

ASA should be given as soon as possible to any patient with ACS. Heparin therapy is indicated in patients with likely or definite ACS. The combination of heparin and ASA reduces the incidence of MI during the in-hospital period and reduces the need for CABG. Low-molecular-weight heparin (LMWH) is superior to unfractionated heparin (UFH) in this setting.

LMWH has greater bioavailability and a more predictable dose response as compared to UFH, but LMWH should be used carefully in the morbidly obese patients, and dosage adjustment is required in renal insufficiency. Clopidogrel should be considered in patients with ACS who are unable to take ASA and in high-risk patients in whom PCI is planned. Clopidogrel, a more potent antiplatelet agent than ASA, provides additional antiplatelet activity when added to ASA. It should be withheld if CABG is a possibility due to the increased risk of perioperative bleeding. Glycoprotein IIb/IIIa receptor antagonists (eg, abciximab, tirofiban) inhibit the cross-bridging of platelets secondary to fibrinogen binding to the activated glycoprotein IIb/IIIa receptor. Glycoprotein IIb/IIIa antagonists should be considered in addition to ASA and heparin in patients with non-STEMI and as adjunctive therapy in patients with STEMI undergoing angioplasty.

β-Blockers

Early intravenous β-blocker therapy (ie, atenolol, metoprolol, carvedilol) reduces infarct size, decreases the frequency of recurrent myocardial ischemia, and improves short-term and long-term survival. β-Blockers diminish myocardial oxygen demand by reducing the heart rate, lowering BP, and myocardial contractility. β-Blocker prolongs diastole, which augments perfusion to injured myocardium, and can be used in left ventricular dysfunction if CHF status is stable.

ACE Inhibitors

An angiotensin-converting enzyme (ACE) inhibitor should be administered early in the course of ACS in most patients. ACE inhibitor therapy can attenuate ventricular remodeling, resulting in a reduction in the development of heart failure and death. ACE inhibitor therapy reduces the risk of recurrent MI and other vascular events. In patients who cannot tolerate an ACE inhibitor due to coughing, an angiotensin-receptor blocker (ARB) is an alternative. Statin therapy improves endothelial function and reduces the risk of future coronary events. A single study showed a reduction in recurrent ischemia when a high-dose statin was administered within 24 to 96 hours of hospital admission. The concept of statin therapy suggests that there is an emerging benefit to statins in ACS beyond a reduction in LDL cholesterol.

Aldosterone Blockers

Eplerenone is a selective aldosterone blocker that limits collagen formation and ventricular remodeling after acute MI. It also has a favorable effect on the neurohormonal profile. Eplerenone reduces mortality when started 3 to 14 days after MI in patients with ejection fractions (EFs) ≤40% and clinical heart failure or diabetes. Aldosterone antagonists should be used with great caution or avoided in patients with renal insufficiency (creatinine >2.5 mg/dL) or preexisting hyperkalemia (>5.0 mEq/L).

Percutaneous Angioplasty and Stent Placement

Percutaneous angioplasty (PCA) and stent placement is the preferred therapy in specific subsets of ACS patients (STEMI, new LBBB, or true posterior MI). **PCI is associated with a lower 30-day mortality rate compared with TPA.** The incorporation of drug-eluting stents has further increased the clinical advantage of PCI over TPA. Angioplasty is indicated in patients with a contraindication to TPA or in patients with coronary spasm (CS). Angioplasty is most effective within 12 hours of the onset of chest pain; but the earlier the intervention, the better the outcome. Prompt transfer of the patient to angiography lab for primary PCI may be beneficial but is contingent upon the transfer occurring within 2 to 3 hours of initial hospital arrival. TPA is an alternative to PCI in suitable candidates with STEMI. By lysing the clot, TPA restores perfusion to the ischemic area, reduces infarct size, and improves survival.

Bypass Surgery

The role of CABG in the treatment of ACS is evolving. **Bypass surgery is preferred in patients who have a large amount of myocardium at ischemic risk due to**

proximal left main disease, or multi-vessel disease, especially with decreased left ventricular EF. CABG may be preferred in patients with diabetes mellitus because of better long-term vessel patency and improved clinical outcomes. There is increasing evidence that drug-eluting stents may produce outcomes comparable to CABG. An IABP is indicated for treatment of ACS with cardiogenic shock, unresponsive to medical therapy, for acute mitral regurgitation secondary to papillary muscle dysfunction, ventricular septal rupture, or refractory angina. The IABP reduces afterload during ventricular systole and increases coronary perfusion during diastole. Patients with refractory CS who are treated with an IABP have a lower in-hospital mortality rate than patients who are not treated with this device.

Follow-Up

Following an acute MI, early cardiac catheterization during hospitalization should be considered for patients with recurrent ischemic symptoms, serious complications, or other intermediate- to high-risk features (eg, CHF, left ventricular dysfunction, ventricular arrhythmias). These complications of ACS are associated with more severe CAD and subsequent cardiac events. **Exercise testing** in post-MI patients without high-risk features is performed as a prognostic assessment. Early stress testing following an MI allows the clinician to assess functional capacity, evaluate efficacy of the patient's current medical regimen, and risk-stratify the patient according to the likelihood of future cardiac events. **Patients with depressed left-ventricular systolic function are at increased risk for subsequent ventricular tachyarrhythmias.** The finding of unsustained ventricular tachycardia more than 48 hours after MI, particularly in patients with EF of <35%, usually prompts electrophysiological testing or implantation of a cardioverter-defibrillator. High-risk patients typically do better with an implantable cardioverter-defibrillator than with antiarrhythmic therapy.

Management of hypertension, diabetes, lipid levels, cessation of smoking, and inauguration of an exercise program are essential. Patients should continue therapy ASA, β-blockers, ACE-inhibitors, statins, and nitrates as prescribed. Approximately 20% of patients experience depression after acute infarction which is associated with an increased risk for recurrent hospitalization and death. Thus, post-infarction patients should be screened for depression. In patients with acute ischemia with hemodynamic instability, intra-aortic balloon pump (IABP) counterpulsation can be used for circulatory support during revascularization. The decision to proceed with invasive interventions aimed at revascularization in addition to medical management is best accomplished with the assistance of cardiology consultation. Patients with unstable angina and non-STEMI with refractory angina despite optimal medical therapy or hemodynamic instability benefit from early invasive strategies. Both survival and QOL improved with early invasive therapy. Invasive intervention should be avoided in patients with significant comorbidities in whom the risks outweigh the potential benefits. In the perioperative setting, the risk of bleeding often precludes the institution of aggressive anticoagulation needed for revascularization.

CLINICAL CASE CORRELATION

- **See also Case 4 (Hemodynamic Monitoring), Case 15 (Cardiac Arrhythmias), Case 16 (Acute Cardiac Failure).**

COMPREHENSION QUESTIONS

14.1 A 73-year-old woman is evaluated in the ED and transferred to the ICU because of chest pain of 4 hours' duration. Her medical history includes a 20-year history of hypertension and Type 2 diabetes mellitus. Her medications include metformin, atenolol, and ASA. On physical examination, her blood pressure is 130/84 mm Hg and her heart rate is 87 beats/minute and regular. Her jugular vein is distended to 5 cm while the patient is upright. She has a faint left carotid bruit, bibasilar crackles to one quarter up from the lung bases. A normal S_1 and S_2 is heard, with a grade 2/6 holosystolic murmur heard best at the apex to the axilla. An electrocardiogram from 6 months ago was normal. The ECG in Figure 14–2 was seen during the chest pain. The initial serum troponin measurement is elevated. She is now admitted to the ICU for an MI. She is free of chest pain while on IV nitroglycerin and her vital signs are stable. Which of the following is the most likely ECG diagnosis.

A. Left bundle branch block with normal sinus rhythm
B. Idioventricular tachycardia
C. Right bundle branch block
D. Third-degree atrioventricular block (complete heart block)
E. Mobitz type II second-degree atrioventricular block

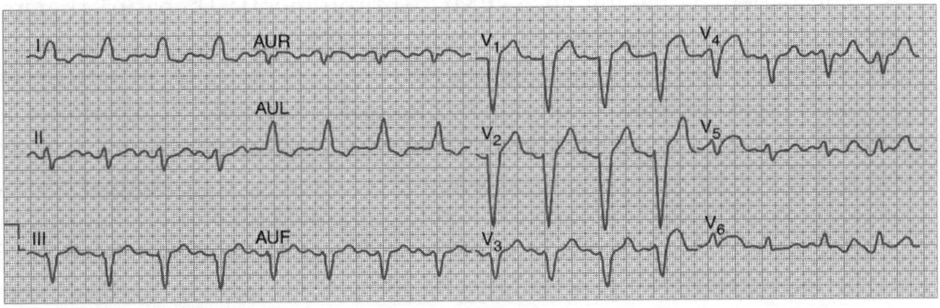

Figure 14–2. 12 lead ECG.

14.2 A 55-year-old man presents with ACS, with 2 mm of ST elevation on the leads II, III, and aVF to the ICU. The troponins are positive. The blood pressure is 130/70 mm Hg on a nitroglycerin drip at 5 μg/kg/min keeping the patient chest pain free, but ECG changes persist and only a 1 mm of ST elevation is seen. There is no lower extremity edema. The patient was given ASA upon entry into the ED. What is/are the best next steps in the management of this patient?

A. Anticoagulation, IV β-blocker, ACE inhibitor, nitroglycerin, and alert catheterization lab

B. Give tissue plasminogen activator (TPA)

C. Increase nitroglycerin to 10 μg/kg/min

D. Get β-natriuretic peptide (BNP) level

E. Call cardiac surgeon for stat CABG post-PCI

ANSWERS TO QUESTIONS

14.1 **A.** LBBB is associated with absent Q waves in leads I, aVL, and V_6; a large, wide, and positive R wave in leads I, aVL, and V_6 ("tombstone" R waves); and prolongation of the QRS complex to >0.12 seconds. The chest pain, elevated cardiac biomarkers, and new-onset left bundle branch block are considered equivalent to having an ST-elevation myocardial infarction (STEMI). Repolarization abnormalities are present consisting of ST segment and T wave vectors directed opposite to the QRS complex. The presentation of ACS with new left bundle branch block should be considered equivalent to an STEMI and true posterior wall MI, with management including early coronary intervention. The maximum benefit is provided by reperfusion within 12 hours of the onset of symptoms. The QRS complex is >0.12 seconds in BBB.

14.2 **A.** The patient is having an STEMI. Antithrombotic (heparin) therapy is indicated. The combination of heparin and ASA reduces the incidence of MI. When administered immediately, ASA reduces mortality in patients with unstable angina or acute infarction by diminishing platelet aggregation. Clopidogrel should be considered in patients with ACS who are unable to take ASA and in high-risk patients in whom Percutaneous transluminal coronary angioplasty (PTCA) is planned. Clopidogrel provides additional antiplatelet activity when added to ASA. It should be withheld if CABG is a possibility due to the increased risk of perioperative bleeding. Glycoprotein IIb/IIIa receptor antagonists inhibit the cross-bridging of platelets secondary to binding fibrinogen. Early intravenous β-blocker therapy reduces infarct size, decreases the frequency of recurrent myocardial ischemia, and improves survival. β-Blockers diminish myocardial oxygen demand by reducing heart rate, systemic arterial pressure, and myocardial contractility. An ACE inhibitor should be administered early in the course of ACS in most patients. ACE inhibitor therapy may also reduce the risk of recurrent infarction. In patients who cannot tolerate an ACE inhibitor, an ARB is an alternative. Statin therapy appears to improve endothelial function and reduce the risk of future ACS.

CLINICAL PEARLS

- ACS include STEMI, unstable angina, and non-ST elevation MI (non-STEMI).
- Atypical symptoms are found in 25% of ACS patients, especially women, diabetics, and the elderly.
- Non-STEMI is associated with elevated cardiac biomarkers while unstable angina is not.
- ICU patients, comorbidities, and instability usually preclude acute CABG or PCI.
- Therapy of MI includes β-blockade, statins, ASA, and ACE inhibitors.
- Troponin elevations are common in ICU patients. Although not always due to myocardial ischemia or infarction, such elevations are associated with poor outcomes.

REFERENCES

Grech ED, Ramsdale DR. Acute coronary syndrome: unstable angina and non-ST segment elevation myocardial infarction. *BMJ*. 2003;326:1259-1261.

Loscalzo J. *Harrison's Pulmonary and Critical Care Medicine*. 2nd ed. New York, NY: McGraw-Hill; 2010.

Panju AA, Hemmelgarn BR, Guyatt GH, Simel DL. Is this patient having a myocardial infarction? *JAMA*. 1998;280:1256-1263.

Toy EC, Simon B, Takenaka K, Liu T, Rosh A. *Case Files Emergency Medicine*. 2nd ed. New York: McGraw-Hill, Lange, 2009.

CASE 15

A 25-year-old man complains of palpitations and tachycardia with skipped heart beats. He is found to be diaphoretic following a brief episode of syncope accompanied by urinary incontinence after participating in a pick-up basketball game. He went to the emergency department (ED) because the palpitations would not subside. The patient's older male sibling also suffers from the same condition. The patient's neurological examination is unremarkable. A magnified snapshot of the ECG tracing is shown (Figure 15–1). These episodes have occurred twice before, after similar physical stimuli. At the last occasion, the tachycardia terminated after a bout of hiccups. His vital signs are: respiratory rate (RR) 22 breaths/minute, blood pressure (BP) 100/50 mm Hg, and heart rate (HR) of 150 beats/minute and regular. His oxygen saturation (O_2sat) is 94% on ambient air (RA). Other values include temperature of 98°F, weight 70 kg, height 72 in. His electrolyte levels were: sodium (Na^+) 140 mEq/L, potassium (K^+) 4 mEq/L, chloride (Cl^-) 105 mEq/L, bicarbonate (HCO_3^-) 23 mEq/L.

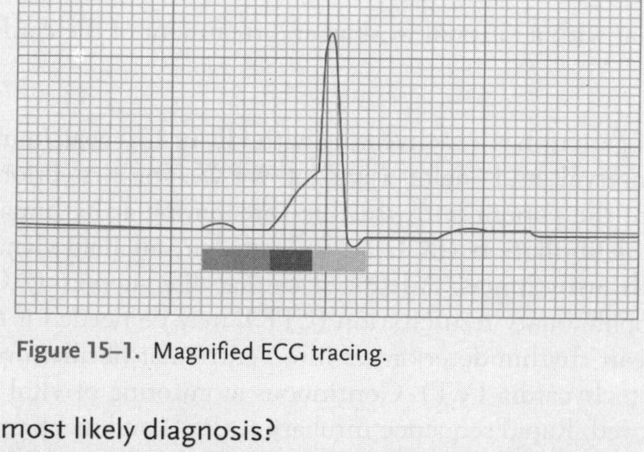

Figure 15–1. Magnified ECG tracing.

- ► What is the most likely diagnosis?
- ► Why is the diagnosis so important for correct treatment?
- ► What is the next step in therapy?

ANSWERS TO CASE 15:
Cardiac Arrhythmias

Summary: A 25-year-old man has palpitations, tachycardia with HR of 150 beats/minute, and a QRS complex with a slurred upstroke of the R wave representing Wolff-Parkinson-White syndrome (WPW), a life-threatening supraventricular arrhythmia. He has a normal blood pressure.

- **Most likely diagnosis:** WPW. The classical findings of short PR interval (rapid AV conduction via accessory pathway) and a "delta wave" (representing pre-excitation of the portion of the ventricle that begins to depolorize by the bypass tract).
- **Importance of diagnosis:** This is an important diagnosis since the usual treatments for supraventricular tachycardias such as blocking the AV node will make the WPW arrhythmia worse, which can lead to the patient's death.
- **Treatment**: The drugs of choice are adenosine, procainamide, or amiodarone, which prolong conduction in the aberrant track and slow repolarization; adenosine may also be used with pure WFW but is contraindicated with concomitant **atrial fibrillation**.

ANALYSIS

Objectives

1. To develop an approach to diagnosing the different types of cardiac arrhythmias.
2. To recognize the most common types of supraventricular and ventricular arrhythmias.
3. To be familiar with a rational workup and treatment of the cardiac arrhythmia.

Considerations

This 25-year-old patient has a tachycardia with HR of 150 beats/minute, the classic shortened PR interval, and "delta wave" of WPW. The first priority is to recognize and stabilize the patient with this life-threatening arrhythmia. Synchronized electric cardiac defibrillation (ECD) is indicated in all hemodynamically unstable patients with arrhythmias. Advanced cardiac life support (ACLS) measures, including cardiopulmonary resuscitation (CPR), may be needed if the patient fails ECD and the heart rhythm deteriorates into ventricular fibrillation (VF) or pulseless ventricular tachycardia (VT). Continuous monitoring of vital signs and ECG should be employed. Rapid sequence intubation (RSI) and mechanical ventilation (MV) and pacing with an external on IV pacemaker may be required. Replacement of intravascular volume, usually with intravenous (IV) normal saline (NS), will increase preload and ventricular volume, BP, and CO. The electrolyte levels should be assessed and corrected if abnormal. Continuous infusion of antiarrhythmic drugs may be employed in order to maintain normal sinus rhythm (NSR). The next priority is to determine the etiology of the cardiac arrhythmia. Electrical activity occurs

Table 15–1 • NORMAL ECG INTERVALS AND DURATIONS

Interval	Time in Seconds	1 Small ECG Box = 0.04 seconds (s)
PR interval	0.12-0.20 s	3-5 small ECG boxes or 1 large box on ECG
QRS	<0.12 s	3 small ECG boxes
QTc	<0.44 s	Variable length, depending on HR

before mechanical activity in the heart; P waves occur before atrial contraction; QRS complex occurs prior to each ventricular contraction, and T waves occur prior to each ventricular repolarization. The accepted duration or interval time of these waves is seen in Table 15–1.

The morphology of P waves can also suggest certain atrial diseases such as the P mitrale. Abnormal P-wave morphology may be seen in mitral valve regurgitation, or the peak in the second half of the P wave seen in left atrial enlargement. The early, tall notch in first half of P wave is seen in right atrial enlargement or P pulmonale. The morphology of the P wave can be upright, biphasic, or inverted in the inferior leads (II, III, aVF) and is best seen in those leads. The inferior leads are looking directly at the atria. A large negative P wave seen in lead V_1 is also indicative of left atrial enlargement.

Drugs such as digoxin, β-blockers (BBs), and calcium channel blockers (CCBs) are used to treat the more common supraventricular arrhythmias (SVTs). These agents block the AV node and are contraindicated in WPW. **The drugs of choice for treating WPW are adenosine, procainamide, or amiodarone** which prolong conduction in the aberrant track and slow repolarization; adenosine is contraindicated with atrial fibrillation. In unstable patients, immediate ECD should be used. Hypoxemia and any electrolyte imbalances, especially of K^+ and Mg^+ should be corrected. Atrial tachycardia may arise from any area of the right or left atrium and the most common arrhythmic pathway is reentry. Reentrant tachycardia is associated with structural heart disease such as Ebstein anomaly but also seen with digitalis toxicity. Atrial fibrillation (AF) in WPW can lead to a rapid rhythm, which may degenerate into ventricular fibrillation (VF). Sudden death may occur in 0.2% of affected individuals over 3 to 10 years.

APPROACH TO: Cardiac Arrhythmias

Arrhythmias can be classified according to their origin. Supraventricular arrhythmias (SVTs) usually have a narrow QRS with visible retrograde P waves (P waves seen after the QRS complex) and originate above the AV node. P waves may also appear to be absent because they become buried in the QRS complex. Ventricular arrhythmias generally have a wide QRS complex (>0.12 ms) similar to a bundle branch block pattern with AV disassociation and can be monomorphic or polymorphic. Arrhythmias are also classified according to rate. Tachycardia is defined as a rate >100 beats/minute. Bradycardia is classified as a rate <60 beats/minute. Common signs and symptoms of these arrhythmias are palpitations, lightheadedness, dyspnea, chest pain, syncope or presyncope, and fatigue. Syncope requires a loss of blood flow to both cerebral hemispheres at the same time. Evaluation of an arrhythmia is based on a recent ECG, an old ECG if available for comparison, a CBC, electrolyte determinations, TSH, ABG or O_2sat, glucose, BUN, and creatinine levels. ECD is indicated for hemodynamically unstable patients regardless of the rhythm.

SUPRAVENTRICULAR ARRHYTHMIAS

Tachyarrhythmias (>100 beats/minute)

- **Sinus tachycardia:** Normal sinus rhythm (NSR) is defined as an SA nodal rhythm with a frequency of 60 to 100 beats/minute. Heart rates >100 beats/minute originating in the SA node are defined as a sinus tachycardia (ST). ST is associated with anxiety, pain, fever, dehydration, stress, and drugs both therapeutic and recreational. Atrial tachycardias arise from ectopic atrial foci and/or the pulmonary veins. Valsalva maneuvers and/or carotid massage can terminate the SVTs. ST, as in multifocal atrial tachycardia (MAT), is defined as an ectopic atrial rhythm with >2 different P-wave morphologies at a rate >100 beats/minute. MAT is typically seen in patients with COPD or other pulmonary disease processes. MAT responds to treatment of the underlying COPD, especially hypoxia with hypercapnia. Antiarrhythmic therapy area is usually unnecessary since MAT is self-limiting and responds to treatment of the underlying cause.

  Supraventricular tachycardia (SVT): SVT is a regular and rapid rhythm with a narrow QRS, with rates between 160 and 180 beats/minute. The most common type, atrioventricular nodal reentry tachycardia (AVNRT), involves reentry electrical activity within the atrioventricular node (AVN). A late P wave can be seen in the final portion of the QRS complex, which is consistent with retrograde P-wave conduction via the AVN. SVT is a benign rhythm in the absence of structural disease. A true SVT should respond to treatment with IV adenosine if it is unresponsive to vagal maneuvers. Adenosine breaks the arrhythmia and causes a long pause in the electrical activity, which resets the AV node for normal AVN conduction (see Figure 15–2).

- **Atrial flutter:** Atrial flutter is recognized by sawtooth P waves with a regular pattern. All P waves have the same morphology and are conducted at regular rates. The P-wave rate and pulse rate varies from 240 to 350 beats/minute. Conduction of P waves to QRS varies from 2 to 1 or 3 to 1 P waves for every QRS complex conduction leading to a heart rate of 100 to 150 beats/minute. Flutter may turn into AF over time. One must rule out secondary noncardiac causes of atrial flutter such as hyperthyroidism, high caffeine intake, overuse of vasoconstricting nasal sprays, β_2 agonists, theophylline, and substance abuse with alcohol, cocaine, or amphetamines.

- **Atrial fibrillation:** AF is the **most common sustained ectopic atrial tachyarrhythmia.** AF is an **irregularly irregular rhythm** on ECG without any discernible P waves being recognized (chaotic pattern as atria fibrillate).

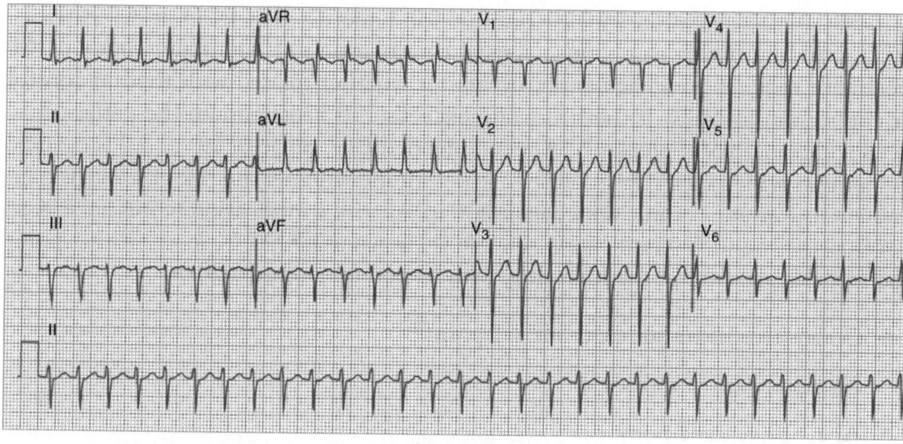

Figure 15–2. AV nodal reentrant tachycardia. HR of 150 beats/minute with narrow complex tachycardia. (Reproduced, with permission, from Longo DL, Fauci AS, Kasper DL, et al. *Harrison's Principles of Internal Medicine*. 18th ed. New York, NY: McGraw-Hill Education; 2012. Figure e30–13.)

Regularization of the R-R interval (becomes less irregular) in AF at heart rates of <60 can be a sign of digoxin toxicity. AF can be classified as:

1. Acute <48 hours
2. Chronic AF persisting for >48 hours
3. Paroxysmal AF
4. Indeterminate AF

This classification helps choose treatment options. Treatment of AF requires anticoagulation with warfarin (Coumadin) to reduce stroke rates in patients who have a $CHADS_2$ score >2. In patients whose $CHADS_2$ score is <2, treatment with ASA is recommended. Stools should be checked for occult blood or any signs of active bleeding before starting heparin or warfarin (Coumadin). **Dabigatran**, a new oral direct thrombin inhibitor, can be used as an alternative to warfarin in nonvalvular AF. Dabigatran does not require frequent blood tests for international normalized ratio (INR) or prothrombin time (PT) monitoring.

An **echocardiogram or a transesophageal echo study is excellent for the evaluation of valvular disease causing AF.** The identification of **intracardiac thrombi** must be excluded prior to cardioversion. Clots in the left atrial appendage are commonly found. When clots are present, anticoagulation is needed for a period of 4 weeks prior to performing elective ECD. Over 80% of patients with AF have some form of underlying heart disease, frequently atrial septal defects are found. In the elderly the primary underlying cause is hypertension. To treat AF or any SVT, Valsalva maneuvers or carotid massage should be attempted to increase vagal tone, to slow AVN conduction, and to cause increased refractoriness. ECD is used in all unstable patients regardless of tachyarrhythmia. IV heparin should be given for any AF of unknown duration, and an evaluation for intracardiac thrombi should be done before attempting ECD to NSR. Anticoagulation should continue for 1 month post ECD in AF patients. ECD is an alternative to pharmacological cardioversion of AF of any duration. AF treatment requires anticoagulation, no matter whether treated with rhythm control or conversion to NSR. If the heart rate exceeds 110 beats/minute the patient may need additional AVN blockade. A recommended INR range of 2.0 to 3.0 is optimal for patients with a $CHADS_2$ score >2. To determine whether the risk of stroke is high enough to warrant chronic anticoagulation in AF, risk stratification scores have been developed. One such stratification scheme is known as $CHADS_2$ score (with 1 point each for the presence of the following, with a maximum score of 6):

- **C**ongestive heart failure (CHF)–1 point
- **H**ypertension–1 point
- **A**ge >75 years–1 point
- **D**iabetes–1 point
- **S**troke or transient ischemic attack (TIA)–2 point

Patients are given 2 points for a history of stroke or TIA (the strongest risk factors) and 1 point for all other risk factors. The risk of stroke is the lowest in patients with a $CHADS_2$ score of 0 (1.2%). The risk is 18% per year for a $CHADS_2$ score of 6 (maximum score). Patients with a $CHADS_2$ score of ≥3 and patients with a history of stroke are at high risk and should be considered for chronic anticoagulation dosing with warfarin. Patients with a $CHADS_2$ score of 1 or 2 should be assessed on an individual basis for ASA versus warfarin therapy. Cerebrovascular accident (CVA) rate in nonrheumatic AF is 5%. Risk factors for stroke are a history of previous TIA or CVA, an MI, hypertension, age >65 years, diabetes, left atrial enlargement, and left ventricular dysfunction.

In nonvalvular AF, the use of warfarin with a target INR of 2 to 3 reduces the stroke risk by 68%, which usually outweighs the bleeding risk. In patients without risk factors, ASA may be sufficient and will decrease the stroke rate by 42%. In patients older than 65, heart rate control may be the best, especially when compared to the expected side effects of antiarrhythmic drugs used to maintain rhythm control. The goal is to maintain a heart rate <100 beats/minute. BBs and CCBs are the drugs of choice for this purpose. Digoxin is not recommended as a single agent especially when the heart rate activity becomes uncontrolled during exercise. Oral or IV agents can lead to cardioversion in 70% to 90% of those cases with the onset of AF within the past 48 hours, but are less effective in treating chronic AF cases appearing after 48 hours. Amiodarone and dronedarone are useful medications when any structural heart disease is present, otherwise propafenone or flecainide is used. Most antiarrhythmic drugs are also proarrhythmic on their own. IV heparin should be started immediately in patients with newly diagnosed AF. Risks of ECD in AF include thromboembolism, tachyarrhythmias, and bradyarrhythmias.

Surgical procedures. Catheter ablation is now frequently done to eliminate the aberrant conducting pathway. This is 99% effective with a mortality of only 1% to 3%. The Maze surgical procedure, in which a series of incisions are made in a maze-like pattern to reduce effective atrial size and prevent reformation of AF waves.

BRADYARRYHTHMIAS (<70 BEATS/MINUTE)

Atrioventricular Nodal Block (AVNB)

- **First-degree heart block:** The PR interval is >0.20 seconds on the ECG. All P waves are conducted and this condition requires no specific treatment. It is benign in most patients.
- **Second-degree heart block:** This heart block is characterized by intermittent nonconduction of P waves and "dropped" ventricular beats. Second-degree heart block is of 2 types, Mobitz I and Mobitz II.
- **Mobitz type I second-degree heart block:** Mobitz type I second-degree heart block is characterized by a progressive prolongation of the PR interval until a dropped beat occurs (also called Wenckebach block) and does not progress to complete heart block. It is transient and usually requires no treatment. Type I may be associated with a bradycardia.
- **Mobitz type II:** Mobitz II second-degree heart block is characterized by nonconduction of P waves and subsequent "dropped" ventricular beats without the progressive prolongation of the PR interval (see Figure 15–3). This is considered **malignant** since it tends to proceed to complete heart block or third-degree heart block. Mobitz II heart block is associated with evidence of additional disease in the conduction system, such as bundle branch block (BBB) or bifascicular or trifascicular block. Mobitz type II heart block suddenly and unpredictably progresses to complete heart block and is usually treated with a pacemaker.
- **Third-degree heart block:** Third-degree heart block is also referred to as complete heart block or atrioventricular disassociation (AVD). In third-degree

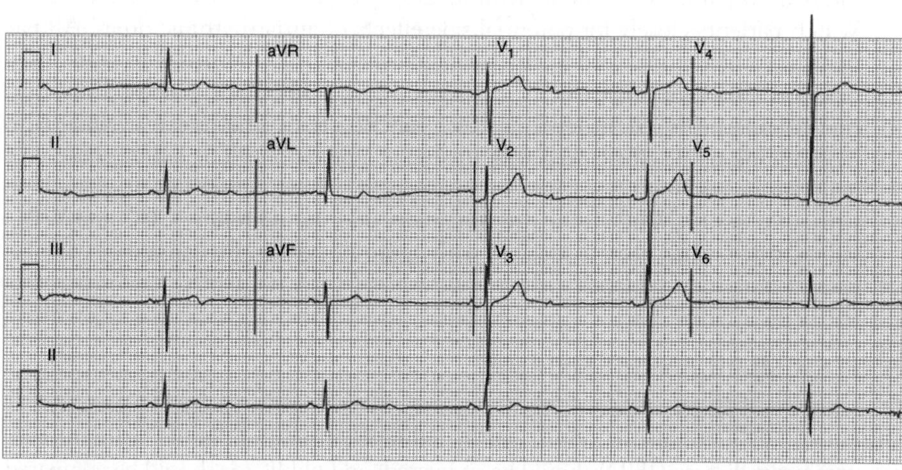

Figure 15–3. Second-degree heart block with bradycardia with ventricular HR of 30 beats/minute. This is Mobitz II heart block with P waves of 60 beats/minute. (Reproduced, with permission, from Longo DL, Fauci AS, Kasper DL, et al. *Harrison's Principles of Internal Medicine.* 18th ed. New York, NY: McGraw-Hill Education; 2012. Figure e30–3.)

heart block, the P rate is higher than the QRS rate and marches at the same interval through the rhythm. Insertion of a pacemaker is usually required for relief of third-degree heart block.

Sinus node dysfunction

Sinus node dysfunction (SND) has also been called sick sinus syndrome (SSS), and refers to abnormalities in the formation of sinus node impulses. These conditions include sinus bradycardia, sinus pause/arrest, chronotropic incompetence, and sinoatrial exit block. SND is frequently associated with various SVTs, such as AF and atrial flutter. When associated with SVTs, SND is often termed tachy-brady syndrome or SSS, is seen frequently in the elderly, and is a common cause for the insertion of a pacemaker.

Treatment: The treatment of bradycardia begins with removing all drugs that are capable of causing a bradycardia. **Atropine** is used in an emergency or cases of symptomatic bradycardia. Atropine IV therapy and external or internal pacing are the main treatment options. Vagal maneuvers and constipation (straining) should be avoided since they can worsen bradycardia. Pacing is indicated for the treatment of symptomatic bradycardia, tachy-brady syndrome, complete heart block, and asymptomatic patients with asystolic pauses >3 seconds or ventricular escape rhythms of <40 beats/minute. Permanent pacing improves survival in complete heart block especially if syncope has occurred previously.

Drug therapy: One should consider a BB or CCB such as verapamil to treat AVN reentrant tachycardia. CCBs slow calcium channel influx and decrease AVN conduction and increase AVN refractoriness. **Amiodarone has the least proarrhythmic effect and is the drug of choice for any patient with LV dysfunction or structural heart disease.** Dronedarone has a similar therapeutic effect as amiodarone without the iodine load of amiodarone. One should monitor the QT interval on patients on antiarrhythmic drugs and compare it to baseline ECGs. Watch patients closely for potential side effects of antiarrhythmic drugs. All patients on amiodarone need to be evaluated every 6 to 12 months with pulmonary function tests, diffusing capacity for carbon monoxide (DLCO), chest x-ray, thyroid-stimulating hormone level, and liver function tests. This testing evaluates the most common side effects seen with the use of amiodarone. The iodine content of amiodarone is so high that CT scans may appear to have contrast even when done without contrast. When using **procainamide, one should follow CBC and WBC values since it has been associated with agranulocytosis.** Procainamide can also cause a drug-induced lupus with positive ANA (RNA not DNA) values.

VENTRICULAR ARRHYTHMIAS

To evaluate and diagnose an arrhythmia, one needs to obtain a 12-lead ECG as well as continuous ECG monitoring. Vital signs including O_2 saturation should be monitored. Ischemic heart disease (IHD) should be suspected, and old ECGs should be compared with the current ones. Reversible causes of ventricular arrhythmias such as drugs, electrolyte abnormalities, CAD, ischemia, IHD, hypoxia, or drug toxicity should be sought.

Ventricular Tachycardia

Ventricular tachycardia (VT) is defined both as a wide- or narrow-complex tachycardia with continuous rapid depolarizing bursts in the ventricular His-Purkinje system. VT needs rapid attention and reversal with ECD as **it is the main cause of sudden death.** VT is a reentrant pathway arrhythmia with abnormal impulse conduction. It is often comorbid with underlying structural heart disease, most commonly ischemic heart disease (IHD), electrolyte imbalances such as ↓ K^+ and ↓ Mg^+, drug toxicity with QT-prolonging drugs (psychiatric medications), prolonged QT syndrome, valvular heart disease, nonischemic cardiomyopathy (viral, alcohol, etc). VT is subdivided into sustained VT lasting >30 seconds or requiring termination with ECD and nonsustained VT consisting of 3 straight PVCs with PVCs being <30 seconds. The morphology of the QRS can also be used to evaluate the origin and cause of VT. Concurrent treatment for IHD and CAD is begun because of their high correlation as underlying disorders in VT.

In families with a history of VT and death, one must consider a history of long QT syndrome. VT is also seen in arrhythmogenic right ventricular dysplasia and Brugada syndrome with RBBB. The symptoms and presentation that patients display depend upon the ventricular rate, duration of the arrhythmia, and presence of underlying heart disease.

Patients with nonsustained VT are usually asymptomatic but may complain of palpitations. Patients with sustained VT may present with syncope or near-syncope or sudden death. VT includes as a group VT, VF, and TdP or long QT syndrome arrhythmias. It is characterized by wide-complex QRS >0.12 seconds and ventricular rate >100 beats/minute (see Figure 15–4). In VT, these rates are typically from 140 to 250 beats/minute, in VF rates are >300 beats/minute, and in TdP rates are 200 to 300 beats/minute. When comparing SVT with aberrancy versus VT, **a history of structural or ischemic heart disease suggests that**

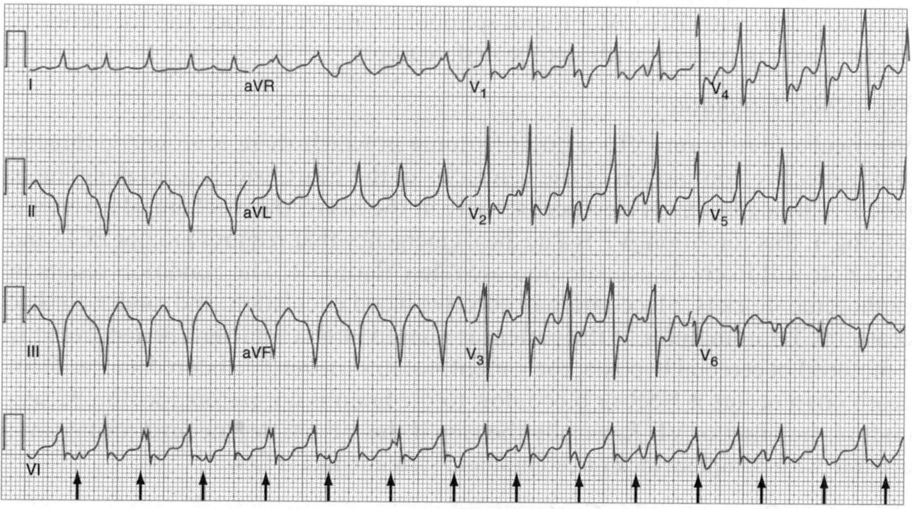

Figure 15–4. Ventricular tachycardia. ECG showing AV dissociation (arrows mark P waves), wide-complex QRS. (Reproduced, with permission, from Longo DL, Fauci AS, Kasper DL, et al. *Harrison's Principles of Internal Medicine.* 18th ed. New York, NY: McGraw-Hill Education; 2012. Figure 233–10.)

the arrhythmia is most likely VT. The presence of AV disassociation or third-degree block also suggests VT. An RBBB morphology QRS >0.14 seconds or an LBBB morphology QRS >0.16 seconds are also more likely to be VT than SVT with aberrancy. A regular R-R interval in VT is more common than SVT with aberrancy. The presence of MI or CAD is almost diagnostic of VT. Profound depression in hemodynamics also point to a VT, but a BP near 100 mm Hg does not exclude it. Large "cannon" a waves of atrial contraction against a closed tricuspid valve caused by the disassociation effect of the third-degree heart block are seen on physical examination.

In unstable patients, VT should be assumed and treated with ECD, delivered in synchronized mode if a pulse is present and in a nonsynchronized mode if a pulse is not present. Definitive treatment of arrhythmias due to reentrant pathways is ablation of those pathways. In the absence of structural heart disease, ablation is the treatment of choice. If structural heart disease is present with an EF <35%, an implanted cardiac defibrillator (ICD) is recommended. ICD use decreased mortality regardless of the etiology in all VT patients with EF <35%.

Drug Therapy

Antiarrhythmic IV drug therapy for VT/VF serves to terminate arrhythmias, to prevent recurrence of arrhythmia, and to prevent life-threatening arrhythmia such as VF (with insertion of an ICD). **For acute treatment of sustained monomorphic VT, IV lidocaine, procainamide, or amiodarone may be used.** Patients with recurrent VT need chronic therapy. Drug treatment of patients with VT and structural heart disease is inferior to implantation of an ICD. Drugs are used as adjuncts when ICD implantation is contraindicated. Pharmacological treatment for nonsustained VT can be avoided unless there is a history of structural heart disease or long QT syndrome. Here procainamide is the drug of choice. IV magnesium sulfate can be used to suppress polymorphic VT in patients with prolonged QT intervals. Treatment for CHF with BBs, ACEI, and spironolactone will reduce the incidence of sudden death in patients with systolic dysfunction.

Ventricular Fibrillation

Ventricular fibrillation (VF) is an arrhythmia in which there is an uncoordinated and ineffective contraction of the ventricles in the heart, which stops pumping of blood. Although there is electrical activity in the heart, the mechanical activity is missing in this condition. VF is a medical emergency that requires prompt ECD and ACLS. It will likely degenerate into asystole ("flatline"). The condition results in cardiogenic shock (CS), cessation of effective blood circulation, and sudden cardiac death (SCD) in minutes. If the patient is revived after a sufficient period (roughly 5 minutes) of cerebral hypoxia, the patient sustains irreversible brain damage. Brain death often occurs if NSR or blood flow to the brain is not restored within 90 seconds of the onset of VF. Especially the case if the VF has degenerated further into asystole with complete lack of cerebral and systemic blood flow.

Premature Pre-ventricular Contractions

Premature pre-ventricular contractions (PVCs) originate from the ventricle (wide QRS) and are always followed by a compensatory pause as the electrical system resets.

A premature atrial contraction (PAC) with aberrancy can mimic a PVC but there is no compensatory pause. PVCs and arrhythmia rates increase as we age. PVCs appear to be benign unless an underlying left ventricular dysfunction is present. In patients with increased left ventricular dysfunction, PVCs are associated with an increased mortality, while reducing PVC frequency does not reduce mortality. SVT with wide QRS due to a BBB or preexcitation syndrome such as WPW can mimic VT.

Arrhythmias Associated with Long QT

Many common drugs cause TdP. The QT period is rate-dependent. Risk factors for TdP are female sex, hypokalemia, hypomagnesemia, structural heart disease, and a history of long QT or drug-induced arrhythmias.

Torsade de pointes (TdP)

Torsade de pointes (TdP) is a form of polymorphic VT associated with a prolonged QT syndrome. For those patients who receive QT-prolonging drugs in the hospital, ECG monitoring of prolonged QT intervals is indicated. TdP should be avoidable if there is an awareness of individual risk factors and ECG signs of drug-induced long QT syndrome (LQTS) are seen. ECG risk factors for TdP include marked QT prolongation to >500 ms (with the exception of amiodarone- or verapamil-induced QT prolongation). Recognition of these ECG harbingers of TdP allows for treatment with IV magnesium, removal of the offending agent, and correction of electrolyte abnormalities. Other exacerbating factors include the prevention of bradycardia and long pauses where temporary pacing will be necessary.

CLINICAL CASE CORRELATION

- **See also Case 4 (Hemodynamic Monitoring), Case 5 (Vasoactive Drugs and Pharmacology), and Case 16 (Acute Cardiac Failure).**

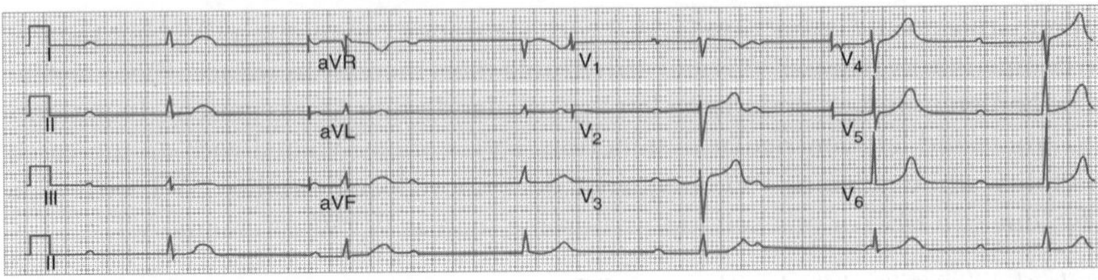

Figure 15–5. EKG.

COMPREHENSION QUESTIONS

15.1 A 73-year-old woman is evaluated in the ICU. She has a history of CAD, and has a near-syncopal episode. Her medications include levothyroxine and hydrochlorothiazide. An ECG 2 years ago was normal. On physical examination, her heart rate is 42 beats/minute and regular. The remainder of the examination is normal. Her TSH level is normal. An ECG obtained as part of the current evaluation is shown (Figure 15–5). Of the following diagnoses, which does the ECG in this case confirm?

A. First-degree atrioventricular heart block

B. Mobitz type I second-degree atrioventricular block

C. Mobitz type II second-degree atrioventricular block

D. Third-degree atrioventricular block (complete heart block)

E. AV nodal atrioventricular heart block

15.2 Which of the following is the best treatment for the patient in Question 15.1?

A. Amiodarone

B. β-Blocker therapy

C. Implantable pacemaker

D. Procainamide

E. Lidocaine

ANSWERS TO QUESTIONS

15.1 **D.** The third-degree AV block, or complete heart block, refers to a lack of AV conduction, and lack of conduction of all atrial impulses (P waves) to the ventricles, as seen in this patient's ECG. Mobitz type II second-degree heart block is characterized by a regularly dropped beat without progressive prolongation of the PR interval and is associated with evidence of additional disease in the conduction system, such as BBB or bifascicular or trifascicular block. Mobitz type II heart block suddenly progresses to complete heart block and is usually treated with a pacemaker.

15.2 **C.** A pacemaker is indicated in patients who have acquired third-degree AV block. Many patients with complete heart block are symptomatic and are treated with a pacemaker. Pacemaker implantation may improve survival for patients with asymptomatic complete heart block; therefore, all patients with complete heart block should be treated with pacemaker implantation.

CLINICAL PEARLS

- The younger the patient with an arrhythmia, the more likely a congenital accessory pathway is present.
- In WPW, the treatment of choice is ablation of the accessory pathway.
- Regularization of AF (at heart rates of 60 beats/minute) can be a sign of digoxin toxicity.
- In nonvalvular AF, warfarin with a target INR of 2.0 to 3.0 decreases stroke risk by 62%.
- Pacemaker insertion improves survival for patients with asymptomatic complete heart block.
- Patients with VT and structural heart disease is ideally treated with an ICD.
- Mobitz type II heart block progresses to complete heart block and is treated by a pacemaker.
- The longer the QT interval, the more the likelihood of an arrhythmia.
- Antiarrhythmic medications are proarrhythmic themselves.
- Where the pulmonary veins enter the left atrium, it appears to be a major site for origin of AF.
- Procainamide is a classic medication causing drug-induced lupus and a positive ANA.

REFERENCES

Dubin D. *Rapid Interpretation of EKGs*. 6th ed. Tampa, FL: Cover Publication Company; October 15, 2000.

Loscalzo J. *Harrison's Pulmonary and Critical Care Medicine*. McGraw-Hill; 2010.

Toy E, Simon B, Takenaka K, Liu T, Rosh A. *Case Files Emergency Medicine*. 2nd ed. New York, NY: McGraw-Hill, Lange.

CASE 16

A 56-year-old man with long-standing ischemic cardiomyopathy (ischemic heart disease [IHD]) was admitted to the intensive care unit (ICU) 24 hours previously. He had hypotension, dyspnea, and respiratory distress. His condition deteriorated following 48 hours of overeating and drinking beer during the Super Bowl Sunday weekend. He has been given intravenous (IV) furosemide without improvement. IV angiotensin-converting enzyme (ACE) inhibitor and IV β-blocker (BB) have also been administered. To improve his respiratory distress, noninvasive ventilation (NIV) has been initiated. Early today, he developed worsening chest pain, shortness of breath, and has become acutely lethargic. On physical examination, his temperature is 99°F, heart rate is 130 beats/minute, blood pressure is 90/50 mm Hg, and respiratory rate is 25 breaths/minute. His jugular venous pressure is elevated while sitting at 45 degrees upright. Lung rales are noted two-thirds up from the bases. The heart rhythm is regular with normal S_1 and S_2 heart sounds; the presence of a new S_3 heart sound is noted. A new 4/6 holosystolic murmur is now heard best at the apex of the point of maximum impulse (PMI) and radiates to the axilla. There is bilateral peripheral edema to the thighs, and his extremities are cool. His central venous pressure (CVP) is 22 mm Hg (normal, 0-5 mm Hg) with a venous O_2 saturation (O_2sat) of 60% versus 98% on arterial O_2 saturation. The laboratory reported his hemoglobin as 13 g/dL.

- What is the most likely diagnosis?
- What complications should be anticipated in this patient?
- What treatment modalities should be initiated?

ANSWER TO CASE 16:

Acute Cardiac Failure

Summary: This is a 56-year-old man with acute decompensating heart failure (ADHF) with cardiogenic shock (CS). The central venous line (CVP) pressure is markedly increased and the cardiac output (CO) is decreased as evidenced by the cool extremities and low SVO_2 saturation. Distention of the jugular vein is the most sensitive clinical sign for ADHF. This patient has a history of CHF aggravated initially by fluid and sodium overload. He deteriorated when he suffered a myocardial infarction (MI), complicated by papillary muscle dysfunction, and acute mitral insufficiency. There is a decreased CO with hypotension and evidence of organ hypoperfusion based on his mental status change and cool extremities, all are compatible with shock.

- **Most likely diagnosis:** Severe CHF with acute decompensated heart failure and cardiogenic shock.
- **Likely complications:** Fluid and sodium overload, MI, papillary muscle dysfunction or rupture, cardiac arrhythmias, pulmonary embolism.
- **Treatment modalities to initiate:** Noninvasive ventilation (NIV) or endotracheal intubation (ETI) and mechanical ventilation (MV), IV ACE inhibitors, IV nitroglycerin, β-blockers, furosemide, and anticoagulation are all indicated. An aortic balloon pump (IABP) should be considered to bridge the patient to a PCI or CABG to reverse the papillary muscle dysfunction. IV nitroprusside and dobutamine are added for improvement of CO by afterload reduction and positive inotropic effect.

ANALYSIS

Objectives

1. To understand how to diagnose acute cardiac failure.
2. To understand which drugs are effective in treating cardiac failure.
3. To understand the underlying causes for acute and chronic cardiac failure.

Considerations

This 56-year-old man with a long-standing IHD was admitted to the ICU 24 hours previously with cardiogenic shock, now has an acute change in mental status and new-onset chest pain. This is indicative of worsening cardiogenic shock. He requires an intra-aortic balloon pump (IABP) to improve CO, BP, and flow to the coronary arteries. Vasopressors are also needed to improve the hemodynamic status. The new holosystolic murmur indicates mitral valve papillary muscle rupture or dysfunction leading to mitral regurgitation. Mechanical ventilation may be required to decrease the work of breathing and respiratory failure. A definitive procedure such as CABG or PTCA will be required since all other measures are simply temporary. This patient's condition is an emergency, and requires urgent intervention.

APPROACH TO: Acute Heart Failure

DEFINITIONS

CONGESTIVE HEART FAILURE (CHF): It is defined as the inability of the heart to supply sufficient substrate to meet the needs of the body.

CARDIOGENIC SHOCK (CS): It is end-stage CHF and is a largely irreversible condition and as such is more often fatal than not.

PULMONARY EDEMA: Accumulation of fluid in the pulmonary air spaces and the interstitial spaces of the lungs, which inhibits oxygen and carbon dioxide diffusion, leading to impaired gas exchange and respiratory failure.

CLINICAL APPROACH

The main cause of CHF is an ischemic cardiac event. Acute MI is the most common cause of CHF and may necessitate emergent revascularization with thrombolytic therapy (rTpa), percutaneous coronary intervention (PCI), or coronary artery bypass graft surgery (CABG). Other causes of CHF include anemia, hyperthyroidism, arrhythmia, and NSAIDs. **Worsening CHF is a side effect of oral hypoglycemic drugs in the thiazolidinedione class (also known as glitazones), making these drugs contraindicated in patients with CHF** (see Table 16–1). ADHD, pulmonary edema, and CHF are all multifactorial syndromes that result from CO impairment. In systolic heart failure, the heart cannot contract adequately, leading to fluid retention. Both the kidneys and vascular baroreceptors sense the decrease in CO inducing an increase in the renin-angiotensin-aldosterone system and the sympathetic system. This increase ultimately leads to **irreversible cardiac dilatation (remodeling)** and further fluid overload by a decreasing CO.

DIAGNOSIS

Symptoms of **acute decompensated heart failure (ADHF)** include dyspnea, fatigue, orthopnea, dyspnea on exertion, and paroxysmal nocturnal dyspnea. CHF can present atypically in patients with nonspecific complaints such as insomnia, nocturia, irritability, anorexia, fatigue, and depression. β-Type natriuretic peptide (BNP) is released by the atria when it becomes acutely dilated, a reflection of increased preload. **An elevated BNP level in the absence of renal failure is suggestive of CHF and is used to diagnose CHF and to follow the effectiveness of treatment.** An increase in BNP induces diuresis and helps decrease fluid levels. A BNP value of <100 pg/mL is useful in ruling out CHF. It is important to distinguish between the 2 types of CHF, **diastolic versus systolic**, since the treatment differs. This can be done via transesophageal echocardiogram (TEE) or transthoracic echocardiograms (TE).

The functional capacity in CHF can serve as a guideline for a stepwise strategy of treatment. A common classification scheme for CHF is that of the New York Heart

Table 16–1 • DIFFERENTIAL DIAGNOSIS OF CHF

Disease	Clinical Findings
Ischemic heart disease (CAD)	History of myocardial infarction, presence of infarction pattern on (ECG), risk factors for coronary artery disease
Idiopathic dilated cardiomyopathy	HF in patients without risk factors or known coronary artery disease
Hypertension	History of poorly controlled hypertension, presence of an S_4, left ventricular hypertrophy on electrocardiogram or ECG
Valvular heart disease	Mitral regurgitation. Aortic stenosis; midsystolic murmur at base that radiates to carotid arteries
Infective endocarditis	Fever, positive blood cultures for typical organisms, risk factors for bacteremia (intravenous drug use, invasive intravenous lines)
Familial dilated cardiomyopathy	Family history of HF or sudden cardiac death
Toxic cardiomyopathies	History of exposure to the toxic agent (ETOH, anthracycline, radiation, cocaine, catecholamines, vitamin deficiencies)
Collagen vascular disease	History of systemic lupus erythematosus, polyarteritis nodosa, scleroderma, dermatomyositis; positive serology results
Endocrinologic disorders	Hyperthyroidism, hypothyroidism, acromegaly, pheochromocytoma, diabetes mellitus
Peripartum cardiomyopathy	HF symptoms with left ventricular dysfunction within 6 mo of a pregnancy
Hypertrophic cardiomyopathies	Family history of hypertrophic cardiomyopathy, ECG findings of ventricular hypertrophy. Outflow tract gradient by physical examination or echocardiography. Only murmur that increase with a Valsalva maneuver (decreased venous return to heart)

Association (NYHA) (Table 16–2). CHF often presents with signs of both left and right heart failure. **The most common cause of right heart failure is left heart failure.** Right heart failure presents with elevated JVD, dependent edema, and ascites but with an absence of pulmonary congestion typical of left heart failure. When evaluating ADHF, one should first obtain a resting 12-lead ECG in all patients. An old ECG is extremely helpful for comparison with the current findings to determine progression of the disease and its time of onset.

Table 16–2 • NEW YORK HEART ASSOCIATION CHF CLASSIFICATION; EFFORT NEEDED TO CAUSE SYMPTOMS

NYHA CHF Class	Description
Class I Stage A	Asymptomatic, left ventricular dysfunction
Class II Stage B	Dyspnea with significant exertion
Class III Stage C	Dyspnea with minimal activity including usual activities of daily living
Class IV Stage D	Dyspnea at rest

A chest x-ray (CXR) often reveals signs of fluid overload and pump failure in the form of pulmonary edema accompanied by cardiomegaly, vascular congestion, Kerley B lines (dilated lymphatics), blunting of costophrenic angles, cephalization of the pulmonary vasculatures, and pleural effusions are common in ADHF/CHF. TE is used to determine the etiology of ADHF. TE evaluations assist in determining whether systolic dysfunction (ejection fraction [EF] <40%) or diastolic dysfunction (normal EF) exists. Significant valvular disease can also be revealed by TE determinations. Left ventricular remodeling with increased left ventricular end diastolic volume and decreased contractility accompanies systolic dysfunction. Coronary artery disease (CAD), the main underlying cause of ADHF in two-thirds of all patients, must be aggressively treated. Patients with post-MI often show evidence of ventricular remodeling.

Diastolic Dysfunction

Patients with diastolic dysfunction have EF values >40% and have normal left ventricular end diastolic volumes. **Left ventricular hypertrophy (LVH) is frequently present with an increased stiffness in the ventricles** and a decreased compliance of the ventricular wall. Diastolic heart failure is common especially in **elderly patients** with the previously described findings, which can be documented by TE/TEE and ECG studies.

TREATMENT

Nonpharmacological Therapy of CHF

When the CHF is compensated, limiting dietary sodium to <2 g/d and limiting fluids to 2 qt/d have decreased hospital readmissions for CHF. Mild exercise, specifically aerobic exercise, is known to improve hemodynamic values in patients with CHF. Exercise also eases the activities of daily living (ADL) and the quality of life (QOL). Identifying sleep disturbances and nighttime hypoxia is also an important step in the management of CHF. Accurately diagnosing and treating obstructive sleep apnea (OSA) can be life saving for these patients. Treatment of OSA will decrease BP, increase the capacity of exercise, decrease hospital admissions and improve QOL. The delivery of positive pressure decreases preload by delivering PEEP. Patients with NYHA class III or class IV (Table 16–2) with a QRS >120 msec should be considered for biventricular pacing. If the EF is <35%, an implantable cardioversion device (ICD) is indicated. Cardiac resynchronization therapy via the pacer and ICD improve the QOL and decrease mortality. Cardiac transplantation improves survival, functional status, and the QOL in patients with NYHA of class III or class IV. Patients on maximal therapy but still displaying ADHF should be considered as subjects for transplantation if <65 years old. Contraindications for transplantation include end organ damage from diabetes, vascular disease, cancer, cerebrovascular accident (CVA), lack of psychological support, or active psychiatric illness.

Drug therapy: CHF patients with systolic dysfunction have improved survival on angiotensin-converting enzyme inhibitors, β-blockers and for some patient groups, aldosterone antagonists. Digitalis used cautiously will decrease hospital readmission for CHF. In **black patients with hypertension and CHF**, adding the combination of **hydralazine and nitrates** to standard therapy **increases survival rates.** Table 16–3 outlines the various pharmacological interventions that should be considered in patients with CHF. In patients with rare forms of CHF, efforts to treat diastolic dysfunction are designed to increase the cardiac output; these interventions include treating the hypertension, maintaining NSR, and treating any form of ischemia.

Table 16–3 • DRUG TREATMENT IN SYSTOLIC DYSFUNCTION

Drug Treatment for Heart Failure Due to Systolic Dysfunction	Drug Actions
Angiotensin-converting enzyme inhibitors (ACE), enalaprilat (IV only), captopril, lisinopril	ACE inhibitors are used for all classes of heart failure. They inhibit angiotensin-converting enzyme, resulting in decreased conversion of angiotensin I to angiotensin II and decreased metabolism of bradykinin. They improve exercise tolerance, hemodynamic status, and survival and may halt progression and cause regression of HF. Avoid in patients with history of ACE inhibitor–induced angioedema.
β-Blockers (carvedilol, metoprolol, bisoprolol)	Used for all classes of CHF. Inhibit adrenergic nervous system and improve survival. Reduce sudden death risk and may halt progression and cause regression of heart failure. Use with caution in patients with NYHA class IV heart failure. Avoid in patients with significant asthma and high-grade conduction system disease.
Aldosterone antagonists (spironolactone, eplerenone)	Improve survival in patients with NYHA II-IV heart failure. Improve survival after MI with left ventricular dysfunction. Follow potassium level closely, especially in patients taking ACE inhibitors and NSAIDs.
Angiotensin-receptor antagonists (losartan, valsartan)	Use in patients who cannot take ACE inhibitors. Inhibit renin-angiotensin system at angiotensin receptor level. Lead to improvement in hemodynamics, symptoms; patients have less incidence of cough
Hydralazine and nitrates (isosorbide dinitrate, isosorbide mononitrate)	Reserved for patients intolerant to ACE inhibitors and angiotensin receptor blocker (ARB). Reduce afterload and preload. Improve survival in patients with heart failure but not so well as ACE inhibitors. Indicated to reduce mortality in black patients when added to ACE inhibitors and β-blockers.
Digitalis glycoside (digoxin)	Positive inotropic agent. Slows heart rate through vagal effects, improves exercise tolerance, and reduces hospitalizations. No survival benefit. Aim for level <2.0 ng/mL. Use lower dose in elderly and in patients with renal insufficiency. Avoid hypokalemia.
Loop diuretics	Palliative in patients with congestive symptoms. No survival benefit.
Positive inotropic agents (dobutamine, milrinone)	Used to improve hemodynamics in patients with severe CHF and maintain patients until cardiac transplant; can be used continuously at home in nontransplant candidates for palliation. Arrhythmogenic; no survival benefit

Management of right ventricular failure: Definitive therapy for an acutely decompensated right ventricular failure (RVF) requires primary treatment of the underlying condition in addition to hemodynamic support. Patients with right ventricular failure can be very resilient and they can recover substantially if the underlying causes are successfully treated. Treatment options include percutaneous coronary intervention for RV infarction. Thrombolytic therapy should be applied if catheterization is not available. Open surgical embolectomy may be required for massive pulmonary emboli (PE) with heart failure due to acute pump failure.

Oxygen: Oxygen should be administered to all CHF patients whether the patient is hypoxic or not. This decreases the anxiety which usually accompanies CHF. The minimal FIO_2 is one that achieves an O_2sat of 92% or greater. NIV and MV may be needed to assist the ventilatory and oxygenation requirements. The application of PEEP should also be considered.

Noninvasive ventilation (NIV): NIV is a perfect treatment modality for ADHF. It decreases the work in breathing, improves oxygenation and ventilation, and decreases preload. NIV may be helpful in pre-oxygenating patients with hypoxemic respiratory failure before ETI. NIV is increasing in ICUs throughout Europe and the United States. Closely monitor for mask tolerance and leaks, alterations in the respiratory rate, the use of accessory muscles, and their synchrony with the ventilator. Within 1 to 2 hours of admission, determine the success or failure of NIV use. (see NIV Chapter 12).

Surgical treatment: Coronary artery bypass graft (CABG) surgery is the removal of an autologous vein and using it to replace the blocked coronary artery in the heart. When the valve responsible for CHF requires modification due to excess valve tissue, valve repair is considered. In some cases, annuloplasty is required to replace the ring around the valve. If repair of the valve is not possible, it should be replaced with an artificial heart valve. The last level in the treatment of CHF is replacement of the heart. When severe heart failure is present and medication or other procedures are not effective, the diseased heart needs to be replaced or augmented. Unfortunately, the number of patients that qualify for heart replacement outnumber the supply of available donors.

Pacemaker: Pacemakers function by sending electric pulses to the heart forcing it to beat at a rate that is considered normal or required by the patient. Pacemakers with sensory capacity can adjust their output rate depending on the cardiac demand of the patient. These devices are used to treat patients with arrhythmias or rhythm problems such as symptomatic bradycardia and tachycardia.

CARDIOGENIC SHOCK

Management of CS should focus on the augmentation of oxygen delivery and BP to maximize tissue perfusion. Delay in the diagnosis or therapy of CS increases mortality. The management of CS can be accomplished by pharmacological and mechanical means, or by revascularization.

Pharmacologic therapy: The **initial treatment for patients with CS focuses on the restoration of normal hemodynamics, oxygenation, and reestablishment of**

a normal heart rhythm. In patients without significant pulmonary edema, **a fluid challenge** before vasopressor therapy is advised to improve splanchnic blood flow. If pulmonary edema is present or there is a lack of response to the fluid challenge, pharmacologic therapy should be initiated. The initial therapy should include medications that have both a **positive inotropic and vasopressor effect**. Cardiogenic shock requires both rapid diagnosis and appropriate therapy. ICU patients often have multiple-organ failure, and differentiating CS from other forms of shock can be difficult. Drugs considered for use as first-line treatments include norepinephrine, dopamine, dobutamine, epinephrine, and phenylephrine. In patients with heart failure, an increased mortality has been described in those given adrenergic inotropic agents. The improved hemodynamics resulting from the use of these agents comes at the cost of increased myocardial consumption of oxygen.

Using vasopressin instead of epinephrine resulted in similar hemodynamic effects via a direct effect on vasopressin receptors. **Vasopressin has been recommended as the drug of first choice to be given during cardiac arrest, supplanting epinephrine.** Therapy with phosphodiesterase inhibitors (eg, milrinone) may be considered, particularly in cases with right ventricular dysfunction, although the hemodynamically unstable patient often poorly tolerates the resultant decrease in SVR. Levosimendan, an investigational calcium sensitizer that also promotes coronary vasodilation, continues to show promise as a novel treatment for CS. The maintenance of normal physiologic parameters (eg, MAP, cardiac index) should be the goal of therapy with any drug intended to correct CS, although high-dose vasopressor treatment has been associated with poorer patient survival.

Mechanical therapy: In patients who are unresponsive to pharmacologic therapy, mechanical augmentation of blood flow may be of benefit. **The placement of an IABP in patients with CS decreases the 6-month mortality.** IABP counterpulsation devices can be put in place at the bedside to improve diastolic pressure, simultaneously reducing left ventricular afterload without increasing myocardial oxygen demand. The incidence of major complications (eg, arterial injury and perforation, limb ischemia, visceral ischemia) associated with IABP insertion is 3%. IABP is contraindicated in patients with severe aortic insufficiency, severe peripheral vascular disease, and aortic aneurysm or dissection. In these conditions the placement of a ventricular assist device (VAD) may be considered.

Other potentially useful procedures include extracorporeal membrane oxygenation (ECMO) and placement of an artificial heart. These have varying degrees of success. Newer percutaneous VADs are a more feasible choice in smaller medical-surgical centers. Patients with LVAD demonstrated significant improvement in hemodynamics, renal function, and in the clearance of serum lactate compared to the use of IABP. There are a limited number of centers that have access to such technology. Experiences in the placement of LVAD devices and in hemodynamic management are necessary to achieve an optimal benefit for patients. The use of IABP was independently associated with survival in the centers most experienced in its use. These devices are intended to serve as a bridge to cardiac transplantation, and resources must be available to continue this, often lengthy, workup.

Revascularization therapy: Because AMI is frequently the cause of CS, reestablishing blood flow to the affected myocardial area is critically important and decreases mortality. Reestablishing coronary arterial flow by the administration of **thrombolytic** agents works, but the preferred modality of revascularization remains **either PCI or CABG**. Thrombolytic therapy for CS after STEMI is only for patients in whom definitive therapy is contraindicated or unavailable. **Fibrinolytic agents may still be considered in those situations in which PCI is not attainable for >90 minutes or patients within 3 hours of their MI, and free of contraindications.** Early revascularization reduces mortality by 22% in patients with CS and by 16% in those who developed CS subsequent to admission. Early revascularization therapy is recommended for patients <75 years with complications of ACS. Revascularization in NSTEMI did result in a significant decrease in mortality. Therefore it is not as important to revascularize NSTEMI patients. Both acute hemodialysis and ultrafiltration are used to remove the overload of fluid, especially in renal compromised patients.

Prevention

Long-standing hypertension is associated with both systolic and diastolic ventricular dysfunction leading to CHF. Hypertension is an independent risk factor for CAD. Controlling hypertension markedly lowers the mortality and the risk for developing CHF. **Diabetics** suffer from increased cardiac events, independent of CAD and hypertension. Diabetes is also associated with LVH and arterial vessel wall stiffening. Aggressive BP control and lipid control with statins have beneficial effects in diabetic patients beyond those seen in the general population. Patients with CHF should avoid exposure to cardiotoxins such as alcohol, smoking, and illicit drugs. Smoking markedly increases the risk of CAD. Cocaine use has both direct and indirect cardiac effects that increase the risk for CHF and sudden cardiac death.

Other common occurrences that lead to ADHF include myocardial ischemia, arrhythmias, AF, severe hypertension, renal dysfunction, unbalanced diet, and noncompliance with treatment. An elevated heart rate can lead to ADHF; thus, causes of tachycardia such as fever, anemia, hyperthyroidism, and infection should be addressed. In CHF the use of BB is indicated in almost all patients. Tachycardia in CHF decreases LV filling time, leading to a drop in CO. Patients with CHF frequently use concomitant medications such as NSAIDs and thiazolidinediones. Thiazolidinedione use for the control of diabetes is contraindicated in patients with CHF.

Daily weight determination at home is still the best evaluator of overall fluid volume. The actual weight is not important but rather the difference from the last measurements and an increased trend in weight is important. The patient or the doctor may increase or decrease the diuretic therapy. Electrolyte imbalances in CHF are mostly related to its treatment. A blood Na^+ level ≤134 mEq/L is an independent risk for mortality and Na^+ levels must be monitored in patients with CHF.

CLINICAL CASE CORRELATION

- **See also Case 4 (Hemodynamic Monitoring), Case 5 (Vasoactive Drugs and Pharmacology), Case 14 (Acute Coronary Syndromes), and Case 15 (Cardiac Arrhythmias).**

COMPREHENSION QUESTIONS

16.1 A 60-year-old man is evaluated in the ICU for chest discomfort that has been present intermittently for 6 hours. The patient was treated with ASA, a β-blocker, and nitroglycerin. The ECG revealed an inferior wall STEMI. Troponins were elevated. On physical examination, the heart rate was 60 beats/minute with a BP of 78/60 mm Hg. The JVD was elevated to the angle of the jaw. Lung auscultation was clear. A parasternal RV lift was present. A right-sided S_3 was heard. Which of the following is the most likely cause for this patient's findings?

A. Acute cardiac tamponade
B. Aortic dissection
C. Left ventricular free-wall rupture
D. Right ventricular myocardial infarction
E. Atrial rupture

16.2 A 68-year-old woman is in the ICU with palpitations and shortness of breath. She has a history of hypertension and chronic AF. Her medications are furosemide, candesartan, and warfarin. On physical examination, her heart rate is 120 beats/minute with an irregular rhythm, and her BP is 130/80 mm Hg. She has an elevated jugular venous pressure, rales in both lungs, and marked pitting edema of the lower extremities. Echocardiography shows LVH, an ejection fraction of 70%, and no significant valvular disease. After IV diuretics were begun, the patient's symptoms improved. Her heart rate is now 90 beats/minute and the BP is 120/75 mm Hg. Which of the following is the most likely primary mechanism causing her heart failure?

A. Constrictive pericarditis
B. Diastolic dysfunction
C. Systolic dysfunction
D. Valvular disease
E. Mixed dysfunction

ANSWERS TO QUESTIONS

16.1 **D.** Right ventricular MI should be suspected in patients with inferior ECG ischemic changes who present with hypotension, clear lung fields, and elevated JVD. An RV lift is present, and tricuspid valve regurgitation is audible. RV dysfunction causes right-sided cardiac enlargement with tricuspid annular dilatation. The ECG demonstrates inferior (leads II, III, aVF) and ST changes indicative of acute ischemia in the region of the right coronary artery. Acute cardiac tamponade and left ventricular free wall rupture are also unlikely in this patient; both are rare late manifestations of MI.

16.2 **B.** The diagnosis of diastolic heart failure is generally made when signs and symptoms of systolic heart failure are present but the transthoracic echocardiogram (TTE) shows a normal EF and an absence of significant valvular abnormalities. This patient has a history and echocardiographic findings consistent with diastolic dysfunction. She has hypertension, which predisposes one to the development of LVH and impaired ventricular relaxation. Although she presented with evidence of CHF, the echocardiogram demonstrated normal systolic function and no significant valvular abnormalities that could account for the CHF. Constrictive pericarditis is unlikely in the absence of pulsus paradoxus and when there is no echocardiographic evidence of pericardial abnormalities. The goals in patients with diastolic heart failure are to optimize diastolic filling by slowing the heart rate with β-blockers. There have been no medications identified that reduce the morbidity or mortality in patients with diastolic dysfunction.

CLINICAL PEARLS

- Jugular venous distention is the most sensitive clinical sign of acute cardiac decompensation.
- Echocardiography confirms the diagnosis of ADHF and aids in directing its management.
- In patients with right ventricular MI, echocardiography demonstrates right ventricular enlargement with reduced systolic function.
- The use of IABP in severe ADHF serves as a bridge to surgery or angioplasty.
- Medications have not lowered morbidity or mortality in CHF secondary to diastolic dysfunction.
- In CHF, reversible factors that can cause exacerbations should be identified and treated. A sodium concentration <134 mEq/L is an independent risk factor for greater mortality in CHF.
- When ECG changes suggest myocardial ischemia, early revascularization is needed.
- Vasopressin can be added to dobutamine and norepinephrine for improvement in MAP.

REFERENCES

Chinnaiyan KM, Alexander D, Maddens M, McCullough PA. Curriculum in cardiology: integrated diagnosis and management of diastolic heart failure. *Am Heart J.* 2007;153:189-200.

Loscalzo J. *Harrison's Pulmonary and Critical Care Medicine.* New York, NY: McGraw-Hill; 2010.

Toy E, Simon B, Takenaka K, Liu T, Rosh A. *Case Files Emergency Medicine.* 2nd ed. New York, NY: McGraw-Hill, Lange; 2009.

CASE 17

A 45-year-old male resident of Minnesota was brought to the emergency department (ED) in January because of fever, confusion, and "inability to talk." His wife reported that he had generalized malaise, headache, and low-grade fever for 3 days with no other specific symptoms. Several hours before coming to the ED, he was noted to have progressive lethargy and confusion and lost his ability to speak. He had not had nausea, vomiting, diarrhea nor focal weakness or seizures. He was previously in good health, took no medications, and denied recent travel outside of the United States. There were no recent insect bites or pet exposures. On physical examination, his temperature was 38.3°C (101°F) and other vital signs were normal. Expressive aphasia was noted, but there were no focal findings or nuchal rigidity and the pupils were equal and reactive to light. There were no petechiae, splinter hemorrhages, subconjunctival hemorrhages, or heart murmurs. The fundi were normal without papilloedema. A lumbar puncture was performed and the findings from the cerebrospinal fluid (CSF) were as follows: leukocyte count 150/μL with 90% lymphocytes, erythrocytes 500/μL, protein 125 mg/dL, glucose 50 mg/dL, and no organisms were seen on a Gram stain. After the lumbar puncture he developed progressive weakness of the right upper extremity.

- What is the most likely diagnosis?
- What is the best treatment for this patient?
- What other diagnostic tests may be performed to support the diagnosis?

ANSWERS TO CASE 17: Meningitis/Encephalitis

Summary: A previously healthy 45-year-old man from Minnesota developed a sudden onset of fever, headache, expressive aphasia, and focal weakness in January. A lumbar puncture reveals no organisms, but elevated protein and leukocytes with lymphocyte predominance. He has progressive weakness of his right upper extremity.

- **Most likely diagnosis:** Herpes simplex virus type 1 (HSV-1) encephalitis.
- **Best treatment:** Admit to the ICU and immediately start intravenous acyclovir.
- **Confirmatory tests:** A brain biopsy is definitive (usually not done if the HSV PCR test is positive and/or empiric acyclovir results in clinical improvement). A PCR on the CSF for HSV-1 should be performed and is often positive. MRI of the brain and EEG added support to the diagnosis.

ANALYSIS

Objectives

1. To describe the most common causes of meningitis and encephalitis.
2. To find the differences in the CSF examination in meningitis and encephalitis etiologic agents.
3. To discuss the options for treating meningitis and encephalitis.

Considerations

This patient has a typical presentation of sporadic HSV-1 encephalitis. His acute onset of low-grade fever, generalized malaise, and headache which progressed to lethargy, aphasia, and then focal weakness of the right upper extremity is strongly suggestive of HSV-1 encephalitis. Seizure is often present. Encephalitis viruses include, Eastern equine encephalitis, St. Louis encephalitis, La Crosse encephalitis, California encephalitis, Powassan fever, and all others, which are less common than West Nile virus (WNV) and HSV-1 encephalitis. In the absence of a known outbreak of WNV, the presentation suggests that the most likely diagnosis is viral encephalitis due to HSV-1. Herpes encephalitis is the most common cause of fatal sporadic encephalitis in the United States and should always be considered in the differential diagnosis "treatable" with antiviral medication. The CSF findings of a lymphocytic pleocytosis with a significant number of RBCs and an elevated protein on LP are suggestive of HSV encephalitis. Decreased CSF glucose levels may also be present in HSV encephalitis, but rarely in other viral encephalitis. A positive PCR for HSV-1 in the CSF would confirm the diagnosis. Supporting information for HSV-1 encephalitis may include CT or MRI of the brain, EEG, brain biopsy, and culture of the CFS for HSV. Other considerations would rickettsia (RMSF); nonspirochetal treponemes (lyme); fungal (cryptococcosis); protozoal (acanthoamoeba, Nagleria); and bacterial etiologies. Therapies should consider geographic exposures, vector exposure (ticks, mosquitoes), occupation, hobbies and immune defects.

APPROACH TO:
Meningitis/Encephalitis

CNS infections are medical emergencies. These include meningitis due to a bacterial or viral infection of tissues surrounding the cerebral cortex (meninges) and encephalitis which is a viral infection of the cerebral cortex. There may be a combination of meningitis and encephalitis (meningoencephalitis) which is most often viral in etiology.

BACTERIAL MENINGITIS

Early diagnosis and appropriate therapy (within 2 hours of presentation) of bacterial meningitis is crucial. More than **75% of all cases of bacterial meningitis in the United States are due to *Streptococcus pneumoniae* or *Neisseria meningitidis*.** Meningitis due to *Haemophilus influenzae* has markedly decreased due to widespread immunization with the Haemophilus B influenza conjugate vaccine. Listeria monocytogenes remains an infection of at-risk patients and infections by this bacterium are sporadic. Less commonly, meningitis due *S. agalactiae* (Group B Streptococcus) and *Escherichia coli* may be seen in at-risk patients (neonates, infants, and immunocompromised patients).

Streptococcus pneumoniae is the most common etiologic agent of community-acquired bacterial meningitis and is often seen in patients with other foci of infection: pneumonia, otitis media, mastoiditis, sinusitis, or endocarditis. It may also be one of the causes of meningitis following **CSF leaks** due to trauma, iatrogenesis, or congenital defects of the meninges. The pneumococcal 13-valent for children and 23-valent vaccine for adults are effective in preventing invasive disease.

Neisseria meningitidis is the second most common sporadic agent of bacterial meningitis and the most common cause of outbreaks and epidemics of bacterial meningitis in the United States. It occurs primarily in children and young adults. Patients with persistent deficiencies in the terminal complement components (C5-C9) are predisposed to infection with *N. meningitidis*. A quadravalent (A, C, Y, or W-135) conjugate vaccine is available, but does not protects against serogroup B, the agent of one-third of cases in the United States. The ACIP has recommended vaccination be used for the prevention of meningococcal disease in the following individuals:

1. Routine vaccination of adolescents at age 11 to 12 years with a booster at age 16
2. A 2-dose primary series administered 2 months apart for persons aged 2 to 54 years with persistent complement deficiency (C5-C9), or functional or anatomic asplenia, or HIV infection

Other less common causes of bacterial meningitis include *Listeria monocytogenes*, Group B streptococci (*S. agalactiae*), aerobic gram-negative bacilli and staphylococcus species. **Listeria monocytogenes meningitis** is associated with **extremes of age**, neonates and persons >50 years of age. Alcoholism, malignancy, immunosuppression, diabetes mellitus, hepatic failure, renal failure, iron overload, collagen vascular disorders, and HIV infection are also predisposing factors. **Group B streptococcal**

meningitis, an important cause of infection in **neonates**, can be seen in adults with the same underlying conditions that predispose to listerial meningitis. **Aerobic gram-negative bacilli** (*Klebsiella* species, *E. coli*, *Serratia marcescens*, and *Pseudomonas aeruginosa*). *Staphylococcus aureus* and *S. epidermidis* may cause meningitis in patients with **head trauma**, subsequent to neurosurgical procedures and placement of CSF shunts, or following bacteremia due to catheters, indwelling devices, and urinary tract infection. **Community-acquired Methicillin-resistant *Staphylococcus aureus*** (CA-MRSA) is an emerging cause of community-acquired meningitis. The differential diagnosis of bacterial meningitis is broad and includes organisms such as mycobacterial, fungal, protozoal, and viral.

Diagnosis of Meningitis

Meningitis should be considered if a patient has **fever, headache, neck stiffness, and altered mental status.** On examination "jolt accentuation" of the headache elicited with rapid horizontal movement of the head is considered to be more sensitive for the diagnosis of meningitis than the traditional Kernig or Brudzinski signs of meningeal irritation. **Nuchal rigidity** is the inability to flex the head forward due to rigidity of the neck muscles. **Kernig sign** is positive when the leg is bent at the hip and knee at an angle of 90 degrees, and subsequent extension of the knee is painful. **Brudzinski sign** is the appearance of involuntary lifting of the legs when the patient's head is lifted from the examining couch when the patient is lying supine. These findings are not specific and may indicate subarachnoid hemorrhage as well as meningitis. Nuchal rigidity, altered mental status, and Kernig and Brudzinski signs may be absent but this should not deter an evaluation for meningitis.

The diagnosis of meningitis is established by the analysis of a CSF specimen (Table 17–1). At times CT imaging may be necessary prior to performing a lumbar puncture to reduce the risk of brain herniation; however, this imaging should not delay empiric antibiotic therapy. **Specific indications for a CT imaging prior to an LP include: focal neurological findings (including seizure), increased intracranial pressure or papilledema, age >65 years, underlying immune deficiency, and coma.** A CSF white cell count ≥500/μL, a CSF lactate acid ≥3.5 mmol/L, or a CSF- to-serum

Table 17–1 • CEREBROSPINAL FLUID FINDINGS IN PATIENTS WITH MENINGITIS

CSF Parameter	Normal	Bacterial	Viral	TB	Cryptococcal
Opening pressure (mm H_2O)	80-200	200-500	≤250	180-300	>200
Leukocyte count (cells/μL)	0-5	1000-5000	50-1000	50-300	20-500
Leukocyte count differential	Lymphs[a]	PMN[b] >80%	Lymphs[a] predominate	Lymphs[a] monocytes	Lymphs[a]
Glucose (mg/dL)	50-70	<40	>45	≤45	<40
Protein (mg/dL)	15-40	100-500	<200	50-100	>45

[a]Lymphocytes.
[b]Polymorphonuclear neutrophils.

glucose ratio ≤0.4 are highly predictive of bacterial meningitis. Latex agglutination testing is available for the evaluation of bacterial meningitis (*H. influenzae* type b; *S. pneumoniae*; *N. meningitidis* groups A, B, C, Y, or W135; *S. agalactiae* and *E. coli* K1; **BD Directigen Meningitis Combo Test**). A polymerase chain reaction (PCR) should be considered as a diagnostic aid especially for meningitis due to enteroviruses which cause about 85% of the viral meningitis seen in the United States (echovirus, coxsackievirus A and B, and the nonpolio enteroviruses).

Tuberculous meningitis can mimic enteroviral and herpes simplex virus infections. IgM antibody capture enzyme-linked immunosorbent assay (ELISA) testing is useful in identifying arbovirus infections especially those due to WNV, St. Louis encephalitis, California encephalitis, Eastern equine encephalitis, La Crosse encephalitis, and Powassan viruses. This is especially important in patients whose CSF evaluation is consistent with aseptic meningitis. Aseptic meningitis is meningeal inflammation without identification of a causative bacterial agent and accompanied by a monocytic pleocytosis of the CSF. Seasonality, geography, exposure to ticks or mosquitoes, and concomitant symptoms and signs are usually helpful in determining the etiology.

The natural history of aseptic meningitis is usually benign and often subclinical or underappreciated due to its low-grade presentation (eg, mumps, enteroviral infections). However, at times, especially WNV can cause devastating effects with severe morbidity and mortality. Testing for fungal, mycobacterial, HIV, and nontreponemal spirochetal agents (Lyme disease) should be performed when clinically indicated (eg, immunosuppression, exposure history) in nonbacterial meningitis. A Venereal Disease Research Laboratory (VDRL) test should be considered on all abnormal CSF samples to exclude syphilis. Noninfectious causes of meningitis should be considered, including drug-induced causes (nonsteroidal anti-inflammatory drug [NSAID] use and collagen vascular diseases, especially systemic lupus erythematosus).

Table 17–2 • EMPIRIC ANTIMICROBIAL THERAPY FOR PURULENT MENINGITIS

Predisposing Factors	Common Bacterial Pathogens	Recommended Antimicrobial Agents
Age 2-50 years	*S. pneumoniae, N. meningitidis*	Vancomycin + a third-generation cephalosporin
Age >50 years	*S. pneumonia, N. meningitidis, L. monocytogenes,*[a] aerobic gram-negative bacilli	Vancomycin + ampicillin + a third-genaration cephalosporin
Basilar skull fracture	*S. pneumonia, H. influenzae,* Group A β-hemolytic streptococci	Vancomycin + a third-generation cephalosporin
Postneuro surgery or head trauma	*S. aureus, S. epidermidis,* aerobic gram-negative bacilli (including *P. aeruginosa*)	Vancomycin + either ceftazidine or cefepime
Cerebrospinal fluid shunt	*S. aureus, S. epidermidis,* aerobic gram-negative bacilli (including *P. aeruginosa*), diphtheroids (including *P. acnes*)	Vancomycin + either ceftazidime or cefepime

[a]Gentamicin may be added for synergy in Listeria, *S. aureus*, and gram-negative meningitis.

Treatment of Meningitis

If the examination of CSF reveals the presence of purulent meningitis and a positive Gram stain suggests a specific etiology, targeted antimicrobial therapy must be initiated as quickly as possible (optimally within 30 minutes of arrival in the ED). If the Gram stain is negative, empiric antibiotic therapy is determined by the patient's age and underlying conditions (Table 17–2). The administration of dexamethasone concomitant with or just prior to the first dose of antimicrobial therapy will attenuate the inflammatory response created by the lysis of certain meningeal pathogens (*H. influenzae*, *Mycobacterium tuberculosis*, *S. pneumoniae*, and *Cryptococcus neoformans*) by antimicrobial agents. If *Listeria monocytogenes* is proven or suspected, ampicillin should be included in the antibacterial regimen to which gentamicin may be added for synergy.

In the treatment of bacterial meningitis, time is of the essence. Antimicrobial treatment should not be delayed while awaiting the results of a CT scan or an MRI. If a CT scan is indicated prior to an LP, antibiotics should be started empirically after an appropriate examination and septic workup.

VIRAL ENCEPHALITIS

Viruses are by far the most common cause of encephalitis. Approximately 20,000 cases of encephalitis occur in the United States each year, with the predominant endemic sporadic cause being the HSV-1. **The most common epidemic cause of viral meningitis is WNV** followed by other sporadic and epidemic viral etiologies. Rabies encephalitis is now rare in North America. Viral encephalitis presents as an acute-onset, febrile illness associated with headache, altered level of consciousness, and occasionally focal neurologic signs. The clinical presentation of encephalitis can be similar to meningitis but the 2 differ in that meningitis is not always characterized by focal neurologic signs and change in mental status. While fever and headache are the principal manifestations of both syndromes, nuchal rigidity is characteristic only of meningitis.

Arboviral diseases such as Eastern equine encephalitis and St. Louis encephalitis have affected humans in the United States for years. These viral infections may be fatal or have significant morbidity, the prevalence in humans has been low and effective treatments and human vaccines have not been developed. This situation changed in 1999 when the first cases of WNV occurred in the United States. The virus spread throughout the United States and has now been diagnosed in thousands of patients annually with significant morbidity and mortality. **WNV encephalitis is most severe in the older age groups with the highest mortality and morbidity rates occurring in those ≥65 years of age.** While most cases of WNV infection are subclinical or mild, the disease can be severe and most often occurs during seasonal outbreaks or epidemic conditions. These severe clinical presentations of WNV include encephalitis, meningitis, flaccid paralysis, and fever. Vaccines have been developed for veterinary use in preventing WNV as early as 2001; however, there are currently no approved vaccines for human use for WNV.

In the United States nonepidemic, sporadic, or focal encephalitis is most frequently due to HSV-1 with one-third of the cases occurring in patients <20 years of age and one-half occurring in those over 50 years old. **HSV-1 encephalitis results from a reactivation of the latent virus in the trigeminal ganglion, resulting in**

inflammatory necrotic lesions in the temporal cortex and limbic system. Most HSV-1 cases occur in the absence of an antecedent illness.

Diagnosis of Encephalitis

After a history and physical examination is completed, CSF analysis should be performed including cell count, glucose, protein, cultures (both viral and bacterial); PCR for specific viral diagnoses including HSV-1, and IgM antibody capture ELISA tests based upon suspected viral etiologies. CSF cultures for HSV-1 and arboviruses are usually negative, but the sensitivity of the PCR for HSV and the arboviral IgM antibody capture ELISA exceeds 90%. **In HSV encephalitis, MRI typically demonstrates unilateral or bilateral abnormalities in the medial and inferior temporal lobes,** which may extend into the frontal lobe. The EEG findings include focal delta activity over the temporal lobes and periodic lateralizing epileptiform discharges (PLEDs). Brain biopsy with fluorescent antibody and histopathology is reserved for patients who do not respond to empiric acyclovir or have negative PCRs of the CSF. CT imaging is not as sensitive as MRI with gadolinium.

The **CSF typically shows a lymphocytic pleocytosis**, an increased number of erythrocytes and an increased concentration of protein; glucose levels are usually normal, but may be low early in the infection. With early HSV-1 encephalitis, the CSF may initially show a PMN predominance which then shifts to a lymphocytosis. Acyclovir should be started immediately when HSV-1 infection is suspected. PCR for HSV-1 DNA in CSF should be obtained but treatment should not be delayed waiting for results. A temporal lobe abnormality on MRI (eg, a hemorrhagic lesion) is considered to be a poor prognostic sign for neurologic recovery, although CMV, EBV, and echoviruses can cause the same syndrome of encephalitis infection.

WNV infection is more frequently associated with a poliomyelitis, Parkinson-like syndrome, or a Guillain-Barre type of presentation. Vector-borne diseases such as WNV infection are unlikely events during a Minnesota winter especially when there is no evidence of an outbreak or epidemic. **The diagnosis of HSV-1 encephalitis is critical because it is the only viral infection of the CNS for which antiviral therapy with acyclovir has been proven effective.** In HSV encephalitis, prompt acyclovir treatment reduces mortality to approximately 25% in adults and older children. Unfortunately over 50% of the patients who survive will have neurologic sequelae.

HIV-RELATED CENTRAL NERVOUS SYSTEM DISEASES

HIV-infected individuals are susceptible to CNS toxoplasmosis infection when their CD4 lymphocyte counts are below 200/μL, and are at high risk with CD4 counts below 50/μL. Localized or focal encephalitis is the most common presentation of toxoplasmosis. **Toxoplasmosis is the most common cause of a CNS mass lesion in AIDS** followed by CNS lymphoma (B cell or non-Hodgkin) which occurs in approximately 2% to 12% of HIV-infected individuals. Unlike the situation in immunocompetent hosts, HIV-associated lymphoma is strongly associated with **Epstein–Barr virus infection.** In patients with AIDS, lymphoma was second only to toxoplasmosis as the most common source of central nervous system mass lesions. A negative PCR for Epstein–Barr virus and the diffuse nature of an MRI abnormality exclude central nervous system lymphoma.

Cryptococcal meningitis (CM) is a subacute infection of the central nervous system associated with a CSF pleocytosis of 40 to 400 cells/μL with lymphocyte predominance and slightly low glucose levels. Diagnosis of cryptococcal CNS infection can be made in >98% of patients by combining the use of rapid antigen detection tests for **cryptococcal antigen, India ink preparation, and CSF cultures for fungi.**

Progressive multifocal leukoencephalopathy (PML) is an opportunistic infection caused by polyomavirus JC, associated with gradual demyelination of the central nervous system and thereby expressed as a progressive neurologic deficit. The lesions of PML are generally bilateral, asymmetric, nonenhancing or with delayed peripheral enhancement, and are periventricular or subcortical in distribution. Radiographic studies reveal no unusual tissue mass effects. This is in contrast to primary central nervous system lymphoma and toxoplasmosis in which mass effect may occur.

Risk factors for AIDS-related opportunistic infections include late-stage HIV infection (CD4 cell count <100/μL), no prior treatment, and the presence of thrush. Patients with PML usually display focal neurologic signs and an MRI will reveal multiple white matter lesions without mass effect, involving the right lateral frontal, right frontoparietal, and left frontal lobes, right pons, bilateral brachium pontis, and right cerebellum. In addition, the PCR is positive for polyomavirus JC in PML. While the gold standard for the diagnosis of PML is brain biopsy, the CNS lesions are usually quite deep and relatively inaccessible. When the preponderance of clinical evidence supports a diagnosis of PML, biopsy can usually be deferred. Approximately 50% of patients with AIDS and PML will survive the PML if highly active antiretroviral therapy is administered, presumably because of the effects of immune reconstitution in arresting the disease process. Neurologic deficits typically persist in survivors proportionate to the disease severity at the time of presentation.

PROTOZOAL MENINGOENCEPHALITIS

Primary amoebic meningoencephalitis may be due to any of the 4 free-living amoebae, for example, *Naegleria fowleri*, *Balamuthia mandrillaris*, *Sappinia diploidea*, and *Acanthoemba castelanii*. Other parasitic infections such as those caused by *Trypanosoma brucei*, *T. cruzi*, and *Toxoplasma gondii* are among those with a protozoan etiology. These pathogens are uncommon causes of CNS infections in North America. *Naegleria fowleri* produces primary amebic meningoencephalitis (PAM) and symptoms of PAM are indistinguishable from acute bacterial meningitis. Other amebae cause granulomatous amebic encephalitis (GAE), which is more apt to be subacute and can present as an indolent or asymptomatic chronic infection. Amebic meningoencephalitis can mimic a brain abscess, aseptic or chronic meningitis, or even a CNS malignancy. Infection with *Strongyloides stercoralis* can lead to a devastating systemic infection often involving the CNS with polymicrobial bacterial meningitis. Termed "hyperinfection syndrome," it is seen in severely immune compromised: HIV, HTLV 1 and 2, and those receiving anti-TNF therapies.

CLINICAL CASE CORRELATION

- **See also Case 18 (Antimicrobial Use in ICU), Case 19 (Sepsis), and Case 20 (Immune-Compromised Patient With Sepsis).**

COMPREHENSION QUESTIONS

17.1 A 44-year-old man who is HIV infected is hospitalized because of a 1-week history of progressive weakness of the left lower extremity and an inability to walk. He has also had a rapid loss of weight, night sweats, and frequent low-grade fever. His CD4 cell count at the time of diagnosis was 88/μL. On physical examination he appears cachectic and chronically ill. His temperature is 38.1°C (100.6°F). Other significant findings included the presence of oral thrush, splenomegaly, bilateral lower extremity weakness, and hyperreflexia. An LP is performed and examination of his CSF shows the following: opening pressure normal; leukocyte count 21/μL with 98% lymphocytes and 2% neutrophils; erythrocyte count 1/μL; protein 85 mg/dL, and glucose 55 mg/dL. The India ink stain, cryptococcal antigen test, and culture for fungi were negative. The PCR was positive for polyomavirus JC and negative for EBV virus. Which of the following is the most likely diagnosis?

A. Cerebral lymphoma

B. Cerebral toxoplasmosis

C. Cryptococcal meningitis

D. Progressive multifocal leukoencephalopathy

E. Tuberculosis

17.2 A 25-year-old man is evaluated in the ED for fever, headache, and mental status changes of 4 hours' duration. He underwent a cadaveric kidney transplantation 10 months ago, and his immunosuppressive regimen includes prednisone and azathioprine. He has no allergies. On physical examination, his temperature is 38.7°C (101.6°F), heart rate is 115 beats/minute, respiratory rate is 25 breaths/minute, and blood pressure is 100/60 mm Hg. He is oriented as to the year and his name but cannot recall the month. His neck is supple, and Kernig and Brudzinski signs are absent. The neurologic examination is normal. His peripheral leukocyte count is 20,000/μL. A CT scan of the head shows no sign of hemorrhage, hydrocephalus, mass effect, or midline shift. An LP is performed and examination of the CSF shows leukocyte count 2000/μL (60% neutrophils, 40% lymphocytes), erythrocyte count 20/μL, glucose 25 mg/dL, protein 150 mg/dL, and a negative Gram stain. The opening spinal pressure is normal. Results of blood, urine, and CSF cultures are pending. Which of the following is the most appropriate empiric antibiotic therapy?

A. Ampicillin and ceftriaxone

B. Ampicillin, ceftriaxone, and vancomycin

C. Ceftriaxone and moxifloxacin

D. Ceftriaxone and vancomycin

E. Moxifloxacin

ANSWERS TO QUESTIONS

17.1 **D.** The most likely diagnosis is PML. PML is an opportunistic infection caused by polyomavirus JC, leading to demyelination of the CNS that causes gradually progressive neurologic deficits. Radiographically, there is no mass effect. The lesions are generally bilateral, asymmetric, nonenhancing, and peri-ventricular or subcortical in distribution. This late-stage HIV infection is based on a CD4 cell count <100/μL The presence of thrush in this patient has a high-risk status for AIDS-related opportunistic infections. He also has focal neurologic signs and an MRI that shows multiple white matter lesions without mass effect involving the right lateral frontal, right frontoparietal, and left frontal lobes and cerebellum. A PCR analysis is positive for polyomavirus JC. The gold standard for diagnosis of PML is a brain biopsy but with the preponderance of evidence supporting a diagnosis of PML, a biopsy can be deferred. If HAART is administered, 50% of AIDS patients will survive PML. Neurologic deficits typically persist in survivors. In patients with HIV infection and CD4 cell counts <200/μL, localized or focal encephalitis is the most common presentation of toxoplasmosis and is the most common CNS system mass lesion. A negative serologic test for toxoplasma-specific IgM would add additional support to the exclusion of toxoplasmic encephalitis. CNS lymphoma occurs in approximately 2% to 12% of HIV-infected individuals. It is strongly associated with Epstein–Barr virus infection. In patients with AIDS, lymphoma was second only to toxoplasmosis as the most common CNS mass lesion.

17.2 **B.** Risk factors for listerial meningitis include immunosuppression, neonatal status or age >50 years, alcoholism, malignancy, diabetes mellitus, hepatic failure, renal failure, iron overload, CVDs, and HIV infection. The most appropriate empiric therapy is ampicillin (the drug of choice for *Listeria*), with ceftriaxone and/or vancomycin. The CSF fluid supports a diagnosis of meningitis. Empiric vancomycin and ceftriaxone are recommended for the treatment of meningitis in patients 2 to 50 years of age. This covers *S. pneumoniae* and *N. meningitidis*, the most common organisms responsible for meningitis in this age group. The analysis of CSF in patients with listerial meningitis often fails to reveal typical gram-positive rods with characteristic "tumbling motility" in wet mount preparations, but often shows pleocytosis and may demonstrate a significant number of lymphocytes in addition to neutrophils. Patients usually have ↑ CSF protein levels; ↓ CSF glucose levels are found less commonly and less profoundly with listerial meningitis. The fluoroquinolones may be effective but do not penetrate the CNS well. Gentamicin is synergistic with ampicillin despite poor CNS penetration.

CLINICAL PEARLS

- Meningitis has a high morbidity and mortality rate, especially in high-risk patients.
- LP and CNS imaging are central to the diagnosis of meningitis and encephalitis.
- Each year 20,000 cases of encephalitis occur in the United States, with the predominant sporadic cause being HSV and the most common epidemic cause being WNV.
- PML is caused by polyomavirus JC, with demyelination of the CNS and neurologic deficits.
- If HART is administered, 50% of patients with AIDS and PML will survive the latter disease.
- HSV is the most common cause of fatal sporadic encephalitis in the United States.
- HSV encephalitis has fever, headache, seizures, focal neurologic signs, and impaired multiple sclerosis (MS).

REFERENCES

Attia J, Hatala R, Cook DJ, Wong JG. The rational clinical examination. Does this adult patient have acute meningitis? *JAMA*. 1999;282:175-181. [PMID:10411200.]

Fitch MT, van de Beek D. Emergency diagnosis and treatment of adult meningitis. *Lancet Infect Dis*. 2007;7:191-200.

Kennedy PG. Viral encephalitis. *J Neurol*. 2005;252:268-272. Epub 2005 Mar 11. [PMID: 15761675.]

CASE 18

A 74-year-old woman has been in the ICU for 8 days for the management of recurrent urinary tract and blood-borne infections. She has a history of a cerebral vascular accident and residual neurological deficits and has been hospitalized for the past 3 weeks. A nurse notifies you for a temperature of 39.4°C (102.92°F). On examination, her pulse rate is100 beats/minute, respiratory rate is 22 breaths/minute, and blood pressure is 110/84 mm Hg. The patient is currently on the third day of ciprofloxacin for empiric treatment of her recurrent urinary tract infection. Her serum creatinine is 2.2 mg/dL. Her urine culture reveals multidrug-resistant (MDR) *Acinetobacter baumannii* and the blood culture reveals the same organism in addition to fungus.

- ▶ What is the most appropriate next step in the management of this patient?
- ▶ What are the underlying processes that predispose to this condition?
- ▶ What are appropriate strategies in the prevention of this problem?

ANSWERS TO CASE 18: Antimicrobial Use in ICU

Summary: An elderly 74-year-old woman with a prolonged hospitalization now has a urinary tract infection and bacteremia with multidrug-resistant (MDR) bacteria. She has an elevated temperature despite antibiotic treatment and has developed fungemia as well.

- **Next step:** Administer appropriate therapy to cover the MDR bacterial infection and fungal infection.
- **Underlying predisposing processes:** The factors in this patient contributing to MDR bacterial and fungal infection are prolonged hospitalization, comorbid conditions, recurrent or persistent infections, relatively immunocompromised state, and previous antibiotic exposures.
- **Prevention of resistance:** Provide prompt broad-spectrum antibiotics for empiric therapy followed by antibiotic de-escalation after culture sensitivities become available and when patient shows good clinical responses to the initial therapy.

ANALYSIS

Objectives

1. To learn the principles of antimicrobial selection and treatment endpoints in ICU patients.
2. To learn antimicrobial treatment strategies that may reduce the occurrence of antimicrobial resistance.
3. To learn the supportive care that may improve responsiveness to antimicrobial treatment in the ICU population.

Considerations

This is a 74-year-old woman with significant residual neurologic deficits and renal insufficiency after suffering from a cerebral vascular accident. She has had a prolonged hospital course and is now in the ICU after contracting a nosocomial infection. She is currently on antibiotics but does not appear to be improving. When a patient does not respond to antimicrobial therapy, it is generally important to determine if another source of infection is present and/or if the antibiotic treatment regimen is inappropriate or insufficient against the microorganisms responsible for the infection. The culture results at this point are helpful in directing her management. Since the same bacteria is isolated from her urine and her blood stream, the infection is severe, systemic, and inadequately controlled with the current antimicrobial regimen. In addition, fungal species isolated on blood culture strongly suggests that fungal sepsis is contributing to the worsening clinical picture. Infection with drug-resistant organisms contributes to prolonged hospitalization, higher hospital costs, and a poorer prognosis. Unfortunately, this patient represents a common clinical scenario in many modern ICUs.

The most important first steps in this patient's management is selection of the correct antimicrobial agents and dosages based on the sensitivity spectrum of the cultured MDR A. *baumannii* and fungal species. Assistance from the institution's microbiology laboratory and infectious disease specialists should be sought out to coordinate the management of her complicated infections. The emergence of antibiotic-resistant bacteria is a significant problem in intensive care units. This resistance makes antimicrobial therapy more difficult as patient's disease process and illness severity continue to increase. The inappropriate administration of broad-spectrum antibiotics can lead to even more difficult-to-treat infections.

DEFINITIONS

NOSOCOMIAL INFECTIONS: Infections acquired in a health-care facility. Generally, the infectious organism is first cultured >48 hours after admission.

HEALTHCARE–ASSOCIATED INFECTIONS: Infections in patients with prior hospitalization for >3 days within the past 90 days, transferred from nursing home, or history of exposure to transfusion/dialysis centers.

EMPIRIC ANTIBIOTIC THERAPY: Antibiotic therapy that is started without culture evidence of infection. The therapy is started based on clinical suspicion of infection based on physiologic parameters.

ANTIMICROBIAL DE-ESCALATION: The goals of the de-escalating strategy are to strike a balance between providing prompt, appropriate initial antimicrobial therapy and minimizing the emergence of antimicrobial resistance. Patients with suspected infections are treated with broad-spectrum antibiotics aimed at most probable organisms that are causing the infections with narrowing (or discontinuing altogether) of the antibiotic coverage as soon as culture results become available, or if no infections are documented. Similarly, duration of treatment may be shortened when patients with uncomplicated infections show clinical improvement/resolution.

ANTIBIOTIC RESISTANCE: The ability of microorganisms to grow in the presence of antibiotic levels that would normally suppress growth or kill susceptible bacteria.

APPROACH TO:
Antimicrobial Use in the ICU

CLINICAL APPROACH

Nosocomial infections affect ICU patients with far greater frequency than patients residing elsewhere in the hospital. Consequently, antibiotics are one of the most common therapies utilized in the intensive care unit. Additionally, up to 70% of all nosocomial infections isolated in the ICU are due to MDR bacteria. The reason for this elevated level of drug-resistant infections is multifactorial. ICU patients have a more severe underlying disease processes, are crowded into small areas of the hospital, and are often malnourished and immunocompromised. They are more likely to be subjected to multiple invasive procedures including endotracheal tubes, indwelling urinary catheters, and central venous lines. In addition to patient-specific risk factors, there are other general factors such as excessive antimicrobial use, poor aseptic technique, and inadequate hand hygiene of health-care providers that contribute to the increased infectious risks. The inappropriate choice and duration of antibiotics therapy can also contribute to the problem by selecting for resistant bacteria overgrowth and infection.

Microbial resistance is increasing in both gram-negative and gram-positive bacteria. These bacteria strains have greater resistance to broad spectrum antibiotics. The inadequate empiric coverage of these resistant bacteria can lead to a higher morbidity and mortality. However, the inappropriate use of broad-spectrum antibiotics can lead to the increase in emergence of resistant bacteria. Thus, the challenge to the physician is to use antibiotics that will cover the resistant bacteria without overtreatment that can lead to resistance.

When a patient is septic, antibiotics must be initiated promptly, preferably, within 1 hour of diagnosis. **Each hour of delay over the next 6 hours has been shown to contribute to a decrease in survival of 7.6%.** For most septic patients, the culture results are not known at the time of the initial presentation; therefore, antibiotics are selected based on clinician's suspicions of the source of infection. The initial choices of the preemptive antimicrobial therapy need to adequately address the potential infective organisms to minimize the mortality associated with the infection. Inadequate initial therapy usually involves either the failure to cover a specific microbe or utilizing antibiotics to which the organism is resistant. Therefore, high-risk patients admitted to the ICU with serious infections should be treated aggressively with broad-spectrum antibiotics until the bacteria cultures are isolated. It is obligatory that before antibiotics are started, cultures should be obtained. Once the culture isolates with their associated antibiotic sensitivities are identified, the antimicrobial therapy should be immediately adjusted to more narrow-coverage antibiotics that have bactericidal activity against the bacteria. This de-escalation therapy allows for treatment of the infection while reducing the risk of antimicrobial resistance. Another key component in the selection of antibiotic choice is based on the basic pharmacokinetics (necessary dosage to achieve adequate levels, tissue penetrance, etc). This is important so that under-dosing does not occur, as this can lead to an increase in the emergence of resistant organisms. This is particularly important in patients with renal insufficiency; adjustments of drug dosing and frequency of administrations are often needed when patient are receiving hemodialysis.

Recognizing when patients are at high risk for developing MDR infections is important in selecting appropriate initial broad-spectrum antibiotics, and these high-risk patients include those who have had prior antibiotics treatments during their hospitalization, prolonged hospitalization, and indwelling devices (such as endotracheal tubes, central venous catheters, and urinary catheters). Infected high-risk patients should be started on combination broad-spectrum antibiotics based on presumed infectious sources and local antibiograms (Table 18–1).

Initial antibiotics are selected based on knowledge of the infection source. Antibiotics have different tissue penetrations and should be taken into account when treating infections. Source control of the infection, such as abscess drainage, should be performed immediately. The choice of antibiotics is somewhat dependent

Table 18–1 • INITIAL EMPIRIC ANTIBIOTIC COMBINATIONS FOR HOSPITAL-ACQUIRED PNEUMONIA

Common Pathogens	Antibiotic Choices
• Methicillin-sensitive *S. aureus* • *Streptococcus pneumoniae* • *Haemophilus influenza* **Antibiotic-sensitive enteric gram-negative bacilli:** • *Escherichia coli* • *Enterobacter spp.* • *Klebsiella* • *Proteus spp.* • *Serratia*	Ceftriaxone or levofloxacin, moxifloxacin, or ciprofloxacin or ampicillin/sulbactam or ertapenem
Possible MDR bacteria: • *Pseudomonas aeruginosa* • *Klebsiella* • *Acinetobacter* • *Methicillin-resistant S. aureus*	Antipseudomonal cephalosporin (cefepime, ceftazidime) *or* antipseudomonal carbepenem (imipenem or meropenem) *or* β-lactam/β-lactamase inhibitor (piperacillin–tazobactam) *plus* antipseudomonal fluoroquinolone (ciprofloxacin or levofloxacin) *or* aminoglycoside (amikacin, gentamicin, or tobramycin) *plus* linezolid or vancomycin

on the local hospital flora. Different resistance rates are found at different hospitals, so antibiograms that show local antibiotic susceptibility should be used as a guide for initiating therapy that will cover local resistance. Once the cultures return with antibiotic susceptibility, antibiotic therapy should be de-escalated in spectrum and duration.

If no organism is isolated after 72 hours, serious consideration should be given to stopping the antibiotic administration. In a study evaluating the duration of therapy in treating patients with ventilator-associated pneumonia (VAP), it was determined that treating patients for 8 days instead of the standard 15 days had no difference in mortality, but significantly reduced the incidence of MDR bacterial infection. Patients with spontaneous bacterial peritonitis receive no additional benefits from being treated for more than 5 days with cefotaxime (Claforan). For all other isolated organisms, the antibiotics should be stopped after a predetermined time course. This allows for shorter therapy with decreased likelihood of selecting resistant organisms. It is also more economical to not provide prolonged, unnecessary antibiotic therapy. However, these maneuvers must all be undertaken after taking into consideration with the patient's clinical status. If the patient continues to remain septic, or is clinically deteriorating, antibiotic administration can be prolonged. Likewise, patients who are immunocompromised or elderly may benefit from longer durations of antibiotics therapy.

There are other strategies that are used in the ICU to decrease infection rates. **Specific strategies that have been shown to decrease the rate of central-line–associated bloodstream infections (CLABSI) when used in combination include hand hygiene, the use of full sterile barriers during central-line insertion, skin**

antisepsis with 2% chlorhexidine solution, subclavian vein insertion site, chorhexidine-impregnated sponge dressings at the line sites, centralizing equipment in a central-line carts during catheter insertion, and daily assessment of central-line necessity. Strategies that may reduce ventilator-associated pneumonias include the elevation of the head of bed, protocols for sedation medications, and ventilation, which are associated with reduced ventilation days.

The early administration of enteral nutritional support also seems to decrease infection rates, allowing for less use of antibiotics. Studies comparing enteral feeding versus parental feeding indicate that there is a decrease in overall infections. Additionally, the use of enteral feeding allows for maintenance of nonspecific mechanisms of immune protection by maintaining gut epithelium. Normal gut epithelium provides for absorption of nutrients, exclusion of pathogenic organisms, production of mucus, and maintenance of normal gap junctions. These mechanisms all protect against potentially harmful bacteria. Not only does enteral feeding aid in nonspecific immune protection, but it also helps provide continued function of gut-associated lymphoid tissue (GALT) which is home to lymphocytes that can produce cytokines and immunoglobulins. All of these factors help provide improved immune function, thus decreasing the need for antibiotics.

CLINICAL CASE CORRELATION

- **See also Case 17 (Meningitis/Encephalitis), Case 19 (Sepsis), and Case 20 (Immune-Compromised Patient With Sepsis).**

COMPREHENSION QUESTIONS

18.1 An 82-year-old woman is admitted to the ICU for presumed urosepsis. Her initial blood pressure is 80/50 mm Hg, heart rate is 110 beats/minute, and oxygen saturation is 100% on 2 L nasal cannula. Urine, blood, and sputum cultures were drawn in the emergency department. Her hemodynamics improve to 120/80 mm Hg and heart rate of 80 bpm after administration of 2 L of normal saline and remain stable. She is started on IV vancomycin. Three days later, all of her cultures return with no growth to date. The next step in management should be:

A. Continue IV vancomycin for 8 more days
B. Continue IV vancomycin for 3 more days
C. Switch to ciprofloxacin PO for 3 days
D. Discontinue antibiotics completely
E. Re-culture the patient

18.2 A 34-year-old man is seen in the emergency department with fever, chills, nausea, and vomiting 2 days after injecting heroin intravenously. Which of the following is the correct order of antibiotic management?

A. Obtain cultures, start specific monotherapy antibiotic, change to broad-spectrum antibiotics if resistant bacteria are found.

B. Start broad-spectrum antibiotics, pan culture (blood, urine, sputum), narrow coverage after 72 hours.

C. Start broad-spectrum antibiotics, culture in 3 days if no improvement, de-escalate antibiotics based on culture results.

D. Obtain blood cultures and obtain a CT scan of the abdomen. If the CT is normal, observe the patient until cultures become available.

E. Pan culture, start broad-spectrum antibiotics, de-escalate after culture results return.

18.3 Which of the following measures decreases the risk of developing antibiotic resistance in the ICU?

A. Central-line skin preparation using povidone-iodine (Betadine)

B. Antibiotic de-escalation

C. Restricting broad-spectrum antibiotics usage

D. Continued antibiotic administration for 2 weeks

E. Using peripherally inserted central venous catheters (PICC) rather than standard central venous catheters

18.4 A 32-year-old woman with a history of poorly controlled Type 1 diabetes had a below knee amputation 2 months ago for gangrene of her foot. Her postoperative course was complicated by a UTI and pneumonia. Her amputation wound spontaneously opened 2 days ago and she was pan-cultured. Her wound was satisfactorily debrided in the operating room and she was started on IV vancomycin and IV piperacillin and tazobactam (Zosyn). She is now being transferred to the ICU for worsening hyperglycemia and dehydration. Her wound culture has grown methicillin-resistant *Staphylococcus aureus* (MRSA) that is sensitive to vancomycin. All other cultures were negative. What is the next step in management?

A. Glucose control and narrow her current coverage to vancomycin.

B. Glucose control; continue her current antibiotics and add cefepime.

C. Glucose control and continue her current regimen.

D. Stop her current antibiotics and perform above knee amputation for source control.

E. Continue current antibiotics and obtain additional cultures.

18.5 An 89-year-old woman who is significantly malnourished is in the ICU with *Pseudomonas aeuriginosa* pneumonia. She has received 5 days of antibiotics, but still has copious amounts of sputum and is continuing to require a significant amount of ventilatory support. The most appropriate course of action is:

A. Continue her current regimen, but re-culture for any spikes in temperature.

B. Discontinue her antibiotics on day 8 of therapy.

C. Broaden her antibiotics for the next 24 hours and then stop antibiotics.

D. Stop antibiotics, re-culture, and await culture results before re-starting antibiotic therapy.

E. Empirically add an antifungal agent.

ANSWERS TO QUESTIONS

18.1 **D.** This patient presented to the emergency department hypotensive and tachycardic and although it was initially thought that she might be septic, none of her cultures returned with any bacteria. Additionally, she improved with simple rehydration, indicating that she was possibly just dehydrated. Thus, there is no need of continuing her antibiotics. The continuation of her antibiotics could also lead to the formation of resistant bacteria.

18.2 **E.** It is essential to obtain cultures prior to starting antibiotic therapy for presumed sepsis. Although the unnecessary use of broad-spectrum antibiotics can lead to increased antimicrobial resistance, it is important that all bacteria are initially covered when starting empiric antibiotic therapy. Once the bacterial cultures return, the antibiotics can be de-escalated to the appropriate monotherapy.

18.3 **B.** The use of broad-spectrum antibiotics for prolonged duration contributes to the increase in antimicrobial resistance. However, their use is necessary in the initial empiric therapy to cover the majority of probable pathogens. Once the cultures have returned, the therapy can be de-escalated, so that the patient's infection can be appropriately treated and broad-spectrum antibiotics use can be limited. Using aseptic technique and limiting the duration of antibiotic administration also helps reduce antimicrobial proliferation and resistance. Chlorhexidine skin preparations have been shown to cause fewer central-line–associated infections in comparison to povidone-iodine (Betadine) skin preparations. The use of PICC in hospitalized patients has not been shown to be associated with reduced catheter-associated infections in comparison to standard central venous catheters.

18.4 **A.** The hyperglycemia can contribute to poor response to antimicrobial therapy in this patient and needs to be better managed. This patient has multiple risk factors for infection with resistant bacteria. Her wound has grown MRSA that is sensitive to vancomycin. This is the most likely source of her sepsis. The addition of piperacillin and tazobactam (Zosyn) does not provide additional benefits. Her wound has been recently inspected and debrided to satisfaction, therefore there is no indication at this time to perform an above the knee amputation. Fungal infections are reasonably common in relatively immunocompromised patients; however, there is no indication of this process at this time.

18.5 **A.** This is an elderly patient who is being treated for pneumonia. Although she is nearing the end of a standard 8-day course of antibiotics for ventilator-associated pneumonia, she is malnourished and still requires a significant amount of ventilatory support. Because of her age and relative immune-compromised status, it is reasonable to extend her antibiotics past the standard 8 days, with re-culturing if her temperatures spike through her current antibiotic coverage and continued vigilance for other causes of her fever.

CLINICAL PEARLS

- Broad-spectrum antibiotics should be started on septic patients based on presumed location of infection and local antibiograms.
- Once culture sensitivities have returned, de-escalation of antibiotics should be done to minimize the use of broad-spectrum antibiotics.
- The duration of antibiotic administration should be limited to specific time courses. If there is no growth of initial cultures after 72 hours, serious consideration should be given to discontinuing the antibiotics.
- Prolonged administration of antibiotics may be necessary in the elderly, immunocompromised, and clinically deteriorating patient.
- Nonpharmacologic strategies for decreasing need for antibiotics in the ICU include aseptic technique, hand-washing, and early enteral nutrition.

REFERENCES

ATS/IDSA. Guidelines for the management of adults with hospital-acquired, ventilator-associated, and healthcare-associated pneumonia. *Am J Resp Crit Care Med*. 2005;171:388-416.

File TM, Jr. Recommendations for the treatment of hospital-acquired and ventilator-associated pneumonia: review of recent international guidelines. *Clin Infect Dis*. 2010;51 (suppl 1):S42-S47.

Leone M, Martin C. How to break the vicious circle of antibiotic resistances? *Current Opin Crit Care*. 2008;14:587-592.

Masterton RG. Antibiotic de-escalation. *Crit Care Clin*. 2011;27:149-162.

Niederman MS. De-escalation therapy in ventilator-associated pneumonia. *Curr Opin Crit Care*. 2006;12:452-457.

Volles DF, Brana TN. Antibiotics in the ICU: focus on agents for resistant pathogens. *Emerg Med Clin N Am*. 2008;26:813-834.

CASE 19

A 59-year-old woman with a history of Type 2 diabetes mellitus was found unconscious at home by her family members. In the emergency center, she was noted to have a temperature of 38.6°C, pulse rate of 112 beats/minute, blood pressure of 96/50 mm Hg, and respiratory rate of 26 breaths/minute. After 2 L of normal saline, the patient became more alert and began to answer questions more appropriately. Laboratory values reveal WBC 26,000/mm^3, hemoglobin 12 g/dL, normal platelet count, and a serum glucose level of 280 mg/dL. A Foley catheter was placed and showed return of concentrated and cloudy urine. The urinalysis revealed 50 WBC per high-power field. A CT scan of the abdomen without contrast revealed no free fluid in the abdomen and an inflamed right kidney with perinephric fat stranding. Shortly after the patient was transferred to the ICU, her nurse notifies you that her blood pressure is 78/50 mm Hg and heart rate is 120 beats/minute.

- ▶ What is the most likely diagnosis?
- ▶ What are the priorities in this patient's management?
- ▶ How would you monitor and support this patient's status?

ANSWERS TO CASE 19: Sepsis

Summary: A 59-year-old diabetic woman is found to be unconscious, febrile, with tachycardia and hypotension. Laboratory analysis reveals a leukocytosis with likely urinary tract infection, and imaging shows involvement of the upper genitourinary system. In the ICU, she develops sudden hypotension and tachycardia.

- **Most likely diagnosis:** Acute urinary tract infection related sepsis and septic shock.
- **Priorities in management:** Fluid resuscitation and antimicrobial therapy.
- **Monitoring and support of organ perfusion:** Intravascular fluid status can be assessed and monitored with CVP catheters or echocardiography. Mean arterial pressure and mixed-venous O_2 measurements are helpful to determine patient's responses to therapy. The patient's mental status, urine outputs, and serum lactate levels during the course of resuscitation are also useful indicators of response to resuscitation. Specific monitoring and support guidelines are available in the Surviving Sepsis Campaign publications.

ANALYSIS

Objectives

1. To learn the guidelines and principles for the management of septic patients.
2. To learn the monitoring and strategies for patients with septic shock.
3. To learn the pharmacologic support for patients with septic shock.
4. To learn the role of glucocorticoid therapy for septic shock.

Considerations

This patient is suffering from shock. Shock is defined as inadequate oxygen delivery to meet the patient's tissue metabolic demands. Her initial altered mental status and concentrated urine are overt signs of inadequate end organ perfusion. There are many ways to classify shock. One useful way to think about the etiologies of shock is to divide them into hypovolemic, cardiac, or distributive processes. Hypovolemic shock is caused by hemorrhage or dehydration. Cardiac processes include intrinsic cardiac dysfunction as well as extrinsic causes such as tamponade or tension pneumothorax. In contrast, sepsis is a distributive process caused by acute vasodilation without an accompanying increase in fluid volume. The acute vasodilation leads to an increase in the capacitance of the circulatory system without an increase in volume, leading to a relative hypovolemia. Other distributive causes of shock include anaphylaxis, neurogenic shock, and third spacing seen with systemic inflammation. Sepsis is related to the systemic inflammatory response syndrome (SIRS), which is characterized by hypo or hyperthermia (temperature $<36°C$ or $>38°C$), tachycardia, tachypnea, leukocytosis, or leukocytopenia. Sepsis can be diagnosed when the features of SIRS are present and an infection is the suspected cause. The diagnosis of sepsis does not necessarily mean that shock is present. Septic shock is the diagnosis when there is ongoing hypotension despite fluid resuscitation. Antimicrobial therapy should be initiated to address the infectious process. The initial approach toward the correction of hypotension is to restore intravascular volume with crystalloid administration, and once this is accomplished, persistent hypotension is further addressed with the addition of vasoactive pharmacologic agents and corticosteroids as indicated.

APPROACH TO: Sepsis

DEFINITIONS

SHOCK: Inadequate oxygen delivery to meet the needs of the body's tissues.

CENTRAL VENOUS PRESSURE: The pressure measured in the superior vena cava reflecting right ventricle end diastolic pressure. It is measured with a centrally inserted venous catheter usually inserted in the internal jugular or subclavian vein. CVP is used clinically to assess volume status in critically ill patients. The CVP is not reliable in patients with tricuspid valve disease.

SIRS: The systemic inflammatory response is a clinical syndrome describing the derangement of the body's inflammatory response. A patient with 3 or more of the findings below meets criteria for the diagnosis of SIRS:

- Temperature <36°C or >38°C
- Heart rate >90 beats/minute
- Respiratory rate >20 breaths/minute
- White blood cell count >12,000 or <4,000/mm^3

SEPSIS: When the etiology of SIRS is presumed to be infectious in origin, the diagnosis of sepsis is made.

SEVERE SEPSIS: Sepsis with at least 1 organ system dysfunction.

SEPTIC SHOCK: Septic shock is present when there is ongoing hypotension despite fluid resuscitation.

EARLY GOAL-DIRECTED THERAPY: A treatment strategy for sepsis with the goal of rapid restoration of tissue perfusion by manipulation of cardiac preload, afterload, contractility as well as oxygen-carrying capacity.

CLINICAL APPROACH

Guidelines and Principles for the Management of Septic Patients

There is a spectrum of severity of sepsis. Uncomplicated sepsis may be caused by gastroenteritis or influenza, and may only require supportive care with or without antibiotic therapy. **Severe sepsis carries a mortality of 25% to 30%. Septic shock is the most severe form of sepsis where mortality can be as high as 50%.**

There are 2 main treatment goals in the approach of septic shock: (1) address the source of the infection, and (2) restore perfusion to the tissues to prevent reversible and irreversible organ injuries. Addressing issues number 1 and 2 listed above should occur simultaneously and as soon as the patient is encountered. Randomized trials have shown that patient survival is improved with early intervention, so patients who meet criteria for the diagnosis of septic shock should be treated as rapidly as possible even if that means starting treatment in the emergency department rather than in the ICU.

Therapy is guided by the information gained from continuous monitoring. Since the vasodilation associated with sepsis may produce relative hypovolemia and distributive shock, aggressive fluid resuscitation may be needed to restore intravascular volume and blood pressure. **The first goal is to achieve a CVP of 8 to 12 mm Hg, a mean arterial pressure (MAP) of >65 mm Hg, and urine output of > 0.5 mL/kg/h.** Sometimes this can be achieved with fluids alone. However, if fluids alone do not achieve these goals, a vasopressor may be needed. One of the targets of resuscitation is to improve central venous oxygen content (Cvo_2) to >70%; if this target is not achieved with fluids, blood transfusions can be given to maintain an appropriate hematocrit. In some patients with severe primary cardiac dysfunction, dobutamine infusion may be initiated to improve cardiac output, Cvo_2, and tissue oxygen delivery.

While the patient is being resuscitated, the source of their infection needs to be identified. Antibiotics should not be withheld during the investigative period. **Empiric, broad-spectrum antibiotics should be started within 1 hour of recognition of septic shock.** The workup includes obtaining blood, urine, and sputum cultures as well as any other appropriate cultures. Imaging may be required to identify other etiologies such as pneumonia or intra-abdominal infections. Once the source of the infection is identified, antibiotic therapy can be tailored based on cultures and antibiotic-resistance profiles.

Monitoring and Strategies for Patients with Septic Shock

The treatment of shock requires continuous monitoring of the hemodynamic status. A central venous catheter can monitor central venous pressure (CVP) as well as Cvo_2 which reflects overall oxygen demand and consumption. A low Cvo_2 suggests inadequate oxygen delivery to the tissue beds. An arterial catheter is often placed to monitor blood pressure and more specifically mean arterial pressure. Finally a Foley catheter is used to ensure adequate urine output, which reflects end organ perfusion.

In some instances a Swan-Ganz catheter, also known as a pulmonary artery catheter (PAC) may be used to obtain more information about cardiac status. For instance the PAC can be used to determine the cardiac filling pressures, cardiac output, and systemic vascular resistance. **The utility of PAC in critically ill patients is controversial, specifically whether it improves survival.** Some of the variables obtained by the PAC can also be determined by echocardiography. Laboratory analysis can also help determine the adequacy of resuscitation. For instance, serial blood lactate levels can be used to monitor the response to treatment. Decreasing trend in lactate levels may indicate that tissue oxygenation is being restored. Similarly, base excess on the arterial blood gas should normalize if oxygen delivery to the tissues is improving.

Pharmacologic Support for Patients with Septic Shock

A primary therapeutic goal in the treatment of septic shock is to restore tissue oxygenation. This is achieved through optimization of preload, cardiac contractility, afterload, and oxygen-carrying capacity. While fluid resuscitation and blood transfusions can improve preload and oxygen-carrying capacity, in severe cases additional pharmacologic support may be required to improve cardiac contractility and afterload.

In hypotension that is unresponsive to fluids, vasopressor therapy is needed. When the MAP is low, auto-regulation of blood pressure to the tissue beds is impaired such that perfusion is entirely dependent on the blood pressure. A vasopressor can improve perfusion pressure and maintain blood flow to the tissues. The **Surviving Sepsis Campaign recommends norepinephrine (Levophed) or dopamine at the lowest dose necessary to maintain tissue perfusion.** Epinephrine may be given if an additional agent is needed. The assessment of the adequacy of tissue perfusion can be determined using blood pressure, Cvo_2, urine output, normalization of blood lactate concentrations, and normalization of base excess on arterial blood gas. Some patients with septic shock do not respond to vasopressors due to relative vasopressin deficiency and would benefit from the **addition of vasopressin** at a constant infusion rate of 0.03 U/min. **Dobutamine** is a β-agonist that increases cardiac contractility and therefore increases cardiac output. Dobutamine is given when the Cvo_2 is low or when myocardial dysfunction is suspected based on elevated filling pressures or low cardiac output. By increasing cardiac output, oxygen delivery to the tissues may be improved in these individuals.

The Role of Glucocorticoid Therapy in Septic Shock

Some critically ill patients have a relative adrenal insufficiency and may benefit from glucocorticoid supplementation. The randomized controlled French multicenter trial involving septic patients with persistent hypotension after appropriate fluid and vasopressor therapy demonstrated improvements in shock reversal and a reduction in mortality when patients received corticosteroids. It is not necessary to prove that a patient has adrenal insufficiency with cortisol stimulation testing prior to giving supplementation. Subsequently, another large European randomized controlled trial (CORTICUS) showed that septic patients who did not require vasopressors did not benefit from corticosteroids treatments, therefore suggesting that **patient selection criteria for corticosteroids treatment in the ICU are very important.**

CLINICAL CASE CORRELATION

- **See also Case 3 (Scoring System/Patient Prognosis), Case 17 (Meningitis/Encephalitis), Case 18 (Antibiotics), and Case 20 (Immune-Compromised Patient With Sepsis).**

COMPREHENSION QUESTIONS

19.1 A 52-year-old man presents with right upper quadrant pain and jaundice. In the emergency department he is found to have a fever of 39.2°C, a heart rate of 112 beats/minute, and a blood pressure of 92/40 mm Hg. He has not urinated for 12 hours. He is tender in the right upper quadrant and has a leukocytosis of 19,000/mm^3. Which of the following is the best next step in his treatment?

A. Admission to the intensive care unit

B. Right upper quadrant ultrasound

C. Intravenous fluid administration

D. Placement of a pulmonary artery catheter

E. Place a Foley catheter for urine output monitoring

19.2 A 56-year-old woman is admitted with pneumonia and suspected sepsis. Which of the following is the most appropriate set of therapeutic endpoint in the treatment of sepsis?

A. Central venous oxygen >70%, urine output >0.5 mL/kg/h, mean arterial pressure of >85 mm Hg

B. Central venous pressure of >4 mm Hg, urine output >0.5 mL/kg/h, mean arterial pressure >55 mm Hg

C. Central venous oxygen >70%, urine output >10 mL/kg/h, central venous pressure 8 to 12 mm Hg

D. Central venous pressure of 8 to 12 mm Hg, temperature <38.5°C, mean arterial pressure >55 mm Hg

E. Central venous pressure of 8 to 12 mm Hg, urine output >0.5 mL/kg/h, mean arterial pressure >65 mm Hg

19.3 A 62-year-old woman is diagnosed with sepsis due to an intra-abdominal abscess from perforated diverticulitis. While awaiting CT-guided drainage of the abscess what is the best way to treat her infection?

A. Start broad-spectrum antibiotics now.

B. Start antibiotics based on Gram stain from the abscess fluid.

C. Wait to start antibiotics until blood culture results return.

D. Only give antibiotics if she does not improve after drainage of the abscess.

E. Once CT-guided drainage is performed, there would be no need for antibiotics therapy.

ANSWERS TO QUESTIONS

19.1 **C.** This patient meets the criteria for the diagnosis of SIRS given his fever, tachycardia, hypotension, and leukocytosis. Additionally his clinical presentation is consistent with infectious cholangitis. Since he meets the criteria for SIRS and an infection is suspected, the diagnosis of sepsis should be made, furthermore his ongoing hypotension and low urine output indicate that he is in septic shock. Early goal-directed therapy with the goal of restoring tissue oxygen delivery improves survival from sepsis, so the first step in the treatment of this patient should be fluid resuscitation. Antibiotics should be initiated within 1 hour of presentation. After fluids have been started, monitors for CVP and blood pressure can be placed. Diagnosing the source of his infection should be done as well but a right upper quadrant ultrasound is not the initial step in his treatment. While he may ultimately require admission to the ICU, therapy should not be delayed while awaiting transfer to the ICU.

19.2 **E.** The goals of therapy for early goal-directed treatment of sepsis reflect the need to restore oxygen delivery to the tissues. Temperature is not an endpoint used to measure the adequacy of tissue oxygenation. Central venous pressure allows for an assessment of overall fluid status, a CVP <8 is consistent with hypovolemia, whereas a CVP of 8 to 12 mm Hg is desired. Adequate urine output (>0.5 mL/kg/h) indicates good end organ perfusion. Normal central venous oxygen saturation (>70%) similarly implies adequate oxygen delivery to the end organs. A mean arterial pressure of >65 mm Hg is the target.

19.3 **A.** In septic patients, institution of early antibiotic therapy, within 1 hour of diagnosis, is very important. While cultures should be obtained, it is not necessary to prove that infection exists or to identify the infecting organism before starting therapy. It is better to start broad-spectrum antimicrobials initially and then tailor them when culture data is available or stop them entirely if no source is identified.

CLINICAL PEARLS

- Sepsis is diagnosed when there are 2 or more criteria for SIRS and an infection is suspected.
- Rapid reversal of hypoperfusion improves survival in sepsis.
- Treatment of sepsis involves fluid administration, vasopressor therapy, blood transfusions as needed, antibiotics, and infectious source control.

REFERENCES

Dellinger RP, Levy MM, Carlet JM, et al. Surviving Sepsis Campaign: International guidelines for management of severe sepsis and septic shock: 2008. *Crit Care Med* 2008;36:296-327.

Holcroft JW, Trunkey DD, Carpenter MA. Shock. *American College of Surgeons*. 6th ed. New York, NY: WebMD Publishing; 2007.

Rivers E, Nguyen B, Havstad S, et al. Early goal-directed therapy in the treatment of severe sepsis and septic shock. *N Engl J Med*. 2001;345:1368-1377.

Surviving Sepsis Campaign. http://www.survivingsepsis.org, accessed July 2, 2013.

CASE 20

A 45-year-old renal transplant patient has persistent fevers on ICU day 4. He was diagnosed with pneumonia confirmed by chest x-ray, and his laboratory tests identified neutropenia. He received cyclosporine to prevent rejection of his graft, and he is no longer dependent on hemodialysis since his transplant. His absolute neutrophil count (ANC) is 90 cells/mm^3 (normal >1500 cells/mm^3) with a white blood cell count (WBC) of 1000 cells/mm^3. Reverse isolation (protecting the patient from his environment) and triple antibiotic therapy with IV vancomycin, levofloxacin, and ceftazidime were started empirically. A central line is placed for fluid support. Blood, urine, and sputum specimens were taken for Gram stain, routine culture, acid fast stain and culture, fungus smears and cultures, and cytology. The patient has a history of being purified protein derivative (PPD) positive 20 years ago, and he currently works as a nurse in an acute care hospital. Despite the empiric antimicrobial therapy, he continues to appear ill and has a temperature of 101.3°F.

- ▶ What is the best management for this patient?
- ▶ What is the cause(s) for immunosuppression with this patient?

ANSWERS TO CASE 20:
Sepsis in the Immune-Compromised Patient

Summary: This 45-year-old male renal transplant patient on immunosuppressive therapy (including cyclosporine) is admitted to the ICU with pneumonia and neutropenia. He is a nurse with a history of being PPD positive and is no longer hemodialysis-dependent. Broad-spectrum antimicrobial therapy was started and a CVP was placed. He remains febrile and toxic after 4 days of treatment in the ICU.

- **Best management:** Start IV antifungal therapy. Adjust antimicrobials based on culture reports and clinical response (improvement or lack of improvement).
- **Cause(s) for immunosuppression**: Renal transplant, severe cyclosporine-induced neutropenia, and an indwelling catheter.

ANALYSIS

Objectives

1. To discuss immunosuppression and its causes in the intensive care setting.
2. To know the likely pathogens based on types of immunosuppressed patients in the ICU.
3. To know the immune dysfunction in sepsis and the proinflammatory and anti-inflammatory states.
4. To know the potential methods for monitoring the immune status of a critically ill patient.

Considerations

The patient is an immunosuppressed 45-year-old man with risk factors for infection from antibiotic-resistant bacteria and fungi: renal transplantation and its attendant immunosuppressive therapy, neutropenia, antimicrobial therapy (alteration in flora and potential selection of resistant organisms), indwelling catheters (renal transplant patient with hemodialysis catheter), hospitalization, prior occupational exposure to methicillin-resistant *Staphylococcus aureus* (MRSA), vancomycin-resistant enterococci (VRE), vancomycin-intermediate *Staphylococcus aureus* (VISA) and multidrug-resistant organisms (MDROs) as well as being a practicing nurse. Additionally, he has a positive PPD test. An antifungal agent should be added to this patient's antimicrobial regimen, because of his immunosuppressed status. *Candida* species would be greatest threat, as they are now the fourth leading cause of blood stream infection (BSI) in the ICU. The antibiotics currently used may be adequate to control most bacterial infections in this setting; however, he is at risk for resistant organisms including: MRSA, VISA, VRE, and gram-negative MDROs. The patient is immunosuppressed to assist survival of his renal transplantation, and his persistent neutropenia is due to his therapy (cyclosporine).

Since he has not responded to standard antimicrobial therapy, an antifungal agent (a triazole such as Fluconazole or echinocandin such as Cancidas) should be added while culture reports are pending. His antibiotic regimen should also be reassessed and possibly changed to cover the earlier-noted bacterial organisms, realizing the possibility of treatment failure with the vancomycin, ceftazidime, and levofloxacin. Further, the history of a positive PPD and potential work exposure to tuberculosis puts him at risk for reactivation or possibly a case of primary TB.

APPROACH TO:
Pneumonia and Sepsis in an Immune-Compromised ICU Patient

DEFINITIONS

ABSOLUTE NEUTROPHIL COUNT (ANC): The absolute number of neutrophils per microliter (mm^3) is the percentage of neutrophils in the WBC. ANCs of $<100/mm^3$ is neutropenia and creates a high risk for certain pathogens/opportunistic organisms such as *Aspergillus* sp., especially if neutropenia lasts >7 days.

For example, WBC = 1000/mm^3 with 10% neutrophils = 10% = 1,000 × 0.1 = ANC of 100/mm^3.

IMMUNNOSUPPRESSION: A decreased or lack of host's immune response and ability to fight infection.

OPPORTUNISTIC PATHOGENS (OIs): Organisms (bacterial, viral, fungal, parasitic), which are usually *not* pathogens in immunocompetent hosts.

MRSA: *Staphylococcus aureus* resistant to methicillin due to the presence of β-lactamases.

VISA: *Staphylococcus aureus* which is partially resistant to vancomycin based on decreased penetration of vancomycin across the cell wall.

MDRO: Gram-negative rod-shaped bacteria, which are resistant to multiple antimicrobials. This resistance is usually plasmid mediated (eg, *Klebsiella pneumoniae*, *Pseudomonas aeruginosa*, *Escherichia coli*, *Enterobacter* sp., *Acinetobacter* sp.).

SIRS: SIRS is nonspecific and can be caused by ischemia, inflammation, trauma, infection, or a combination of several insults. SIRS is not always related to infection and is defined as 2 or more of the following variables: fever of more than 38°C or <36°C; heart rate exceeding 90 beats/minute, respiratory rate exceeding 20 breaths/minute or a $PaCO_2$ level of <32 mm Hg, an abnormal white blood cell count (>12,000/μL or <4000/μL or >10% bands).

SEPSIS: Sepsis is a clinical term used to describe SIRS with defined or suspected infection, with or without organ dysfunction. Sepsis is a complex syndrome that is difficult to define, diagnose, and treat. It is a range of clinical conditions caused by the body's systemic response (SIRS) to an infection; if severe sepsis develops, accompanied by single or multiple organ dysfunction or failure, there is a high risk of death.

Sepsis is a major cause of mortality, killing approximately 1400 people worldwide every day.

CLINICAL APPROACH

Immunosuppression may be subdivided into congenital, acquired, and iatrogenic or drug/therapy origins (see Table 20–1). **The most common inherited cause in adults is described as a common variable immunodeficiency (CVI),** where there is insufficient production of antibodies to infectious agents. CVI can be treated with pooled human immune globulin supplementation. Immunosuppression can result from infections such as HIV (the virus that produces AIDS), measles, and cancers. HIV/AIDS and lymphomas can cause significant decreases in T-cell–mediated immunity. **AIDS has emerged as the most common cause of suppressed cell-mediated immunity (CMI).** Fortunately, HAART (highly active anti-retroviral therapy) and the application of antimicrobial prophylaxis have made a deep impact on the survival of AIDS patients. Therapy-induced immunosuppression may be caused by a variety of drugs and treatments. These include corticosteroids, azathioprine, methotrexate, mycophenolate mofetil, cyclophosphamide, infliximab, rituximab, an increasing number of chemotherapeutic agents, and irradiation or radiation therapy, to list a few.

Infection Prevention

The immune system's primary function is to prevent infection. When the immune system is suppressed, dysfunctional, or absent, the patient's ability to combat infections is reduced and the incidence of infections is increased. These infections may arise from microorganisms called **"opportunistic infections" (OI)** that do not normally cause infectious diseases. Infections are usually more severe in immunosuppressed patients, and have a greater potential to result fatally. The best methods to protect these patients are to avoid unnecessary or overly aggressive immunosuppressive therapy as much as possible, avoid exposure to infectious agents, and reconstitute the immune system when possible. Other preventive strategies include appropriate immunizations, prophylactic antimicrobials, and following isolation and handwashing policies.

Table 20–1 • MAJOR TYPES OF IMMUNE DEFECTS: SPECIFIC DEFECTS, CONDITIONS AND DISEASES

- Disruption or inflammation of mucosa and/or skin (including indwelling "lines")
- Phagocytic defects: neutropenia, chemotaxis, killing defects
- Humoral or antibody (B-cell) defects: hypogammaglobulinemia, IgA deficiency
- Complement system defects: low complement deficiencies, C3 and C5 (*S. pneumoniae, Haemophilus influenzae* infection); high complement deficiencies, C5b, C6, C7, C8, C9 (*Neisseria meningitidis, Neisseria gonorrhoeae* infection)
- Cell-mediated (T-cell) defects: eg, HIV/AIDS and lymphoma
- Splenectomy or hyposplenism defects: encapsulated organism, opsonization defects

Improvements in transplantation, HIV therapy, cancer therapy, and prevention in immunosuppression has resulted in better understanding of the diagnosis, prevention, and therapy of those affected in these settings. Travel and immigration has further complicated this venue with the "globalization of infections."

For neutropenic patients, reverse isolation is important. Also raw vegetables should be avoided unless they are irradiated, to prevent the transfer of bacteria to the patient's gastrointestinal system via the food. Indwelling catheters should be avoided and monitored closely when used. Attention to hand washing and the proper use of gloves, facial masks, and clothing is essential. The proper application of hand hygiene is critical in the prevention of these infections, but compliance among health-care workers is below 40%. In some cases, **granulocyte colony-stimulating factor (G-CSF)** is needed. Health-care associated infections are the most common adverse events resulting from hospitalization. Approximately 5% to 10% of hospitalized patients in the developed world acquire such infections.

ICU Care

Improvements in patient survival with comorbid disease and advances in critical care management have resulted in an increase in the number of patients in the ICU who are immunocompromised. An immunocompromised host may have alterations in phagocytic, cellular, or humoral immunity that increase the risk of infectious complications or provide an opportunistic process from a therapy-induced lymphoproliferative disorder or cancer.

Additionally, patients may also become immunocompromised if they have an alteration or breach of their skin or mucosal defense barriers that permits microorganisms to initiate a local or a systemic infection (eg, indwelling vascular catheters, Foley catheters, endotracheal tubes, and erosions of the mucosa or skin). Specific organisms must be considered in the setting of immunosuppression based on the type of defect(s) present.

Specific Organisms

Although the causes of fever in immunocompromised hosts are numerous and often never elucidated, some guidance to therapy is given by knowing the specific immunologic defect or defects present in the patient (Table 20–2). The **duration of immune defense alteration has an extremely important effect on the types of infectious complications** that are likely to occur. This includes ICU patients who are immunocompromised because of cancer or its treatment, those undergoing transplantation of bone marrow or solid organs, patients who have had a splenectomy, and patients with human immunodeficiency virus (HIV) infection or the acquired immunodeficiency syndrome (AIDS). Recognizing specific issues and challenges in the management of immunocompromised patients and focusing on infectious complications is vital in patient survival and well being in the ICU setting (see Table 20–3).

Sepsis

Sepsis is a major cause of morbidity and mortality in intensive care units (ICUs) and accounts for more than 210,000 deaths annually in the United States. The number of septic patients is increasing every year, and the mortality rate from sepsis remains high. Clinically, **sepsis initially presents as a hyperinflammatory response** to the immune system to attenuate the inflammation, and **then progresses to an immune system down-regulation**, which can result in prolonged immune dysfunction.

Table 20–2 • IMMUNE DEFECTS AND COMMONLY ASSOCIATED PATHOGENS

Immune Defect	Commonly Associated Pathogens
Skin and mucosal disruption	*Burns: Pseudomonas aeruginosa, S. aureus*, MRSA, VRE, VISA, trauma: *S. pyogenes, S. epidermidis*
Phagocytic defects: Neutropenia Chemotaxis Killing defects	Gram-positive cocci >GNR ("enteric"), *P. aeruginosa, Aspergillus* and *Candida* sp., *S. aureus*, GNR ("enterics") *S. aureus, Burkholderia cepacia*, GNR, *Aspergillus*
Humoral immunity, hypogammaglobulinemia, IgA deficiency, asplenia, hyposplenism	*S. pneumoniae, H. influenzae* Pyogenic bacteria, *Giardia lamblia* *S. pneumoniae, H. influenzae*
Cell-mediated immunity	Intracellular bacteria (*Listeria monocytogenes*), viruses (HSV, VZV, CMV), fungi (*Candida* sp., *Cryptococcus neoformans* spp.), Parasites (*Toxoplasma gondii*)
Complement defects: C3 or C5, C5b, C6, C7, C8, C9	*S. pneumoniae, H. influenzae* *N. meningitidis, N. gonorrhoeae*

This period of immune hyporesponsiveness, or immunoparalysis, limits host defense against primary infections, thereby predisposing the secondary nosocomial infections, multiorgan dysfunction, and ultimately death. The pathophysiology of these events is still not completely understood.

Host Response

The host response to infection is complex and varies depending on type of infection, the infective dose (bacterial load), and host genetic factors. Microbial invasion of a healthy patient activates both the acquired and innate immune systems. During an infectious process the host's leukocytes (eg, macrophages) respond to exogenous danger signals that are the pathogens-associated molecular patterns (PAMPs). Endogenous mediators released during the anti-microbial response amplify this response. This proinflammatory state helps to localize infections by recruiting phagocytes and immune cells to the area(s) of infection, but when it is exaggerated, septic shock and multi-organ dysfunction syndrome (MODS) can result. Antigen is presented to naïve T-cells in the lymphoid organs. These cells are then primed to differentiate into either helper T (TH) type-1 or -2 cells. TH-1 cells are involved in cell-mediated immunity and secrete interferon-γ (IFN-γ) and IL-2, whereas TH-2 cells participate in humoral-antibody–mediated immunity and secrete IL-10, IL-4, IL-5, and transforming growth factor-β (TGF-β). This shift to TH-2 cells is a hallmark of how the inflammatory response is down-regulated. This has been called the **compensatory anti-inflammatory response syndrome (CARS).** CARS may occur in patients who survive the initial SIRS/sepsis syndrome response when the proinflammatory state resolves and who then enter a state of immune suppression and dysfunction. Most deaths in sepsis occur late in the course of the syndrome

Table 20–3 • CAUSES OF FEVER BY IMMUNOSUPPRESSION AND SITE

Site	Bone Marrow Transplant	Kidney Transplant	Liver Transplant	Lung Transplant	Heart Transplant	Adult HIV Infection/ AIDS
Blood	Bacteremia, fungemia	Bacteremia	Uncommon	Uncommon	Uncommon	*S. pneumoniae*
Lung	Sinusitis, fungal Bacterial/fungal pneumonia with neutropenia Cytomegalovirus 30-60 d after allogenic transplant	Uncommon	Uncommon	Common pneumonia local or diffuse, many are fungal	Common, local or diffuse	Bacterial sinusitis, otitis Pneumonia: *P. jirovecii, S. pneumoniae, Cryptococcus-Pseudomonas*
Liver	Hepatosplenic candidiasis while recovering from neutropenia	Uncommon	Hepatitis, cholangitis, abscess	Uncommon	Uncommon	Hepatitis A, B, and C Perianal herpes simplex
CNS	*Toxoplasma, Nocardia, Cryptococcus* uncommon, *Aspergillosis* sp.	*Listeria*, uncommon	*Listeria*, uncommon	*Listeria*, uncommon	*Listeria*, uncommon	*Toxoplasma*, cryptococcal meningitis, neurosyphilis, cytomegalovirus
Skin	Bone marrow same as high risk	CMV	Uncommon	Uncommon	Uncommon	Herpes simples, cytomegalovirus, varicella zoster virus

Table 20–4 • THE PROINFLAMMATORY AND ANTI-INFLAMMATORY STATES	
Proinflammatory Cytokines "Sepsis/Severe Sepsis Syndrome"	**Compensatory Anti-inflammatory Response Syndrome "CARS"**
TNF-α	TH-2 cells, TH-1 cells, interferon-γ (IFN-γ)
IL-6	IL-10
IL-1	IL-4
Acute phase proteins are released	IL-5

and during the later phase of immune suppression or anti-inflammatory state (Table 20–4).

Posttransplant Immunosuppression

Recent new immunosuppressants have recorded a significant reduction in the incidence of acute graft rejection, and this success has not been accompanied by increases in infection or malignancy. The price for reducing the incidence of allograft rejection by these improved immunosuppressants was anticipated to be a proportional increase in the incidence of infection and malignancy. However, the newer immunosuppressants such as tacrolimus, mycophenolate mofetil (MMF), leflunomide, and sirolimus have actually shown a significant reduction in the incidence of acute rejection free of increases in infection and malignancy (Table 20–5).

Identifying Immune Dysfunction in the Septic Patient

The host immune response to sepsis is complex and involves many circulating mediators and cells. Various cytokines have been studied for their correlation with mortality. **Markedly elevated levels of circulating IL-6 and soluble-TNF receptors are correlated with the severity of disease and the 28-day mortality** from any cause; thus, this information may help determine when anti-inflammatory therapy may be beneficial. Blood levels of anti-inflammatory cytokines may help determine whether a patient is immunosuppressed. **Elevated and sustained levels of IL-10 and high IL-10/TNF-α ratios also were predictive of a poor outcome.** IL-10 and TGF-β are an immunosuppressive cytokine, and its continued presence in the septic patient may contribute to immune dysfunction. IL-10 may prove to be a useful marker of immune dysfunction but this supposition must be supported by larger trials before its clinical application is possible (Table 20–6).

Potential Therapies Aimed at Immune Dysfunction in Sepsis

Anti-inflammatory therapies, including TNF-α antagonists, IL-1 receptor antagonists, anti-endotoxin antibodies, corticosteroids, and granulocyte colony-stimulating factor (G-CSF) have not decreased overall mortality in patients with sepsis. IV immunoglobulin (IVIG) supplies specific antibodies to certain pathologic microbial factors, such as endotoxins, and elevated level of immunoglobulins depressed in sepsis. IVIG may be used as an adjunctive therapy for severe sepsis or septic shock. Activated protein C increases mortality and is no longer used.

Table 20–5 • TREATMENT OF IMMUNOCOMPROMISED PATIENTS WITH NEW FEVER

Condition	Treatment Plan
Low-risk cancer patient	Broad-spectrum antibiotics with a single parenteral agent (levofloxacin and amoxicillin plus clavulanate potassium)
High-risk cancer patient	Same as low risk or use a combination regimen; Consider additional treatment or modification if the patient has a persistent fever or neutropenia
Bone marrow transplantation	**Immediately postoperative:** same as high-risk cancer after receiving transplant; patients are at risk for CMV, *Varicella zoster virus*, other viral syndromes, as well as parasitic, and fungal infections **Greater than 100 days posttransplant (late infection):** likely from encapsulated bacteria, which are managed with antibiotic therapy
Kidney transplantation	Postoperative, treatment should be directed empirically with broad-spectrum antibiotics for septicemia, pyelonephritis, or pneumonia (consider CMV, viral, or parasitic infections)
Liver transplantation	Immediately postoperatively, treatment should be directed empirically for bacteremia, enteric organisms, and ascending cholangitis
Lung transplantation	**Immediately postoperative:** treat for a gram-negative bacteria from pneumonitis. Patients with cystic fibrosis and pseudomonas have a significant risk for this infection. **Late infection:** consider *Aspergillus*
Heart transplantation	**Immediately postoperative:** treat for gram-positive or gram-negative bacteria with a consideration for pneumonia or mediastinitus Common postoperative viral infections are CMV, EBV Common postoperative fungal infections are *Pneumocystis jiroveci* and *Toxoplasma*
Splenectomy	Give antibiotic regimen for encapsulated organisms
HIV/AIDS in children	Focus therapy for specific-site of infection (ie, URI vs UTI, etc). Treatment depends on the age-corrected CD4 count for low CD4 counts. Opportunistic infections: *Pneumocystitis carinii, Mycobacterium avium*, and *Cytomegalovirus* should be considered and treatment should be directed empirically.
HIV in adults	Treatment similar to children; with the exception of *Streptococcus pneumonia,* bacterial infections are less common. When the CD4 count is $<200\ mm^3$, treatment directed toward PCP or Toxoplasomosis With CD4 count $< 50\ mm^3$, treatment should be directed toward M. tuberculosis, *M. avium,* and *Cryptococcus.*

Table 20–6 • POSSIBLE DIAGNOSTIC MARKERS OF IMMUNE DYSFUNCTION
Increased initial and sustained IL-10 levels
High IL-10/TNF-α ratios
Decreased mHLA-DR expression
Interleukin-10 (IL-10); monocyte human leukocyte antigen type (mHLA-DR), tumor necrosis factor-α (TNF-α)

CLINICAL CASE CORRELATION

- **See also Case 17 (Meningitis/Encephalitis), Case 18 (Antibiotics), Case 19 (Sepsis), and Case 33 (Multiorgan Dysfunction)**

COMPREHENSION QUESTIONS

20.1 A previously healthy 27-year-old man was admitted to the ICU after an MVA. He was intubated, given fluid resuscitation, and blood transfusions prior to transfer to the OR for laparotomy due to a ruptured viscus (stomach). After surgery he was managed in the ICU with TPN, Foley catheterization, and completed 4 days of preventive antibiotic therapy for the ruptured viscus. He was extubated on the third day in ICU, but he was maintained on TPN following the laparotomy. On the sixth day in the ICU, his temperature spiked to >102°F. Upon examination he was noted to be toxic but had no identifiable focus of infection. A chest x-ray showed no lung infiltrate. What empiric therapy would you initiate pending the result of cultures for common pathogens?

A. Gram-negative bacterial sepsis following the ruptured viscus. Broad-spectrum antibiotics.

B. Candidemia. Start fluconazole or echinocandin (eg, caspofungin).

C. Influenza, rimantadine

D. Invasive aspergillosis; voriconazole

E. Hospital-acquired pneumonia (HAP); vancomycin and ceftazidime

20.2 A 55-year-old man is transferred to the ICU for evaluation of a fever of 103°F, pleuritic chest pain, shortness of breath, and hemoptysis. He is 21 days status post-allogenic bone marrow transplant (BMT) for acute myelogenous leukemia (AML). Chest x-rays revealed the presence of an infiltrate and a CT of the chest revealed a cavitary lesion with a "halo" sign. He remains profoundly neutropenic (<100 neutrophils/mm^3) and thrombocytopenic (10,000/mm^3). Examination reveals that he is tachypneic and tachycardic. Bronchoscopy shows hyphae budding at 45 degrees. What empiric therapy should be instituted?

A. Amphotericin B given IV. Open lung biopsy or transthoracic biopsy.
B. Voriconazole. Gram stain of sputum, determine galactomannan level.
C. Fluconazole IV. Bronchoscopy with transbronchial biopsy.
D. Echinocandin IV. Video-assisted thoracoscopy with directed biopsy for C and S and silver stain.
E. Treat empirically for tuberculosis.

ANSWERS TO QUESTIONS

20.1 **E.** The patient is at high risk for candidemia due to the ruptured viscus and upper GI surgery, indwelling lines with total parenteral nutrition (TPN), prior use of broad-spectrum antibiotics for the ruptured viscus, and blood transfusion. Other risk factors for candidemia in the ICU include neutropenia, hematologic malignancies, hemodialysis, burns, prior enteric bacteremia, and recent fluconazole use (<30 days). Unstable patients should be started preemptively or empirically on an echinocandin (eg, caspofungin): patient outcomes are related to both the early visit and choice of an effective therapy. Stable patients may be started on fluconazole pending the result of fungal cultures. Over 50% of patients in the ICU who develop candidemia are colonized with nonalbicans species of *Candida* (eg. *Candida glabrata*, *C. parapsilosis*, *C. tropicalis*, and *C. lusitaniae*). In ICU patients with invasive candidiasis/candidemia the removal or replacement of indwelling venous catheters and any other catheters and an evaluation of the importance of TPN should be routine and considered in all patients whenever unless absolutely unfeasible.

20.2 **B.** The patient has had an allogenic bone marrow transplantation (BMT) with prolonged and severe neutropenia. The finding of a "halo" sign, and hyphae budding at 45 degrees is highly consistent with an *Aspergillus* lung infection seen in 10% to 20% of patients with BMT; *Aspergillus* is most prominent due to effective prophylaxis of *Candida* with current protocols. Therapy of suspected *Aspergillus* lung infections must be instituted as early as possible to improve outcomes. Voriconazole is now the DOC for this infection. The diagnosis of pulmonary *Aspergillus* infections is confirmed by demonstrating the branching hyphae at an acute angle in silver stains of tissue biopsy, as it is a vasoinvasive hyphae and has subsequent positive cultures. Finding *Aspergillus* in his sputum and seeing a rise in his baseline galactomannan level (done weekly posttransplant) would be consistent with the diagnosis of IAI.

CLINICAL PEARLS

- Common variable immunodeficiency is the most common inherited immunodeficiency in adults.
- TH-2 cells may be important in transitioning from a hyper-inflammatory state to immune dysfunction in sepsis.
- Most deaths in sepsis occur late in syndrome and survivors show evidence of immune recovery.
- "Profound and prolonged" neutropenia is at a high risk for invasive *Aspergillosis.*
- Hand washing is the most important preventive strategy to reduce hospital-acquired infections.

REFERENCES

Clifford S, Deutschman MS. *Evidence Based Practice of Critical Care*. Philadelphia: Saunders; 2010.

Loscalzo J. *Harrison's Pulmonary and Critical Care Medicine*. New York, NY: McGraw-Hill; 2010.

Pizzo PA. Fever in immunocompromised patients. *N Engl J Med*. Sep 16 1999;341:893-900.

Toy EC, Simon B, Takenaka K, Liu T, Rosh A. *Case Files Emergency Medicine*. 2nd ed, New York: McGraw-Hill, Lange, 2009.

CASE 21

A 63-year-old man was hospitalized 6 days ago for an acute myocardial infarction. Today, he began to complain of vague epigastric pain; however, an ECG and cardiac enzymes test ruled out an MI. Several hours later, he began to feel dizzy and passed a large amount of dark bloody stool per rectum. Shortly thereafter, he vomited approximately 100 mL of blood. At this point, his blood pressure is 90/60 mm Hg and pulse rate is 85 beats/minute. He is transferred to the ICU for further monitoring.

- ▸ What are the priorities in this patient's management?
- ▸ What are the risk factors for this patient's condition?
- ▸ What are the factors that adversely affect the outcome?

ANSWERS TO CASE 21: Gastrointestinal Bleeding

Summary: A 63-year-old man who is hospitalized for a recent myocardial infarction develops signs and symptoms of acute upper GI hemorrhage. His vital signs are concerning for hemorrhagic shock.

Priorities in management: Establishing a secure airway and maintaining adequate circulating blood volume and definitive hemorrhage control. The patient should be resuscitated with the combination of crystalloids and blood products to optimize cardiac function and maintaining a normal coagulation process. This includes potential transfusions of packed red cells, platelets, and fresh-frozen plasma to correct any coagulation defects. Once the patient's physiologic status is stabilized, he should be prepared for upper GI endoscopy to diagnose and potentially treat his gastrointestinal bleeding.

Risk factors for this patient's condition: The patient is recovering from a recent myocardial infarction. The stress related to his current illness is a risk factor. In addition, patients with unstable cardiac conditions often receive antiplatelet therapy, which can increase his risk for bleeding complications.

Factors that adversely affect the outcome: There are many reported clinical and endoscopic factors that influence outcomes, some of which are applicable to this patient.

Clinical contributors to adverse outcome to patients with upper GI hemorrhage include shock on admission, comorbid illnesses, prior history of bleeding requiring transfusion, admission Hgb <8 g/dL, transfusion requirement of >5 U of PRBCs, blood in the NG aspirate that does not clear with lavage, and age > 65.

Endoscopic contributors of adverse outcome in acute upper gastrointestinal hemorrhage: visible vessel in ulcer base (> 50% rebleeding risk), active bleeding from ulcer base, adherent clot at ulcer base, location of ulcer (worse prognosis when located on posterior lesser curvature of stomach or posterior duodenal bulb), and ulcer diameter >2 cm.

ANALYSIS

Objectives

1. To learn the initial management and diagnostic strategy for patients with upper gastrointestinal bleeding.
2. To learn the management of patient with nonvariceal and variceal upper gastrointestinal bleeding.
3. To learn the differences in the management approaches to patients with upper GI bleeding and lower GI bleeding.

Considerations

This patient has acute upper gastrointestinal hemorrhage. He is older and is at an increased risk for a low-flow state due to potentially diminished cardiac output (from his recent myocardial infarction). Additionally, he has been in the hospital for 6 days and is at risk for stress-related ulcer formation and hemorrhage. Antiplatelet therapy has most likely been prescribed for his cardiac condition, which further increases his risk for bleeding complications. The major goal at this time is to optimize the support of his hemodynamic status without creating increased physiological stress. In addition, pharmacological therapy needs to be initiated as his bleeding is determined as most likely nonvariceal or variceal in origin. Appropriate resuscitation followed by timely diagnosis and endoscopy would be important.

APPROACH TO: Gastrointestinal Bleeding

DEFINITIONS

UPPER GI BLEEDING: Bleeding source is proximal to the ligament of Treitz (esophagus, stomach, and duodenum).

LOWER GI BLEEDING: Bleeding source is distal to the ligament of Treitz (jenunum, ileum, colon, and rectum).

OCCULT GI BLEEDING: Slow bleeding originating anywhere along the GI tract. Patients do not complain of bleeding symptoms and commonly present with anemia, fatigue, and hemoccult positive stool.

GASTRODUODENAL ULCERATION: Comprise the majority of upper GI bleeding episodes (50%), usually due to *Helicobacter pylori* (80%-90%).

PORTAL HYPERTENSION–ASSOCIATED BLEEDING: Esophagogastric varices are present in 30% to 60% of patients with cirrhosis. Significant mortality is attributable to the first bleeding episode (30%-50%).

STRESS GASTRITIS: The physiologic stress from trauma, burns, major surgery, or severe medical illness is associated with the development of hemorrhagic gastritis, or stress erosions in the fundus or gastric body.

ESOPHAGITIS: Gastroesophageal reflux disease (GERD) can predispose patients to mucosal ulceration and upper GI bleeding. Bleeding can also occur from erosion by a nasogastric tube (NGT), typically in the chronically hospitalized patient.

NSAID EROSIVE GASTROPATHY: NSAID-related ulcers can develop within 1 to 2 days of treatment and usually appear in the antral portion of the stomach. Ulcers typically present asymptomatically and resolve after cessation of treatment.

GASTRIC ANTRAL VASCULAR ECTASIA (GAVE): GAVE is a rare cause of upper GI bleeding overall. It is commonly referred to as "watermelon stomach" because of the watermelon striped-like appearance of mucosal erythema stemming from the pylorus (usually limited to the antrum). GAVE is associated with bone marrow transplants, scleroderma, and cirrhosis. A direct cause is not identified.

DIEULAFOY LESION: Dieulafoy is a large ectatic submucosal arteriole that erodes through the mucosal layer of the stomach. Most appear in the proximal stomach (up to 95%), predominantly on the lesser curvature and within 6 cm of the gastroesophageal junction.

PERCUTANEOUS TRANSARTERIAL EMBOLIZATION: This interventional radiology approach is an alternative to surgery in patients for whom endoscopic therapy has failed. The rate of technical success has been reported to range from 52% to 98% with recurrent bleeding in 10% to 20% of patients.

CLINICAL APPROACH

The initial management and diagnostic strategy for patients with upper gastrointestinal bleeding is noted in Figure 21–1. The ABC's of resuscitation should be employed for all patients with upper GI bleeding. Hemodynamically unstable patients (SBP ≤90, orthostatic hypotension), those with evidence of severe bleeding (HCT drop of >6%), or those with a transfusion requirement of >2 U PRBCs should be admitted to the ICU for resuscitation and close monitoring. Central venous pressure monitoring should be considered especially in patients with significant cardiopulmonary and renal comorbidities. The decision to initiate blood transfusions for patients should be based on individual patient's underlying conditions, hemodynamic and perfusion statuses rather than any predetermined hemoglobin values.

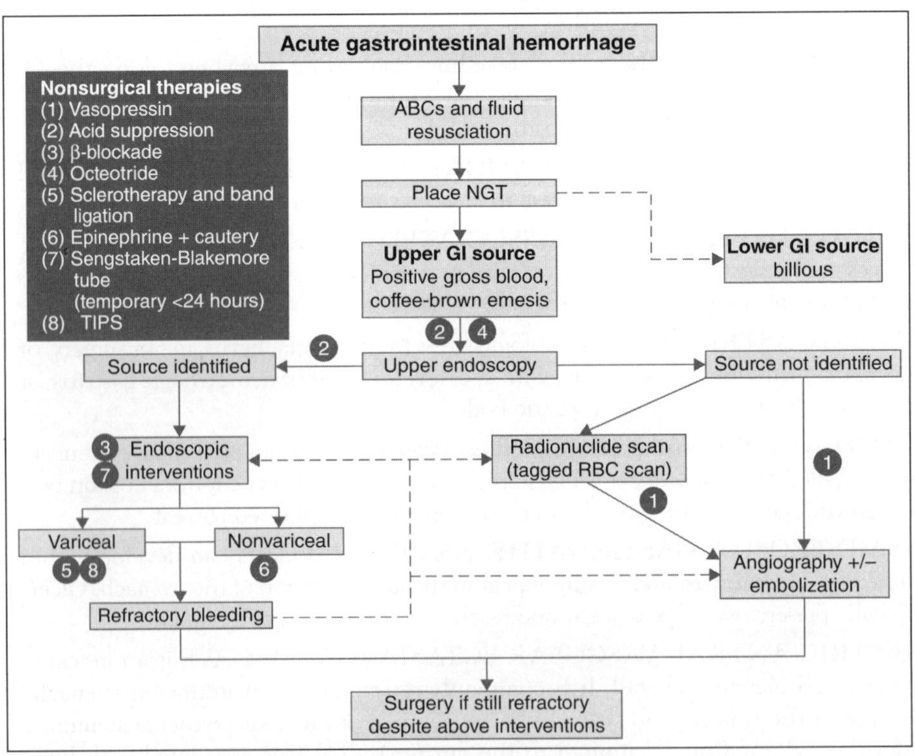

Figure 21–1. Management for acute upper gastrointestinal hemorrhage

Correction of coagulopathy (INR >1.5 or platelet count <50,000/mm^3) with fresh-frozen plasma or platelet transfusions is important in patients with ongoing bleeding. Patients receiving antiplatelet therapy should have platelet transfusions to provide functioning platelets, since numerically normal platelet counts do not necessarily indicate normal platelet functions. Decisions to reinitiate or terminate antiplatelet therapy should be based on the risks/benefits of individual patient's cardiovascular comorbidities versus bleeding risks.

After resuscitation, an initial attempt at determining whether the source is an upper or lower source should be made. In patients with massive upper GI tract bleeding, agitation, or impaired respiratory status, endotracheal intubation should be considered prior to the initiation of endoscopy. After the ABCs are stabilized and resuscitation is underway, an NGT should be placed. If the **aspirate is coffee-ground or bloody in nature, an upper GI source is confirmed.** Even if there is a clear aspirate, there still exists a small possibility that bleeding could be from the duodenum (closed pylorus). **Absence of blood or coffee-ground emesis in the presence of an open pylorus (presence of bilious NG aspirate) localizes bleeding to the lower GI tract.** In upper GI bleeding cases, the patient should proceed to upper endoscopy to definitively localize and potentially treat the lesion.

Upper GI endoscopy can identify the source and status of bleeding in 90% of cases. Early endoscopy (within 12 hours) is recommended for most patients with acute upper gastrointestinal hemorrhage, as it appears to improve the diagnostic sensitivity of the procedure. Endoscopic findings are often helpful to risk-stratify patients to low- or high risk for recurrent or life-threatening hemorrhage. This may assist in selecting patients who may be suitable for early hospital or ICU discharges or, alternatively, further ICU monitoring.

Administration of **intravenous erythromycin (3 mg/kg IV over 20-30 minutes) 30 to 90 minutes prior to endoscopy can often improve visibility, shorten endoscopy time, and reduce the need for second-look endoscopy.** Erythromycin is a motilin agonist in the GI tract, which promotes antegrade flow of gastric and duodenal contents.

Patients who are found to have mucosal ulcerations during esophagogastroduodenoscopy (EGD) should undergo biopsy of the gastric and antral mucosa to evaluate for *H. pylori*. Patients who are positive should receive triple therapy (clarithromycin 500 BID, amoxicillin 1 g BID, and a proton pump inhibitor [PPI]) for at least 1 week. PPI therapy should be stopped 1 week prior to repeat *H. pylori* testing (at 4 weeks) to prevent false-negative results.

In situations where endoscopy fails to identify the site or control the bleeding, angiographic techniques can also be applied to diagnose and treat the upper GI bleeding. Although the role of angiography is better defined for lower GI bleeding, selective angiography is useful for localization and embolization of upper GI bleeding in up to 75% of patients with active bleeding.

Management of Upper GI Bleeding

Medical treatment for both variceal and nonvariceal acute GI hemorrhage:

1. **Vasopressin:** Vasopressin can dramatically decrease the splanchnic blood flow and reduce upper GI bleeding. However, vasopressin and vasopressin analogues are now in disfavor due to the systemic vasoconstrictive effects, and for that

reason octreotide is a preferred adjunctive therapy in conjunction with EGD for variceal upper GI hemorrhage.

2. **Acid suppression:** Acid suppression with high-dose PPIs (pantoprazole 80 mg bolus followed by 8 mg/h infusion) given before or after endoscopy has been shown to significantly reduce the occurrence of rebleeding, decrease hospital stay, reduce the number of actively bleeding ulcers, and reduce transfusion requirements. In patients with NSAID-related ulcers, 4 weeks of outpatient PPI therapy is suggested.

Medical treatment for variceal acute GI hemorrhage:

1. **Octreotide:** Prior to endoscopy, octreotide (loading dose 50 μg, followed by 25-50 μg/h × 5 days) may be administered, which may reduce the risk of bleeding. Octreotide can also be used as adjunctive therapy if endoscopy is unsuccessful, contraindicated, or unavailable. Although it has been best studied in the variceal population, octreotide is also loosely indicated for treatment of acute nonvariceal upper gastrointestinal bleeding.

2. **β-Blockers:** Used as maintenance therapy after acute upper GI bleeding from portal hypertension has been controlled. Oral β-blockade plus endoscopic therapy has been shown to reduce the rebleeding rate over endoscopic therapy alone. Endoscopic band ligation followed by β-blockade is recommended treatment strategy for variceal bleeding.

Interventions for upper GI hemorrhage from variceal sources:

1. **Sclerotherapy and band ligation:** Endoscopic sclerotherapy and/or band ligation for esophageal varices is the mainstay of emergent treatment. However, the risk of rebleeding is significant—up to 50% with sclerotherapy and 35% with band ligation. Some evidence suggests that band ligation, when compared to sclerotherapy, is associated with fewer treatment-related complications. Lower rebleeding rates and improved survival have been reported with band ligation. For nonvariceal bleeding, endoscopic hemostasis may be achieved with the use of epinephrine injections followed by thermal therapy. Permanent hemostasis occurs in roughly 80% to 90% of patients.

2. **Sengstaken-Blakemore tube:** In rare circumstances where bleeding cannot be controlled endoscopically, the Sengstaken-Blakemore (SB) (Minnesota) tube can be used with the caveat that it must not be inflated for >48 hours due to the high risk of tissue necrosis. The gastric balloon is inflated first, and if bleeding is not controlled, the esophageal balloon is inflated. SB tube placement is helpful for the temporary control of bleeding so that arrangements can be made for definitive care (eg, TIPS or endoscopic therapy).

3. **Transjugular intrahepatic portosystemic shunt (TIPS):** Ideally applied in Child-Pugh class B or C cirrhotic patients. TIPS can provide a bridge to liver transplantation. In comparison to sclerotherapy or band ligation, rebleeding rates are lower with TIPS. However, TIPS is associated with an increased occurrence of hepatic encephalopathy but no difference in overall survival. Rebleeding following TIPS can occur when shunt thrombosis occurs.

Surgical treatment for upper GI hemorrhage:

1. **Surgical shunts:** Patients who are Child A are considered for surgical decompression (eg, distal splenorenal shunt) since the likelihood of occlusion for TIPS at 2 years outweighs the potential benefit of TIPS.
2. **Operative exploration:** Operative exploration for upper gastrointestinal hemorrhage is generally reserved for individuals who fail endoscopic treatment. Depending on the source of the hemorrhage, procedures may include bleeding vessel ligation, lesion resection, and/or acid reduction procedures (eg, vagotomy) to prevent future ulcer formation. Transplantation is a rare last resort for Child B and C patients in the emergent setting due to variceal bleeding.

CASE CORRELATION

- **See also Case 4 (Hemodynamic Monitoring), Case 5 (Vasoactive Drugs), Case 33 (Multiorgan Dysfunction), and Case 41 (Hemorrhage and Coagulopathy).**

COMPREHENSION QUESTIONS

21.1 A 55-year-old alcoholic with a history of alcoholic cirrhosis arrives to the ED vomiting copious amounts of blood, hypotensive (BP 88/50 mm Hg), tachycardic (HR 115 beats/minute), and with an O_2 saturation of 95%. He is intubated, resuscitated, and taken to the endoscopy suite for further therapy. Which of the following therapeutic modalities has the highest bleeding recurrence rate for the variceal population after initial endoscopic treatment?

A. Sclerotherapy alone
B. Band ligation alone
C. Sclerotherapy and band ligation
D. TIPS
E. Operative portal-systemic shunt

21.2 A 60-year-old man with a history of *H. pylori* antral ulcer treated with triple therapy 5 weeks ago comes to clinic for follow-up. He says his clinical condition has improved. He continues to take omeprazole for symptoms of GERD (last dose was this morning). What is the best laboratory measure for confirmation of eradication of *H. pylori* in this patient?

A. Repeat endoscopy with histologic examination
B. Anti-IgG against *H. pylori*
C. Urea breath test performed as soon as feasible
D. Campylobacter-like organism (CLO) test
E. Stop omeprazole for a week before urea breath best

21.3 A 65-year-old cirrhotic woman is brought to the emergency department with acute hematemesis and altered mental status. She is hypotensive, tachycardic, and vomiting blood. After intubation and fluid resuscitation, she is taken to the endoscopy suite where multiple large varicosities are seen at the GE junction. The gastroenterologist infuses octreotide and vasopressin, attempts band ligation, sclerotherapy, and a Minnesota tube, all of which slow but do not stop the bleeding. Her laboratory studies reveal the following: Hgb 5.8 g/dL, platelets 90,000/mm^3; INR 2.8; AST/ALT 86/90 IU/L, albumin 1.8 g/L; total bilirubin 2.1 mg/dL; BUN/Cr 80/2.6 mg/dL. After 8 U of PRBCs, 6 U of FFP, and 10 pack of platelets, she remains borderline hypotensive (95/60 mm Hg) and has continued bleeding. What would be the next best intervention?

A. Try another Sengstaken-Blakemore tube
B. Continue fluid resuscitation and transfusion
C. TIPS
D. Hepatic transplantation
E. Distal splenorenal (Warren) shunt

ANSWERS TO QUESTIONS

21.1 **A.** Multiple randomized trials have compared sclerotherapy versus sclerotherapy and band ligation versus band ligation alone. Meta-analyses suggest that rebleeding rates are highest in patients who undergo sclerotherapy alone (particularly patients with large varices). There is no additional benefit with regard to rebleeding if band ligation is accompanied by sclerotherapy in the same setting versus band ligation alone. For this reason, band ligation is the preferred first endoscopic modality, with 35% chance of rebleeding. TIPS is superior to endoscopic therapy, with rebleeding rates far less than band ligation and sclerotherapy. Operative portal-systemic shunts are associated with low rebleeding rates but high procedure-associated mortality.

21.2 **E.** This patient is >4 weeks out of treatment for *H. pylori* but continues to take a PPI which can cause false-negative results. The patient should be instructed to stop taking his omeprazole for a week and then return to clinic to perform a urea breath test to confirm eradication of his infection.

21.3 **C.** TIPS is the best option for this patient who is classified as a Child-Pugh class C cirrhotic. Of the other interventions, option (A) is incorrect because it is a temporizing measure. (B) is incorrect because the patient is likely developing a consumptive coagulopathy and progressing into DIC. (D) is not a good choice because it is not likely for her to receive a donor liver in an acute situation, and (E) is incorrect as Warren shunts are indicated only in Child A patients.

CLINICAL PEARLS

- Incidence of upper GI bleeding is approximately 170/100,000 patients a year, greater than lower GI bleeding.
- The mortality rate of upper GI bleeding is between 5% and 11%.
- Priorities in management for acute upper GI bleeding include securing an airway, volume resuscitation, and early upper endoscopy.
- The majority of upper GI bleeding cases are due to gastroduodenal ulceration, the majority of which can be managed endoscopically.
- Variceal hemorrhage is best managed by endoscopic techniques with TIPS as an alternative. Surgical shunts have fallen out of favor in the acute setting and TIPS is a viable bridge to hepatic transplantation.

REFERENCES

Jutabha R, Jensen D. Approach to upper gastrointestinal bleeding in adults. www.uptodate.com. October 8, 2010, accessed July 2, 2013.

Mulholland MW, Lillemoe KD, Doherty GM, et al. *Greenfield Surgery: Scientific Principles and Practice.* 4th ed. Philadelphia, PA: Williams and Wilkins; 2005.

Shuhart M, Kowldley K, Neighbor B. GI bleeding. http://www.uwgi.org/guidelines/ch_07/ch07txt.htm (Online Review). April 5, 2011, accessed July 2, 2013.

Townsend CM, Beauchamp RD, Evers BM, Mattox KL. *Sabiston Textbook of Surgery*. 18th ed. St. Louis, MO: W.B. Saunders Company; 2008.

CASE 22

A 26-year-old woman was brought to the emergency center after being found to be lethargic and vomiting at home by her roommate. The roommate, who had been on a business trip, had not seen the patient for 1½ days. On examination, the patient appears lethargic and mildly jaundiced. Her CBC is within normal limits. The serum liver transaminases are (ALT): 2500 IU/L and AST: 3100 IU/L. Serum glucose is 50 mg/dL, and total bilirubin is 2.8 mg/dL. Her prothrombin time is 45 seconds (INR 4), creatinine level is 2.6 mg/dL, and her arterial pH is 7.35. The serum acetaminophen concentration is 120 mcg/mL (normal <50 mcg/mL). The patient had an NG tube placed in the ED followed by gastric lavage and evacuation of gastric contents. In addition, she had activated charcoal treatment in the ED. She was later transferred to the ICU.

- What is the next step in treatment?
- What are the complications associated with this process?
- What are other treatment options in addition to medications and supportive measures?

ANSWERS TO CASE 22:
Acute Liver Failure

Summary: A 26-year-old woman is brought to the hospital with vomiting and lethargy. Her laboratory studies demonstrate marked elevation of the serum transaminases, elevation in her serum bilirubin, and creatinine. Her blood glucose and artery pH are low. Her serum acetaminophen level is elevated. Initial treatment with gastric lavage and activated charcoal has already been given prior to her arrival to the ICU. This is consistent with acute acetaminophen toxicity.

- **Next step:** Administer *N*-acetylcysteine (NAC) therapy by mouth. This can be mixed with a carbonated beverage to improve tolerance. The initial loading dose is 140 mg/kg followed by 70 mg/kg every 4 hours for 17 doses or until the INR decreases to <1.5. If the patient is unable to tolerate oral intake, then intravenous *N*-acetylcysteine can be administered.
- **Complications:** Complications that may occur as the result of acute liver failure include cerebral edema, infections (including bacterial and fungal infections), acute kidney injury, high-output hyperdynamic process, and coagulopathy and bleeding complications.
- **Treatments other than medications and supportive measures:** Patients with severe acute liver failures may need liver transplantation. Alternatively, some limited experiences have shown that acellular liver support devices or bioartificial liver support devices may be temporarily implemented to provide support while liver recovery occurs. Alternatively, bioartificial liver devices can also be used as a bridge for the support of patients with fulminant hepatic failure prior to liver transplantation.

ANALYSIS

Objectives

1. To learn the initial evaluation and diagnosis of acute hepatic failure.
2. To learn the causes of acute hepatic failure.
3. To learn the management of acute hepatic failure.
4. To learn to identify patients with acute hepatic failure who may need referral for liver transplantation.

Considerations

This patient's presentation is highly suspicious for acute liver failure due to acetaminophen overdose. However, because the circumstances of this overdose are uncertain, the initial evaluation must also include a toxicology screen for other possible medications and illicit drug-related causes, and a hepatitis screen for viral hepatitis. In addition, appropriate imaging and blood cultures to rule out sepsis as the potential cause of this multiple organ dysfunction are required. Because there were no witnesses to the ingestion, it is difficult to determine the timing of the over-ingestion of acetaminophen; therefore, gastric lavage and activated charcoal therapy provided in the emergency department were appropriate early measures. NAC administration is vital to minimize the liver toxicity in this patient, and this should be initiated as early as possible in the emergency department and continued in the ICU. ICU admission for observation is very appropriate for this patient, given her altered mental status, acute kidney injury, and metabolic acidosis that suggest serious toxicity from ingestion. A detailed neurological examination needs to be completed in addition to a CT scan of the brain, given the patient's initial presentation of lethargy. Her neurological presentation suggests possible grade 2 encephalopathy; in which case, the patient would be considered a potential candidate for referral to a liver transplant center. Even though acetaminophen-induced acute hepatic failure is the most common cause of acute liver failure in the United States, the survival is reported to be reasonably good at 78% to 80%, and >80% when NAC can be administered within 12 hours of ingestion.

APPROACH TO:
The Patient with Acute Hepatic Failure

DEFINITIONS

ACUTE HEPATIC FAILURE: Defined as the development of impaired liver synthetic function, coagulopathy, and hepatic encephalopathy in less than a 2- to 3-month period in a patient without underlying liver disease.

GRADING OF HEPATIC ENCEPHALOPATHY: The West Haven grading system is based on level of impaired autonomy, level of consciousness, intellectual function, and behavior.

GRADE 1: Trivial lack of awareness, shortened attention span, euphoria or anxiety, impaired performance of simple addition or subtraction, minimal change in level of consciousness.

GRADE 2: Lethargy or apathy, disorientation for place or time, subtle personality change, inappropriate behavior, asterixis.

GRADE 3: Somnolence or semi-stupor but with response to verbal stimuli; marked confusion and disorientation.

GRADE 4: Comatose and unresponsive to verbal or noxious stimuli; decorticate or decerebrate posturing.

N-ACETYLCYSTEINE (NAC): NAC helps detoxify the acetaminophen toxic metabolite (NAPQI). Ideally, NAC is given within 8 to 10 hours after ingestion, and protects against NAPGI-induced liver and renal injuries. NAC administration has been demonstrated to reduce the liver injury associated with acetaminophen overdose even when given within 16 hours after ingestion. The recommended dose is 140 mg/kg diluted in oral solution as a loading dose, followed by 70 mg/kg oral doses every 4 hours for 17 doses. Patients who are unable to tolerate oral intake can be given intravenous NAC with an initial loading dose of 150 mg/kg in D_5W over 15 minutes, followed by a maintenance infusion dose of 50 mg/kg over 4 hours, and then 100 mg/kg infusion over the next 16 hours.

LIVER SUPPORT SYSTEMS: Liver support devices are categorized as **acellular systems** that utilize albumin dialysis or **bioartificial liver (BAL) support systems**. The most common acellular system is the molecular reabsorbent and recirculating system (MARS). MARS has been shown to improve hemodynamic status, decrease encephalopathy, decrease intracranial pressure, and decrease serum bilirubin and creatinine. The bioartificial liver support systems are extracorporeal circulatory systems that utilize a veno-venal dialysis concept, where the patient's blood is circulated through a cell-based bioreactor. The bioreactors are loaded with either transformed human hepatocytes or porcine hepatocytes. Application of the BAL essentially provides patients with temporary liver-filtering and biosynthetic functions. Clinical applications of BAL have been shown to improve the 30-day survival of patients with acute liver failure.

KING'S COLLEGE HOSPITAL (KCH) CRITERIA: This is the most widely applied criteria for the selection of patients with acute liver failure for liver transplantation.

The **KCH criteria for acetaminophen-induced failure** are:

1. pH <7.30 after resuscitation, irrespective of encephalopathy grade
2. Prothrombin time >100 seconds and creatinine >300 μmol/L in patients with grade III or grade IV encephalopathy

Modification to include lactate of >3.5 mmol/L after fluid resuscitation has been proposed by some. Patients with acetaminophen toxicity who meet the KCH criteria have a ≥90% mortality without liver transplantation. A recent meta-analysis showed that the KCH criteria are associated with sensitivity of 69% and specificity of 92% in predicting death without transplantation.

The **KCH criteria are different for patients with acute liver failure not induced by acetaminophen, and these** include: prothrombin time >100 seconds or 3 or more of the following criteria:

1. Age less <10 or >40 years
2. Acute liver failure caused by non-A, non-B, non-C hepatitis, halothane hepatitis, or idiosyncratic drug reaction
3. Jaundice present for >1week prior to onset of encephalopathy
4. Prothrombin time >50 seconds
5. Serum bilirubin >17.5 mg/dL

Acute liver failure can be produced by a variety of causes including toxins, viral infections, metabolic causes, vascular causes, and autoimmune causes. Acute liver injuries from these mechanisms can cause damages leading to hepatocyte apoptosis and/or necrosis. Injuries associated with mitochondrial permeability changes typically lead to apoptosis if the cells' ATP stores are preserved; examples include acute Wilson disease and Reye syndrome. When injuries producing mitochondrial permeability changes occur in the face of cellular ATP depletion, cell necrosis occur. The site of injury within the liver architecture is important in determining the potential for cellular regeneration and recovery prognosis. Stem cells are located in the portal tract region, and preservation of these cells is important for regeneration; therefore, injury to the portal zone is associated with lower potential for regeneration and worse prognosis.

CLINICAL APPROACH

Etiologies

Toxin-Induced Injuries **Liver damage caused by acetaminophen is the most common type of toxin-induced injury, and can occur with ingestions of 4 g/d, but more often injuries are caused by the consumption of >10 g/d.** Acetaminophen is metabolized in the hepatocytes by cytochrome enzymes to the toxic metabolite *N*-acetyl *p*-benzoquinone imine (NAP-QI), which is normally detoxified by conjugation with glutathione. Depletion of glutathione can increase the susceptibility of the individual to acetaminophen-induced liver injury. Acetaminophen-induced injuries are typically concentrated in the central zones, where the portal tracts are spared. Based on the architectural site of the injury, the potential for recovery is generally very good.

Amanita **(mushroom) poisoning is more commonly encountered in Western Europe than the United States.** In the United States, *Amanita* species are most frequently encountered in coastal Pacific Northwest, and to lesser extents in the Blue Ridge Mountains, Pennsylvania, New Jersey, and Ohio. Most *Amanitas* are encountered during late summer to early winter. There are over 5000 species of mushrooms; however, only 50 are poisonous to humans. Three of the *Amanita* species are responsible for >90% of all mushroom-related fatalities. Patients with mushroom poisoning typically present with vomiting, crampy abdominal pain, and diarrhea within 10 to 12 hours of ingestion. Clinical and laboratory findings associated with acute liver injury are often not manifested until 2 days after ingestion. Treatment measures include evacuation of duodenal contents by suction to interrupt the enterohepatic circulation of amatoxins. Sodium bicarbonate administration within 2 hours of ingestion may be helpful in elimination of urinary α-amanitin. Hemodialysis or hemoperfusion utilizing a charcoal filter may also be effective in removing amatoxins from the circulation. The overall prognosis of patients with *Amanita* poisoning is not good, because some patients who recover from the acute insult will go on to chronic hepatitis and late liver failure.

Viral Hepatitis–Induced Acute Liver Failure Viral hepatitis caused by hepatitis A, B, and E viruses can produce acute liver injuries, which generally result in spontaneous resolution; however, a small percentage of these patients may go on to develop acute hepatic failure. **Antiviral treatments have not been demonstrated to reduce the occurrence of viral hepatitis–associated acute liver failure.** The acute hepatitis associated with hepatitis B has been shown to be associated with a worse prognosis when coinfection with hepatitis D is present. Antiviral therapy may be indicated for patients with hepatitis B–induced acute liver failure, when the patient is anticipated to require liver transplantation; the use of antiviral therapy in this setting reduces the risk of hepatitis B recurrences in the transplanted liver.

Metabolic Causes of Acute Liver Failure Metabolic causes of acute liver failure include acute fatty liver of pregnancy. This is an unusual metabolic process in which the metabolic abnormality in the fetus causes maternal liver injuries that typically occur during the third trimester of pregnancy, with some patients developing rapid progression of jaundice and liver failure. In approximately 50% of the cases, this process occurs with preeclampsia. Delivery of the fetus is the treatment of choice for most patients. There have been limited reports suggesting that the plasma exchange therapy may also be of benefit in these patients.

Patients with Wilson disease may present with acute liver failure caused by copper toxicosis. Frequently, these patients have underlying chronic liver injuries prior to the onset of the acute injuries. The application of MARS has been shown to reverse some of the acute injuries associated with this process.

Vascular Causes of Acute Liver Failure Acute obstruction of the hepatic veins (Budd–Chiari syndrome) may occur as a result of hypercoagulable states. Once identified, patients may benefit from portal venous decompression procedures such as transhepatic intrahepatic protosystemic shunt (TIPS) or operative portocaval shunts to reduce further liver parenchymal injuries. **Ischemia** is a common cause of acute liver injury, and this is typically described as "shock liver." This type of injury is typically associated with a severe and/or prolonged hypotensive episode, which causes injuries mostly in the central zone. Treatment is to address the underlying condition causing the global hemodynamic compromise.

Evaluation of Patients with Acute Hepatic Failure

Early recognition of the condition is important in improving prognosis, since early recognition permits for the identification of the inciting events, initiation of cause-specific therapies, and early referral to specialty units for specialized support or transplantation. The history is useful to identify and determine possible substance ingestion and timing of ingestion. In addition, history of preexisting liver diseases or risk factors will help determine the chronicity of the liver injury. During the physical examination, the focus is on assessing the liver and spleen sizes, and the presence or absence of stigmatas of chronic liver disease. The neurological evaluation should be thorough noting the papillary sizes and reactivity, deep tendon responses, mental status, and cognitive functions. The **West Haven Criteria and the GCS** are both helpful for quantification of neurological functions. It is important to keep in mind that the neurological status may change as the patient's condition changes; therefore, neurological assessments should be repeated frequently to determine progress. Laboratory evaluations should be performed to determine possible causes of injury, metabolic panels, coagulation panels, complete blood count, and blood and tissue typing if liver transplantation is anticipated. Imaging studies should be performed to assess liver characteristic and size, spleen size, and patency of hepatic vasculature. Management of acute liver failure patients is often optimized when a multidisciplinary team including intensivists, transplant surgeons, transplant hepatologists, and nephrologists are involved in the care of patients with the most severe injuries.

Complications Associated with Acute Hepatic Failure

Cerebral edema leading to intracranial hypertension is one of the most lethal complications associated with acute liver failure. Risk factors associated with this complication include grade 3 or 4 encephalopathy, serum ammonia >150 to 200 μM, rapid progression of encephalopathy, superinfection, requirement for vasopressor support, and requirement for renal replacement therapy. Intracranial hypertension can be identified by CT imaging or intracranial pressure monitoring. Intracranial pressure monitoring is the most reliable way of identifying this complication; however, placement of monitors in these patients can be associated with 10% to 20% risk of bleeding complication. Moderate hypothermia (32°C-33°C) has been shown to be an effective treatment for patients with intracranial hypertension.

Hemodynamic failure is commonly seen in patients with acute liver failure. Typically, it is associated with high cardiac output and low systemic vascular resistance. Because this picture closely resembles the septic response, it is important that all infectious causes are ruled out. Support of the blood pressure is important in these patients to maintain cerebral prefusion and vasopressors are often needed.

Hematologic failure with coagulopathy occurs commonly in patients with acute liver failure. Empiric administration of 10 mg of vitamin K intravenously is recommended because subclinical vitamin K deficiency can contribute to coagulopathy. Prophylactic transfusion of blood products to correct coagulopathy has not been shown to improve outcome; however, for bleeding patients or prior to invasive procedures, transfusion to correct the INR to 1.5 and increase the platelet count to >50,000/mm^3 is recommended. Cryoprecipitate is recommended for bleeding patients with fibrinogen <100 mg/dL. Recombinant factor 7a is sometime helpful when bleeding patients do not respond to FFP transfusions.

Acute kidney injury may accompany acute liver failure. Urinary sodium levels are low in patients who are volume depleted and in patients with hepatorenal syndrome. Volume assessment is important in these patients with either intravascular monitoring devices or echocardiography. Renal replacement therapy is often needed as the acute kidney injury progresses. For patients requiring renal replacement therapy, continuous venovenal hemofiltration with dialysis is often better tolerated than intermittent dialysis.

Infections occur commonly in the acute liver failure patients, and it is the most common cause of death in this patient population. It is believed that these patients have impaired Kuppfer cell function and abnormal clearance of gut bacteria and bacterial product, which render the patients susceptible to bacterial and fungal infections. Although some groups believe that broad-spectrum prophylactic antibiotics should be administered in patients with acute liver failure, survival has not been shown to improve with prophylaxis. Clinicians should maintain high vigilance for possible infections in these patients who have low threshold for treatment.

Catabolism and nutritional failure occurs commonly in this patient population. Oral feeding is advisable until patients develop grade 2 to 3 encephalopathies. Caloric targets for patients should be 25 to 30 kcal/kg. Enteral or parenteral nutrition should be initiated when oral intake is not feasible. Protein intake should be limited to 1 g/kg/d to minimize excess ammonia production. Supplemental glutamine should be avoided as it appears to contribute to excess ammonia production and worsening of cerebral edema.

LIVER TRANSPLANTATION

Patients with acute liver failure who do not recover despite appropriate medical care and supportive care should be referred as early as possible for consideration for liver transplantation. The **King's College Hospital Criteria are the most commonly used criteria for the selection of patients for transplantation referral.** The long-term outcome for patients undergoing transplantation for acute hepatic failure is generally not as good as outcome following liver transplantation for chronic liver diseases. The 1-, 3-, and 5-year graft survival reported are 63%, 58%, and 56%, respectively.

CLINICAL CASE CORRELATION

- **See also Case 3 (Scoring System and Prognosis), Case 30 (Altered Mental Status), Case 33 (Multiorgan Dysfunction), and Case 41 (Hemorrhage and Coagulopathy).**

COMPREHENSION QUESTIONS

22.1 Which of the following statements regarding acetaminophen-induced acute liver failure is most accurate?

A. The recovery/survival is <30%.

B. Hepatocytes in the portal zone are most affected.

C. It is the second most common cause of acute liver failure in the United States behind *Amanita* ingestion.

D. NAC therapy does not provide any benefits when delayed by more than 4 hours after ingestion.

E. Individuals with glutathione depletion have greater susceptibility to toxicity.

22.2 A 32-year-old woman presents with *Amanita*-induced acute liver failure, whose encephalopathy progresses from grade 1 to grade 3 over the course of 6 hours in the ICU. She is intubated in the ICU for airway protection. Which of the following is the most appropriate next step?

A. Initiate hemodialysis to eliminate amatoxins

B. Perform CT of the brain

C. Transfer to a liver transplantation center

D. Initiate broad-spectrum antibiotics

E. Put the patient on vasopressors to increase cerebral perfusion pressure

22.3 A 28-year-old man develops acute fulminant hepatic failure following inadvertent ingestion of poisoned *Amanita*. He is currently undergoing treatment for coagulopathy and respiratory failure that is requiring mechanical ventilation. On day 2 in the ICU, you are notified by his nurse regarding a slight change in his motor response on the left and decreased pupillary responses to light in the right eyes. Which of the following is the most appropriate management at this time?

A. Change the ventilatory settings to keep $PACO_2$ at 35 mm Hg.

B. Placement of ventriculostomy drain.

C. CT scan of the brain.

D. Referral for liver transplantation.

E. Referral for bioartificial liver support.

ANSWERS TO QUESTIONS

22.1 **E.** Glutathione depletion can increase the susceptibility of individuals to acetaminophen toxicity, and this can be seen in fasting patients and patients with chronic alcohol use. Acetaminophen causes predominant injury to hepatocytes in the central zone, while sparing cells in the periportal zones. Based on this distribution, injuries to the stem cells occur less frequently resulting in good potential for recovery. Survival >80% is expected with acetaminophen-induced liver injury. NAC administration has been shown to provide improved liver recovery when given as late as 16 hours after acetaminophen ingestion.

22.2 **B.** For this patient with rapid progression of encephalopathy, intracranial hypertension from increasing cerebral edema is a major concern. A CT of the brain should be obtained immediately to assess the brain. Alternatively, an intracranial pressure monitor can be placed, but this approach carries a bleeding risk of 10% to 20%. This patient ultimately may need to be referred for liver transplantation consideration, but an acute ICP increase need to be addressed first.

22.3 **C.** This patient with acute fulminant hepatic failure is showing signs of right cerebral hemispheric mass effects. The mass effects are likely produced by intracerebral hemorrhage due to coagulopathy related to hepatic failure. Cerebral edema causing intracranial hypertension can also be a cause of these neurological changes; however, cerebral edema–induced changes are unlikely to be limited to the right hemisphere. Ventriculostomy drain could be helpful to directly measure ICP but could also cause bleeding complications and should not be done until a mass lesion is ruled out with CT. The patient's overall poor liver status could make liver transplantation or bioartificial liver support necessary; however, these options should not be entertained until the question regarding his new neurological findings are addressed.

CLINICAL PEARLS

- ▶ Chronic alcohol ingestion stimulates cytochrome CYP-2E1 activity, inhibits the rate of glutathione synthesis, and can increase toxicity to acetaminophen.
- ▶ The 1-, 3-, and 5-year survival following liver transplantation for acute liver failure is 10% to 20% lower than liver transplantation performed for chronic liver diseases.
- ▶ The MARS and bioartificial liver (BAL) are useful for the support of patients while liver recovery is occurring, and these devices can be used as bridge to liver transplantation.
- ▶ In acetaminophen toxicity, NAC helps to detoxify the acetaminophen toxic metabolite (NAPQI). Ideally, when NAC is given within 8 to 10 hours after ingestion it protects against NAPGI-induced liver and renal injuries.

REFERENCES

Chun LJ, Tong MJ, Busuttil RW, Hiatt JR. Acetaminophen hepatotoxicity and acute liver failure. *J Clin Gastroenterol*. 2009;43:342-349.

Schilsky ML, Honiden S, Arnott L, Emre S. ICU management of acute liver failure. *Clin Chest Med*. 2009;30:71-87.

Stravits RT. Critical management decisions in patients with acute liver failure. *Chest*. 2008;134:1092-1102.

Trotter JF. Practical management of acute liver failure in the intensive care unit. *Curr Opin Crit Care*. 2009;15:163-167.

CASE 23

A 57-year-old woman with a history of Type 2 diabetes mellitus and hypertension has been admitted to the ICU for management of acute urinary tract infection sepsis, today being ICU day 3. The patient weighs 63 kg. The patient's laboratory studies demonstrated an increase in serum creatinine from 1.0 mg/dL to 2.1 mg/dL. Her serum electrolytes are within normal limits. Her total urine output for the most recent 24 hours (day 2) is only 650 mL, which is significantly less than the output from the 24 hours before (day 1), recorded as 1100 mL.

- ▶ What is the most likely diagnosis?
- ▶ What are the best next steps in evaluating and managing this patient?

ANSWERS TO CASE 23:
Acute Kidney Injury

Summary: A 57-year-old woman is being managed in the ICU with a new diagnosis of acute urinary tract infection sepsis. On hospital day 3 her urine output drops significantly and her serum creatinine increases from 1.0 mg/dL to 2.1 mg/dL.

- **Most likely diagnosis:** Acute kidney injury with the serum creatinine increasing twofold and associated with decreased urine output.
- **Next step:** Initiate immediate supportive treatment (fluid management, antibiotics directed at source control, vasopressors, and diuretics) and obtain CBC, serum chemistry, urinalysis, and blood and urine cultures if new infection is suspected. Initiate consultation with the renal service for possible renal replacement therapy.

ANALYSIS

Objectives

1. To become familiar with the diagnosis, staging, and treatment of acute kidney injury.
2. To list the causes of acute kidney injury in ICU patients.
3. To understand the indications for emergent renal replacement therapy.

Considerations

The patient's history indicates a known diagnosis of acute urinary tract infection sepsis, which in itself is a potentially life-threatening condition. On her third day of hospitalization, she develops a significant increase in the serum markers of her kidney function, a decrease in urine output, and an abrupt rise in serum creatinine. These markers indicate that her kidney function is compromised and investigation into the cause and initiation of treatment should begin. The initial decline of kidney function may be reversible with treatment; however, the underlying cause of the kidney dysfunction will need to be addressed so that ultimately the urological system can regain normal homeostasis. It is likely that with adequate management, the kidneys' functional status may normalize; however, the possibility of further decompensation may occur, leading to the requirement of renal replacement therapy for patient survival.

APPROACH TO:
Acute Kidney Injury

DEFINITIONS

OLIGURIA: Decrease from the normal level of urine output (<0.5 mL/kg/h).

ANURIA: No urine output in >24 hours, usually irreversible.

RENAL REPLACEMENT THERAPY: Dialysis/hemofiltration, the only FDA-approved therapy for AKI.

CHRONIC KIDNEY DISEASE: An irreversible failure in the homeostasis of the renal filtration system.

SIRS: Systemic inflammatory response syndrome that comprises abnormal body temperature (higher than 38°C or <36°C), heart rate >90 beats/minute, respiration >20 breaths/minute, or arterial partial pressure of CO_2 <32 mm Hg, and deranged white blood cell counts (>12 × 10^3/mm^3, <4 × 10^3/mm^3, or >10% bands).

SEPSIS: SIRS and an identifiable source of infection (or high level of suspicion of an identifiable source of infection).

SEPTIC SHOCK: Meeting the criteria for sepsis with low blood pressure (SBP <90 mm Hg).

UROSEPSIS: Sepsis caused by infection of the urinary tract and/or male genital organs (eg, prostate).

CLINICAL APPROACH

Acute kidney injury (AKI) has now replaced the term acute renal failure. It is now widely agreed that there is a spectrum of the disease extending from less severe forms of injury to that of more advanced injury. The significance of this disease is great, with up to 200,000 people each year in the United States affected and a hospital-acquired prevalence of 7.1%. There is a strong evidence that **sepsis and septic shock are the most important causes of AKI in critically ill patients, accounting for 50% or more of cases of AKI in ICU patients.** It is now recognized that AKI is an independent risk factor for mortality, with experimental models suggesting that AKI is associated with an up-regulation of systemic inflammatory mediator release.

AKI is a clinical diagnosis characterized by rapid reduction in function resulting in inability to maintain electrolyte, fluid and acid–base homeostasis. The mainstay for diagnosis of AKI has been the measurement of urine output over a given time period, as well as a rise in specific biological markers of kidney function, with the most common being serum creatinine (SCr). Specifically, AKI is defined **when 1 of the following criteria is met:**

- SCr rises by ≥26 μmol/L within 48 h
- SCr acutely rises ≥1.5 fold from the reference value (*Note*: Reference SCr should be the lowest creatinine value recorded within 3 months of the event.)
- Urine output is <0.5 mL/kg/h for >6 consecutive hours.

Staging of AKI is useful at the bedside, as AKI is considered a spectrum of severity, and the recognition of disease severity is helpful in the selection of treatments (Table 23–1).

Although urine output and SCr are presently the best biomarkers for AKI, they are not ideal, since kidney injury has already occurred before these values become abnormal; therefore, reliance on these markers may result in delays in disease recognition. This has led to the search for biomarkers enabling early diagnosis of

Table 23–1 • RISK, INJURY, FAILURE, LOSS, AND END-STAGE KIDNEY CLASSIFICATION

Stage/Criteria	Serum Creatinine (SCr) Criteria	Urine Output Criteria
1 (Risk)	SCr × 1.5 from reference SCr	<0.5 mL/kg/h for >6 h
2 (Injury)	SCr × 2 from reference SCr	<0.5 mL/kg/h for >12 h
3 (Failure)	SCr × 3 from reference SCr or SCr ≥4 mg/dL with acute rise >0.5 mg/dL	<0.3 mL/kg/h for >24 h or anuria × 12 h
4 Loss	Complete loss of renal function for >4 weeks	
5 End-stage	End-stage kidney disease >3 months	

kidney insult and earlier treatment. At present, several novel biomarkers are being investigated, and these include neutrophil gelatinase-associated lipocalin (NGAL), kidney injury molecule-1 (KIM-1), interleukin-18 (IL-18), and cystatin C. These biomarkers show early promise for tools for the early detection of AKI.

Management

The first step in the management of AKI is to be aware of **patients at highest risk for the development of AKI. These include age >75 years, chronic kidney disease (CKD, eGFR <60 mL/min/1.73 m^2), cardiac failure, peripheral vascular disease, diabetes mellitus, and those taking nephrotoxic medications. Acute medical conditions that increase the risk of AKI include reduced fluid intake or increased fluid losses (dehydration), urinary tract obstruction or infections, sepsis, myoglobinuria, and recent drug ingestion.**

The urinalysis can provide useful information in determining the cause of AKI. Significant proteinuria (+3 or +4) suggests intrinsic glomerular disease. Hematuria in association with proteinuria may indicate a diagnosis of glomerular disease. Hematuria may also indicate the presence of a tumor in the lower urinary tract. Myoglobinuria produces a positive reagent strip reaction (dipstick) without traces of RBC in the urine. The presence of >5 WBC per high-power field in a patient with AKI suggests the presence of infection, acute interstitial nephritis, or glomerulonephritis. Urine microscopy can also provide useful information regarding AKI causes. Urinary crystals are identified in patients with glycol poisoning, tumor lysis syndrome, or drug exposures (sulfonamides, acyclovir, and triameterene). Other diagnostic tests for patients with AKI include urine osmolality, urine/plasma creatinine and urea ratios, urinary sodium, fractional excretion of sodium (FE_{Na}), fractional excretion of urea, free water clearance, and creatinine clearance. Patients who are prerenal may have increased urinary sodium reabsorption and increased urinary urea reabsorption; therefore, they would exhibit low FE_{NA} and FE_{Urea}. Patients with AKI caused by hepatorenal syndrome have extremely low urinary sodium (<10 mmol/L).

Ultrasound is the most useful diagnostic modality to assess for the possibility of upper urinary tract obstruction. It is important to recognize that hydronephrosis may not be present in patients with urinary tract obstruction and hypovolemia; therefore, patients suspected of obstructive uropathy should undergo a repeat study after repletion of intravascular volumes.

Acute kidney injury can be a potentially reversible disorder if treated in a timely and appropriate manner. Early recognition is important and may improve the chances for full recovery of kidney functions. A patient's supportive measures must be optimized to include appropriate fluid therapy, administration of vasopressor and/or inotropic medicines, and treatment of the underlying illness, particularly sepsis. Accurate measurements of all intake including oral, intravenous rates, and boluses as well as all output (urine, emesis, etc) must be accurately recorded to give the clinician the most complete and accurate assessment of the patient's volume status. This may require the use of an indwelling urine catheter for precise urine output measurement. All medications administered should be interrogated for potential nephrotoxic effects and stopped accordingly. Avoidance of intravenous radiographic contrast will help avoid further injury to the kidneys.

Generally accepted indications for renal replacement therapy (RRT) include **profound acidemia, electrolyte imbalances (eg, hyperkalemia), ingestion or idiopathic overload of toxins/metabolites**, **symptomatic fluid overload**, and **symptomatic uremia** (eg, increased bleeding from platelet dysfunction, pericardial tamponade, and severe mental status change). Ideally, RRT should be initiated once the diagnosis of AKI is certain and unavoidable, yet prior to terminal organ complications.

Venous access for RRT requires planning that takes into consideration the level of irreversible kidney damage and the anticipated duration of therapy. When short-term (temporary) dialysis is anticipated, venovenous access is the preferred route. Venovenous access is established with ultrasound-guided placement of a double lumen catheter into a large central vein (preferably internal jugular or femoral veins). This access may be used for weeks until the patient's physiologic homeostasis will be determined to become normal or if prolonged RRT is required. For patients in whom long-term dialysis is anticipated, planning should be initiated for the placement of arteriovenous access. In comparison to intermittent dialysis, continuous renal replacement therapy may have the advantage of achieving better control of uremia, prevention of hypotension during dialysis, and improved clearance of inflammatory mediators; however, there is no convincing evidence to indicate that continuous RRT provides additional advantages over intermittent RRT. Similarly, clinical evidence does not support the use of high-dose RRT over standard-dose RRT.

All patients who survive AKI but whose kidney function does not return to normal will need planning for CKD management, including but not limited to long-term RRT access. A center for RRT will need to accept the patient and subsequently into the practice of a renal physician. Kidney transplantation is the definitive treatment for those with failed kidneys.

Long-term Prognosis

Despite advances in the supportive care of patient with AKI in the ICU, prognostication of renal recovery continues to be a difficult challenge. Several urinary biomarkers are being investigated for their prognostication value for AKI recovery. These include urinary neutrophil gelatinase-associated lipocalin (uN-GAL), urinary hepatocyte growth factor (uHGF), urinary cystatin C (uCystatin C), and IL-18. Recent clinical studies suggest that patterns of change in these urinary markers may be valuable in predicting recovery in AKI patients.

CLINICAL CASE CORRELATION

- **See also Cases 24 and 25 (Acid–Base Abnormalities I and II), Case 26 (Fluid and Electrolyte Abnormalities), and Case 33 (Multiorgan Dysfunction).**

COMPREHENSION QUESTIONS

23.1 A 58-year-old man with diabetes mellitus presents to hospital with left lower quadrant pain for 2 days. He has had nausea and vomiting with subjective fevers and anorexia. His vital signs are temperature of 100.4°F, pulse of 112 beats/minute, BP of 100/68 mm Hg, respiratory rate of 20 breaths/minute, and oxygen saturation of 99% on room air. His eyes are sunken and abdomen is tender in the left lower quadrant. Laboratory studies are significant for WBC of 15,000 and SCr of 1.68 mg/dL (reference value is 0.95). What is the initial best treatment to prevent further kidney injury?

A. Obtain immediate blood and urine cultures then start empiric antibiotics.

B. Admit to hospital and keep NPO.

C. Obtain CT scan to rule out intraabdominal abscess.

D. Insert 2 large-bore IVs then bolus with 1 to 2 L crystalloid.

E. Insert Foley catheter to measure urine output.

23.2 A 24-year-old man weighing 80 kg is admitted to the intensive care unit following an exploratory laparotomy after a GSW to his lower right hemithorax and abdomen. Intraoperative exploration showed a 1 cm laceration on the dome of the liver, a right diaphragmatic injury, and a transverse colon injury requiring partial colectomy with primary anastomosis. He was also found to have laceration of the left kidney. During the night, his urine output is measured at 60 mL/h for the first 3 hours, 50 mL/h for the fourth hour, and 20 mL/h for the fifth and sixth hours, and the urine appears dark. His heart rate and blood pressure have not changed. What is the next step in his management?

A. Place a central venous catheter for CVP monitoring.

B. Bring the patient back into the operating room for reexploration.

C. Obtain CT imaging of the abdomen and pelvis.

D. Transfuse packed red blood cells.

E. Bolus the patient intravenous fluids.

23.3 You are managing patients in the intensive care unit, and you are concerned that one of your patients with sepsis due to a lung infection has developed fluid overload secondary to stage 3 AKI and may not recover her normal kidney function. What is the best plan for instituting appropriate care for this patient?

A. Obtain urinary electrolyte measurement.

B. Obtain measurement of the patient's platelet count.

C. Insert a venovenous access catheter for RRT.

D. Refer patient for renal transplantation consideration.

E. Increase the dose of her loop diuretic medication.

23.4 A 43-year-old man with AKI had a venovenous catheter placed for urgent RRT. He is now in his hospital bed and his wound bandages are saturated with blood. You notice that he is also bleeding from his peripheral IV sites. What is the definitive treatment?

A. Transfusion of red blood cells.

B. Transfusion of platelets.

C. Initiate RRT.

D. Administer DDAVP.

E. Give intravenous calcium.

ANSWERS TO QUESTIONS

23.1 **D.** This patient is presenting with signs and symptoms concerning for the diagnosis of acute diverticulitis and septic shock. His presenting SCr of 1.68 is >1.5 that of his baseline and thus meets the criteria of AKI. This patient has intravascular volume depletion from his illness. Fluid resuscitation is the first step in early goal-directed therapy of sepsis and will subsequently yield benefit for the hypoperfusion state of his kidneys. Oxygen therapy should be given along with fluid resuscitation, followed with blood cultures and the appropriate antibiotic initiated for his presumed intraabdominal sepsis. Imaging may be helpful to guide therapy but only after the patient is hemodynamically stable. A Foley catheter should be placed to determine fluid volume status and guide the clinician on management of fluid therapy.

23.2 **A.** This patient does not meet the definitions of AKI but is in danger of its development. One criteria for AKI is urine output (UOP) <0.5 mL/kg/h for >6 hours. This patient would be of concern for AKI if his UOP is <40 mL/h, which he has had for the last 2 hours. Given his injuries and recent operation, his low urine output is likely secondary to intravascular volume depletion. The next step in management would therefore be to confirm this diagnosis with the placement of a CVP line, and then to replete his volume as necessary.

23.3 **C.** Studies have demonstrated that for acute RRT, venovenous access is the modality of choice, especially given that this patient is fluid overloaded at this time. Urinary electrolytes are not helpful at this time to further define the patient's kidney functions. Referral for renal transplantation is premature, as the patient's renal functions may eventually recover from her stage 3 AKI. Increasing the dose of her loop diuretics is an option; however, given the patient's fluid status and ongoing pulmonary problem, dialysis may be the more effective strategy for this patient at this time.

23.4 **C.** This patient has platelet dysfunction due to uremia from kidney failure. The definitive treatment is RRT. Administering blood products will not achieve the desired hemostasis that is required. Calcium is often needed as a replacement for patients receiving red blood cell transfusions, as calcium is sequestered by the high amounts of citrate in the fluid. DDAVP, also known as vasopressin arginine, can improve the binding of platelets in clot formation. It can be used as temporizing first-line treatment for uremic bleeding if there is a delay before the patient can receive RRT.

CLINICAL PEARLS

- Urine output and serum creatinine are the best biomarkers for acute kidney injury.
- AKI is potentially reversible with the appropriate measures if performed early; however, some patients may evolve to develop CKD.
- RRT may be needed for both short- and long-term therapy with kidney injury.

REFERENCES

Chuasuwan A, Kellum JA. Acute kidney injury and its management. *Contrib Nephrol*. 2011;171:218-225.

Florian ME, Pilatz A, Weidner W. Optimal management of urosepsis from the urological perspective. *International J Antimicrob Agents*. 2007:390-397.

Lewington A, Kanagasundaram S. Renal association clinical practice guidelines on acute kidney injury. *Nephron Clin Pract*. 2011;118(suppl 1):c349-c390.

Srisawat N, Wen X, Lee M, et al. Urinary biomarkers predict renal recovery in critically ill patients with renal support. *Clin J Am Soc Nephrol*. 2011;6: 1815-1823.

Zarjou A, Agarwal A. Sepsis and acute kidney injury. *J Am Soc Nephrol*. 2011;22(6):999-1006.

Liu KD, Brakeman PR. Renal repair and recovery. *Crit Care Med*. 2008;36(4 suppl):S187-S192.

CASE 24

A 56-year-old female patient with an overdose from an unknown drug is admitted to the ICU with respiratory failure and a change in mental status. A drug screen is pending. She has a long psychiatric history. Arterial blood gas (ABG) showed a pH of 7.43, a $Pa\text{CO}_2$ of 32 mm Hg, and a $P\text{AO}_2$ of 100 mm Hg on a fractional inspired oxygen concentration ($F\text{IO}_2$) of 30%. The electrolyte levels were: sodium (Na+) 145 mEq/L, potassium (K+) 4 mEq/L, chloride (Cl–) 105 mEq/L, bicarbonate (HCO_3) 20 mEq/L. Other blood values were blood urea nitrogen (BUN) 35 mg/dL, creatinine (Cr) 1.3 mg/d, and serum albumin 4 g/L.

- ▶ What is the most likely diagnosis?
- ▶ What is the acid–base abnormality?
- ▶ What is the best initial therapy for this disorder?

ANSWERS TO CASE 24: Acid–Base Abnormalities Part I

Summary: This 56-year-old woman has taken a medication overdose and is admitted to the ICU. Arterial blood gas (ABG) shows a pH of 7.43, a $PaCO_2$ of 32 mm Hg, and a PaO_2 of 100 mm Hg on fractional inspired oxygen concentration (FiO_2) of 30%. The electrolyte levels were sodium (Na+) 145 mEq/L, potassium (K+) 4 mEq/L, chloride (Cl–) 105 mEq/L, and bicarbonate (HCO_3) 20 mEq/L.

- **Most likely diagnosis:** Aspirin (ASA) overdose.
- **Acid–base disorder:** Metabolic acidosis with respiratory alkalosis.
- **Initial therapy:** Hydration with normal saline and fluids containing bicarbonate, with alkalinization of urine and increasing excretion of acidic aspirin.

ANALYSIS

Objectives

1. To describe the pathophysiology of ASA toxicity.
2. To describe a systematic approach to acid–base interpretation.
3. To understand how to treat ASA toxicity.

Considerations

This patient has a classical acid–base disorder of metabolic acidosis with a respiratory alkalosis. The bicarbonate level is 20 mEq/L, indicating a metabolic acidosis process; however, the PCO_2 is 32 mm Hg and pH is 7.43 indicating a respiratory alkalosis. Also, the patient's CNS signs and symptoms are very suggestive for ASA overdose. ASA overdose starts with tinnitus, advances to hyperventilation, and finally progresses to metabolic acidosis. This is confirmed with an ASA level. Other drugs should be evaluated as well since patients often take multiple agents in overdose situations. Gastric lavage and activated charcoal are useful in acute ingestion. Severe metabolic derangements can occur, uncoupling oxidative phosphorylation; CNS dysfunction or injury is the most serious and can lead to mental status changes, delirium, or even coma. Severe hypoxemia may result from ASA-related pulmonary edema. Adequate fluid replacement without causing pulmonary edema is prudent. Alkalinization of the urine is important to facilitate urinary excretion of the ASA; this can be accomplished with judicious sodium bicarbonate in the IV fluids. Hemodialysis is indicated for severe toxicity, refractory acidosis, coma or seizures, noncardiogenic pulmonary edema, and renal failure.

APPROACH TO:
Acid–Base Abnormalities

DEFINITIONS

ANION GAP = [Na+] – ([Cl–] + [HCO_3^-]) Normal 12 ± 2
WINTERS FORMULA: Expected $PACO_2$ = 1.5 × [HCO_3^-] + 8 ± 2 mm Hg
CORRECTED HCO_3 = [measured HCO_3] + ([measured anion-gap] – 12)
PLASMA OSMOLALITY = 2 × (Na+) + (glucose/18) + (blood urea nitrogen/2.8)
OSMOLAL GAP = Measured osmolality – calculated osmolality

(If >10 difference indicates presence of unmeasured osmoles)

CLINICAL APPROACH

The best approach to potential acid–base alterations is a stepwise approach outlined in the following manner:

Ask and answer the following questions

- Is the patient acidemic or alkalemic? Acidemic if <7.38 or alkalemic if >7.42.
- Is the acid–base disorder primarily metabolic (HCO_3) or respiratory/ventilatory ($PACO_2$)?
- What is the anion gap? Sodium – (Chloride + HCO_3) = <12 ± 2 (albumin >4 G).
- If a metabolic/respiratory acidosis exists, is there appropriate metabolic/respiratory compensation? See expected compensation Table 24–1.
- If an anion-gap acidemia is present, is there another preexisting metabolic disturbance?

Use Δ Gap Δ HCO_3 or calculated HCO_3 or Δ/Δ ratio.

Application of the stepwise approach to the clinical scenario above:

- Is the patient acidemic or alkalemic? **Alkalemic.**
- Is the acid–base disorder primarily metabolic, HCO_3 or respiratory, CO_2? **Metabolic acidosis (low HCO_3 with gap) caused by ASA is the secondary disorder; a primary respiratory alkalosis (earlier onset) is still present.**
- What is the anion gap? 145 – (105 + 20) = **20 (normal 12 ± 2) = YES**
- If a metabolic/respiratory acidosis exists, is there an appropriate metabolic/respiratory compensation? No, $PACO_2$ by Winters formula is 20 × 1.5 + 8 (±2) = 38 (±2) = 36 to 40
- The $PACO_2$ is 32 and less than expected range of 36 to 40, showing **a respiratory alkalosis.**
- If an anion-gap acidemia is present, is there a complicating metabolic disturbance? **No.**

Table 24–1 • PREDICTION OF COMPENSATORY RESPONSES ON SIMPLE ACID–BASE DISTURBANCES AND PATTERN OF CHANGES

		Range of Values		
Disorder	**Prediction of Compensation**	**pH**	**HCO_3^-**	**Pa_{CO_2}**
Metabolic acidosis	$Pa_{CO_2} = (1.5 \times HCO_3^-) + 8 \pm 2$ *or* Pa_{CO_2} will ↓ 1.25 mmHg per mmol/L ↓ in HCO_3^- *or* $Pa_{CO_2} = HCO_3^- + 15$	Low	Low	Low
Metabolic alkalosis	Pa_{CO_2} will ↑ 0.75 mmHg per mmol/L ↑ in HCO_3^- *or* Pa_{CO_2} will ↑ 6 mmHg per 10 mmol/L ↑ in HCO_3^- *or* $Pa_{CO_2} = HCO_3^- + 15$	High	High	High
Respiratory alkalosis Acute Chronic	 HCO_3^- will ↓ 0.2 mmol/L per mmHg ↓ in Pa_{CO_2} HCO_3^- will ↓ 0.4 mmol/L per mmHg ↓ in Pa_{CO_2}	High	Low	Low
Respiratory acidosis Acute Chronic	 HCO_3^- will ↑ 0.1 mmol/L per mmHg ↑ in Pa_{CO_2} HCO_3^- will ↑ 0.4 mmol/L per mmHg ↑ in Pa_{CO_2}	Low	High	High

(Reproduced, with permission, from Longo DL, Fauci AS, Kasper DL, et al. *Harrison's Principles of Internal Medicine.* 18th ed. New York, NY: McGraw-Hill Education; 2012. Table 40-1.)

In metabolic acidosis, the anion gap guides one to the cause and treatment of the acidosis. Metabolic acidosis can be calculated from the amount of HCO_3 consumed with a positive anion gap versus the amount of loss of HCO_3 with a negative anion gap (Table 24–1).

Example 1: A 47-year-old man with a 3-day history of severe diarrhea is evaluated because of muscle weakness and dizziness. Laboratory studies show sodium 140 mEq/L, potassium 3.2 mEq/L, chloride 120 mEq/L, and bicarbonate 14 mEq/L. Arterial blood gas studies on room air pH 7.27, $PaCO_2$ 27 mm Hg, PaO_2 77 mm Hg.

What is the acid–base derangement?

A common sense systematic approach to solving acid–base problems involves answering 5 questions:

- Is the patient acidemic or alkalemic? **Acidemic**
- Is the acid–base disorder primarily metabolic or respiratory? **Metabolic acidosis**
- What is the anion gap?

$$140 - (120 + 14) = \mathbf{06} \text{ (normal } 12 \pm 2)$$

- If a metabolic/respiratory acidosis exists, is there appropriate metabolic/respiratory compensation? **Yes.** Using Winters formula the predicted $PaCO_2$ for HCO_3 of 14 is

$$14 \times 1.5 + 8 = 29 \pm 2$$

equaling a predicted compensated $PACO_2$ 27 to 31 mm Hg. Here the $PACO_2$ of 27 mm Hg is in the expected range, so we have a correct amount of respiratory compensation and thus a simple nongap metabolic acidosis.

- If an anion-gap acidemia is present, is there a complicating metabolic disturbance? **No.**

  Δ gap $12 - 06 = 6$. Δ HCO_3 $24 - 14 = 10$. $10 - 6 = 4$ (normal ± 6)

  If the Δ gap is greater than +6 a preexisting metabolic alkalosis was present, whereas if the Δ gap is less than −6, then a preexisting metabolic acidosis is present.

  Corrected HCO_3 24 ± 6 = [measured HCO_3 (14)] + ([measured anion gap (06)] − 12) = 22

Answer: Non–anion-gap metabolic acidosis with appropriate respiratory alkalosis compensation.

In Example 1, the anion gap = 130 − (100 + 10) = 20, indicates an ion-gap metabolic acidosis. If the primary disturbance is a condition other than metabolic acidosis, the presence of an anion gap reveals a "hidden" metabolic acidosis. Negative charges on proteins account for the missing unmeasured anions (mainly albumin at 4 g = −12 of an anion gap). The presence of either a low albumin level (an anion) or an unmeasured cationic light chain (eg, multiple myeloma) result in a low anion gap. When the primary disturbance is a metabolic acidosis, the anion gap helps narrow the diagnostic possibilities to an anion-gap acidosis or a non–anion-gap acidosis. Healthy individuals have an anion gap of 12 ±2 mEq/L. The normal anion gap of 12 is represented by the negative charge of the normal 4 g of albumin or a charge of −3 anions per gram of albumin. The compensatory response to a primary disturbance is predictable and brings the pH back toward normal.

Compensation may be appropriate even if the pH is abnormal. The assessment of compensation helps detect mixed respiratory and metabolic acid–base disturbances. In example 1, the expected $PACO_2 = [(1.5 \times 10) + 8] = 23$ (± 2). Because the measured $PACO_2$ is 23 mm Hg and within the predicted range, respiratory compensation is appropriate, making the diagnosis a metabolic acidosis with appropriate respiratory compensation. If the $PACO_2$ is lower than expected, a secondary respiratory alkalosis is diagnosed; if the $PACO_2$ is higher than expected, a secondary respiratory acidosis is diagnosed. The process for diagnosing a coexisting metabolic disturbance involves calculating the "corrected HCO_3." If the corrected HCO_3 is $<24 \pm 6$ mEq/L, a coexisting non–anion-gap metabolic acidosis is present. If the corrected HCO_3 is $>24 \pm 6$ mEq/L, a coexisting metabolic alkalosis is present.

This formula is based upon the assumption that the measured anion gap represents in part the bicarbonate that was consumed compensating for the acidosis. If the anion gap is added to the measured bicarbonate concentration and the "normal" anion gap of 12 is subtracted, the result represents the bicarbonate concentration if the anion-gap acidosis were not present.

Anion-Gap Metabolic Acidosis

Anion-gap metabolic acidosis exists when acids associated with an unmeasured anion (such as lactate) are produced or gained from an exogenous source. Common causes of high anion-gap metabolic acidosis include lactic acidosis, ketoacidosis (ethanol, starvation, and diabetes), uremia, methanol, ethylene glycol, and ASA poisonings. A decrease in bicarbonate concentration and resultant anion-gap metabolic acidosis occur when lactic acid accumulates, as seen in states of tissue hypoperfusion. Drug-induced mitochondrial dysfunction, associated with nucleoside therapy in the treatment of AIDS, can lead to lactic acidosis in the absence of obvious tissue hypoxia (called type 2 lactic acidosis). Tonic-clonic seizures, which are associated with an increased metabolic rate, result in a lactic acidosis that quickly reverses; thus, administration of HCO_3 is not needed. Ethylene glycol poisoning causes an anion-gap acidosis and acute renal failure. Clues to ethylene glycol poisoning include an osmolal gap (>10 difference between measured and calculated osmolality) and urinary calcium oxalate crystals as the cause for the renal failure. Methanol poisoning causes an anion-gap acidosis, osmolal gap, and optic nerve toxicity (formic acid toxicity). Isopropyl alcohol poisoning causes an osmolal gap but no acidosis. An osmolal gap is present when the measured plasma osmolality exceeds the calculated plasma osmolality by >10 mOsm/kg.

When glucose is in short supply or cannot be utilized, the liver converts free fatty acids into ketones to be used as an alternative energy source. In diabetic ketoacidosis, the decreased insulin activity and increased glucagon activity lead to the formation of aceto acetic acid and β-hydroxybutyric acid, both of which are ketones. The presence of these ketoacids decreases the serum bicarbonate concentration and increases the anion gap. Treatment of anion-gap metabolic acidosis requires reversing the condition that led to the excess acid production. Treatment with bicarbonate is unnecessary, except in extreme cases of acidosis when the pH is <7.20, a level at which dysrhythmia becomes likely and cardiac contractility and responsiveness to catecholamines and medications are impaired (Table 24–2).

Non–Anion-Gap Metabolic Acidosis

Non–anion-gap metabolic acidosis is also called hyperchloremic metabolic acidosis. This develops because fluids containing sodium bicarbonate are lost or hydrogen chloride (or potential hydrogen chloride) is added to the extracellular fluid. The ensuing hyperchloremic metabolic acidosis will not change the anion gap, because the reduction in the bicarbonate concentration is offset by the increase in chloride. The most common cause of non–anion-gap metabolic acidosis is diarrhea. Diarrhea leads to loss of bicarbonate because the intestinal fluid below the stomach is relatively alkaline. All types of renal tubular acidosis (RTA) cause hyperchloremic nongap metabolic acidosis.

Proximal (type 2) RTA is caused by a reduced capacity of the kidney to reabsorb bicarbonate. **Distal (type 1) RTA** results from an inability of the renal tubules to generate a normal pH gradient (normal urinary pH <5.5) due to an inability to excrete hydrogen ions.

Table 24–2 • CAUSES OF HIGH ANION-GAP ACIDOSIS
Lactic acidosis
Ketoacidosis (diabetes, alcohol, starvation)
Toxins (ethylene glycol, salicylates, methanol, propylene glycol)
Renal failure

Type 4 RTA, commonly associated with diabetes, is a hyperkalemic hyperchloremic metabolic acidosis that is due to hypoaldosteronism or an inadequate renal tubular response to aldosterone. This leads to a reduction in the urinary excretion of potassium and hyperkalemia, which interferes with the renal production of NH4+. The inhibition of renal hydrogen ion excretion caused by aldosterone deficiency leads to a nongap metabolic acidosis.

Bicarbonate therapy is generally indicated in non–anion-gap acidosis, whereas correction of the underlying cause is the primary concern in anion-gap acidosis. Oral bicarbonate (oral citrate solution) is the preferred agent for chronic therapy of non–anion-gap acidosis. The preferred bicarbonate salt for treating hypokalemic RTA is potassium bicarbonate or potassium citrate. For acute presentations, especially in patients with concomitant impaired respiratory function, intravenous bicarbonate therapy may be indicated.

Example 2: A 36-year-old woman is evaluated because of generalized weakness. Laboratory show BUN of 40 mg/dL, creatinine 1.9 mg/dL, Na 130 mEq/L, K 3.0 mEq/L, Cl 85 mEq/L, and HCO_3 36 mEq/L. ABG studies on room air reveal pH of 7.58, P_{ACO_2} of 42 mm Hg, and P_{AO_2} of 90 mm Hg. Urinary electrolytes showed Na 50 mEq/L, K 30 mEq/L, and Cl concentration of 10 mEq/L.

What is the acid–base derangement?

- Is the patient acidemic or alkalemic? Alkalemic
- Is the acid–base disorder primarily metabolic or respiratory? Metabolic (high HCO_3)
- What is the anion gap? $130 - (85 + 36) = 9$
- If a metabolic/respiratory acidosis exists, is there appropriate metabolic/respiratory compensation? **No**, predicted P_{ACO_2} is $(36 - 24) = 12 \times 0.7 = 8.4 + 40 =$ P_{ACO_2} of 48.4. The actual P_{ACO_2} is 42 and below the predicted 48, so there is an accompanying respiratory alkalosis.
- If an anion-gap acidemia is present, is there a complicating metabolic disturbance? **No, since this is an alkalotic process.**

Answer: Combined metabolic and respiratory alkalosis. The elevated arterial pH and HCO_3 are consistent with a primary metabolic alkalosis. The arterial P_{ACO_2} is inappropriately low for the degree of metabolic alkalosis. Therefore, **both metabolic alkalosis and respiratory alkalosis are present.**

Metabolic Alkalosis

A primary increase in HCO_3 concentration can result from a loss of hydrogen chloride or less commonly, the addition of bicarbonate. This metabolic alkalosis is corrected through urinary excretion of the excess bicarbonate. Increased reabsorption is caused by a contraction of extracellular fluid (ECF), chloride depletion, hypokalemia, or elevated mineralocorticoid activity. The most common causes of metabolic alkalosis are vomiting, nasogastric suction, and diuretic therapy. Table 24–2.

For those cases, which are classified as chloride responsive, the administration of sodium chloride reverses the alkalosis by expanding the intravascular volume and reducing the activity of the renin-angiotensin-aldosterone axis. This process generates hypokalemia and maintains the metabolic alkalosis. The very low urinary chloride concentration in Example 2 suggests vomiting or remote diuretic ingestion that are correctable by sodium chloride volume expansion. Less commonly, metabolic alkalosis is maintained in the absence of volume depletion. This condition is recognized by a high urinary chloride level (>20 mEq/L) related to an elevated mineralocorticoid effect. Consequently, these disorders are also called chloride unresponsive or chloride-resistant metabolic alkalosis. H_2 blockers and proton pump inhibitors may help to decrease losses of hydrogen ions in patients with prolonged gastric suction or chronic vomiting. Potassium chloride is almost always indicated for the treatment of hypokalemia. In very severe metabolic alkalosis (pH > 7.6), hemodialysis is the preferred treatment. Infusion of acidic solutions is rarely indicated.

CLINICAL CASE CORRELATION

- **See also Case 25 (Acid–Base Abnormalities II) and Case 37 (Poisoning).**

COMPREHENSION QUESTIONS

24.1 While on call, you are paged by the nurse to evaluate an obese 48-year-old woman admitted for intractable diarrhea and severe dehydration due to *Clostridium difficile* colitis and exacerbation of her COPD. Her laboratory values were pH 7.27, $PACO_2$ 44 mm Hg, PAO_2 50 mm Hg, O_2sat 85% (on FIO_2 of 28%). Na 140 mEqL, K 3.6 mEqL , Cl– 118 mEqL, HCO_3 18 mEq/L, BUN 45, and creatinine of 1 mg/dL. Urinary chloride is 10 mEq/L. What is the acid–base disturbance?

A. Normal anion-gap metabolic acidosis

B. Chronic respiratory acidosis with metabolic alkalosis

C. Acute respiratory acidosis, uncompensated

D. Acute respiratory acidosis, compensated

E. Metabolic acidosis with hyperosmolar state

24.2 A 64-year-old man is admitted to the intensive care unit with pneumonia and septic shock. Over the past 4 days, he has had an increasing shortness of breath and fever. His only medical problem prior to hospitalization was hypertension. His significant surgical history includes a cholecystectomy. His medications are amlodipine and hydrochlorothiazide. On physical examination, his temperature is 38.8°C (101.8°F), heart rate is 110 beats/minute, respiration rate is 22 breaths/minute, and blood pressure is 85/50 mm Hg. Other than tachycardia, his cardiac examination is normal. On pulmonary examination, there are crackles over the entire right lung field. Laboratory studies on admission: sodium 136 mEq/L, potassium 4.8 mEq/L, chloride 100 mEq/L, bicarbonate 10 mEq/L. Arterial blood gas studies (on room air): pH 6.94, PCO_2 48 mm Hg, PO_2 51 mm Hg. Which of the following acid–base conditions is most likely present in this patient?

A. Anion-gap metabolic acidosis
B. Mixed anion-gap metabolic acidosis and respiratory acidosis
C. Mixed anion-gap metabolic acidosis and respiratory alkalosis
D. Mixed non–anion-gap metabolic acidosis and respiratory acidosis
E. Mixed non–anion-gap metabolic acidosis and respiratory alkalosis

ANSWERS TO QUESTIONS

24.1 **A. Normal anion-gap metabolic acidosis (without respiratory compensation)**

- Is the patient acidemic or alkalemic? Acidemic
- Is the acid–base disorder primarily metabolic or respiratory? Metabolic (low HCO_3)
- What is the anion gap? $140 - (118 + 18) = 4$
- If a metabolic/respiratory acidosis exists, is there appropriate metabolic/respiratory compensation? No, predicted $PACO_2$ is $18 \times 1.5 = 27 + 8 = 35 \pm 2$ (33 to 37) The actual $PACO_2$ is 44 and above the predicted range of 33 to 37 (using Winters formula), so there is an accompanying respiratory acidosis.
- If an anion-gap acidemia is present, is there a complicating metabolic disturbance?

Remember, $PACO_2$ and HCO_3^- move in the same direction sine they compensate for each other, $PACO_2$ is an acid, HCO_3 is a base. The normal $PACO_2$ level is 40 mm Hg and the normal $PACO_2$ level is 44 mm Hg. The HCO_3 is lower than 24 without an anion gap, so a nongap hyperchloremic metabolic acidosis is present. The urine chloride is 10 mEq/L. This type of acidosis should respond to aggressive hydration with normal saline. The saline will increase intravascular fluid, which will decrease reabsorption of HCO_3 by the proximal tubule.

24.2 **B.** Mixed anion-gap metabolic and respiratory acidosis. A decrease in the pH and bicarbonate level is consistent with a primary metabolic acidosis. In a patient with a primary metabolic acidosis, a P_{CO_2} that is higher than expected indicates a mixed metabolic and respiratory acidosis. This patient has a mixed anion-gap metabolic acidosis and respiratory acidosis. The pH of 6.94 indicates a life-threatening acidosis. This patient requires immediate intubation with mechanical ventilation for oxygenation, and adequate ventilation, since that is the quickest and most reliable means to decrease the P_{ACO_2} and increase the pH to a goal of >7.20. The decreased bicarbonate level accompanied by an elevated anion gap is consistent with an anion-gap metabolic acidosis, most likely due to septic shock–associated lactic acidosis. Winters formula can be used to estimate the expected P_{CO_2} for the degree of acidosis.

CLINICAL PEARLS

- In metabolic acidosis the difference of an anion-gap acidosis from a nongap acidosis directs the treatment.
- The treatment of positive-gap acidosis requires a reversal of the underlying condition.
- The treatment of nongap metabolic acidosis depends upon a replenishing of the HCO_3 loss.
- In type 1 RTA, the distal tubule inability to excrete H+ ions causes loss of urinary HCO_3.
- Type 2 RTA affects the proximal tubule where HCO_3^- fails to be reabsorbed.
- In osmolal gaps >10 Osm, consider ethanol, methanol, ethylene glycol, and isopropyl alcohol.
- Methanol causes anion-gap hyperosmolal metabolic acidosis and blindness by formic acid.
- Ethylene glycol causes anion-gap hyperosmolal metabolic acidosis with renal failure and the formation of calcium oxalate stones.
- Isopropyl or rubbing alcohol causes a hyperosmolal state but without acidosis.

REFERENCES

Adrogué HJ, Madias NE. Management of life-threatening acid-base disorders. Part I. *N Engl J Med.* 1998;338:26-34.

American College of Physicians. *Medical Knowledge Self-Assessment Program 14*. Philadelphia, PA: American College of Physicians; 2006.

American College of Physicians and the Clerkship Directors in Internal Medicine. *Internal Medicine Essentials for Clerkship Students*. Philadelphia: ACP Press; 2007-2008.

Loscalzo J. *Harrison's Pulmonary and Critical Care Medicine*. New York, NY: McGrawHill; 2011.

Toy EC, Simon B, Takenaka K, Liu T, Rosh A. *Case Files Emergency Medicine*. 2nd ed. New York: McGraw-Hill Publishers, 2009.

CASE 25

A 44-year-old man who was diagnosed with cryptogenic cirrhosis 2 years ago is now being hospitalized for a fractured left hip sustained after a car accident. He also has a pulmonary emboli, is in respiratory distress, and is admitted to the ICU for monitoring. He is currently on the waiting list for a liver transplant. He has a 25-pack-year smoking history but does not drink alcoholic beverages and has not used illicit drugs for the past 10 years. His current medications include aspirin, spironolactone, lactulose, propranolol, and furosemide. On physical examination, his temperature is 36°C (96.8°F), heart rate is 92 beats/minute, respiration rate is 28 breaths/minute, and blood pressure is 98/55 mm Hg. He is cachectic and has scleral icterus and palmar erythema. His mentation appears normal, and asterixis are absent. The cardiac examination reveals no heart murmurs or rubs, and his lungs are clear. The abdomen is distended but is not tender. Peripheral edema is present in both lower extremities. The laboratory reports the following values: sodium 134 mEq/L, potassium 3.3 mEq/L, chloride 107 mEq/L, bicarbonate 18 mEq/L. Arterial blood gas studies (on room air) show a pH 7.48, a P_{ACO_2} of 25 mm Hg and a P_{AO_2} of 92 mm Hg, bicarbonate level of 18 mEq/L.

- ▶ What is this patient's acid–base disorder?
- ▶ What is the best treatment for this patient?

ANSWERS TO CASE 25:

Acid–Base Abnormalities Part II

Summary: This is a 44-year-old man with a history of cryptogenic cirrhosis who underwent a motor vehicle accident and developed a pulmonary embolism. He is noted to have an arterial pH of 7.48, $PACO_2$ of 25 mm Hg, PAO_2 of 92 mm Hg, and bicarbonate level of 18 mEq/L.

- **Acid–base disorder:** Respiratory alkalosis with appropriate partial metabolic compensation
- **Treatment options:** Adequate pain control avoiding respiratory depression. BiPAP may be indicated to address the respiratory distress. If the ascites is under tension, a high-volume paracentesis may be performed to alleviate the pressure on the diaphragms. This increased respiratory drive is due to restriction imposed on the lungs by the diaphragm elevation. Pleural effusions secondary to the ascites further exacerbate the situation. The ascitic fluid should be sent for a CBC and culture in search for spontaneous bacterial peritonitis, which is commonly seen in patients with ascites.

ANALYSIS

Objectives

1. To use a common stepwise approach to acid–base evaluation.
2. To understand the respiratory effects on acid–base disorders.
3. To understand the most common causes of respiratory disorders, related to an acid–base imbalance.

Considerations

This patient has end-stage liver disease. Respiratory alkalosis often develops in patients with end-stage liver disease, and the partial metabolic acidosis compensation (decreased bicarbonate level) speaks for a chronic respiratory alkalosis. This likely is due to an increased minute ventilation (V_E). One speculated mechanism is that diminished hepatic steroid metabolism leads to elevated serum progesterone levels, which stimulate respiratory drive. Additionally, the patient has acute pulmonary embolism, which leads to a VQ mismatch, stimulating an acute increase in minute ventilation.

APPROACH TO:

Acid-Base Disorders II

Introduction

Acid–base status can be diagnosed by answering a series of questions (see Case 24): In respiratory disorders, $PACO_2$ and HCO_3 move in the same direction. If the $PACO_2$ decreases, so does the HCO_3; and if the $PACO_2$ falls, the HCO_3 also falls

(Table 24–1). This correlation exists, since the respiratory and metabolic parameters compensate for changes in the other. In pure metabolic disorders, the pH, $PACO_2$ and HCO_3 all point in the same direction. When the $PACO_2$ or HCO_3 move in the opposite direction of the pH, a mixed respiratory and metabolic component is responsible for the disorder.

For example, if the primary respiratory disorder is acute in nature, then the measured HCO_3 should change in coordination with the change in $PACO_2$. For every 10 mm Hg decrease in $PACO_2$, there should be a 2 mEq/L decrease in HCO_3 (normal HCO_3 of 24 mEq/L) in the acute condition, and a fall of 4 mEq/L from the normal HCO_3 in the chronic condition. If the change in HCO_3 is less than expected, then a metabolic acidosis accompanies the respiratory alkalosis. If the HCO_3 is greater than expected, then a concomitant metabolic alkalosis is present.

Respiratory Acidosis

Respiratory acidosis is due to a primary increase in arterial $PACO_2$, which accumulates when the ventilation is inadequate. Hypoventilation can result from neurological disorders (stroke) or medications (narcotics) that affect the respiratory center of the CNS, respiratory muscle weakness (eg, myasthenia gravis or Guillain-Barré syndrome), chest wall deformities (severe kyphoscoliosis), obstruction of airways (COPD), or pulmonary venous thromboembolism. Treatment of respiratory acidosis should focus on addressing the underlying disorder. In patients with acute respiratory acidosis and hypoxemia, supplemental O_2 may be administered carefully, keeping the O_2sat around 90% to avoid further hypercapnia. Aerosolized bronchodilators should be delivered under controlled FIO_2 or compressed ambient air (FIO_2 21%). To increase the effective alveolar ventilation, BiPAP on NIV or endotracheal intubation and mechanical ventilation may be needed.

Example 1: A 47-year-old man with a history of severe COPD is admitted to the ICU for a COPD exacerbation and respiratory distress. He is evaluated because of weakness and dizziness and daytime hypersomnolence. Laboratory studies show serum sodium 140 mEq/L; potassium 5 mEq/L; chloride 100 mEq/L; and serum bicarbonate of 30 mEq/L. Arterial blood gas studies on room air reveal pH, 7.34; $PACO_2$, 55 mm Hg; and bicarbonate, 38 mEq/L.

What is the acid–base disorder?

- Is the patient acidemic or alkalemic? **(pH = 7.34) Acidemic**
- Is the acid–base disorder primarily metabolic or respiratory? **Respiratory acidosis with appropriate compensation (chronic respiratory acidosis)**
- What is the anion gap? 140 – (100 + 30) = **10 mEq/L (normal)**
- If a metabolic/respiratory acidosis exists, is there appropriate metabolic/respiratory compensation? **Yes, expected change** = 1.5 × 4 = 6 + 24 (normal HCO_3) = **30 mEq/L (predicted compensated HCO_3)**
- If an anion-gap acidemia is present, is there a complicating metabolic disturbance? No

Answer: Respiratory acidosis with partial metabolic alkalosis compensation.

Respiratory Alkalosis

Hyperventilation reduces the arterial $PACO_2$, which increases the pH, causing respiratory alkalosis. Common causes of respiratory alkalosis can be sorted by conditions involving the pulmonary vasculature (eg, pulmonary hypertension and venous thromboembolism), pulmonary parenchyma (eg, pulmonary fibrosis, heart failure, and pneumonia), pulmonary airways (asthma) and conditions affecting ventilatory control (eg, anxiety, aspirin toxicity, sepsis, hypoxia, and pregnancy). The expected compensatory responses for acute and chronic respiratory alkalosis are shown in Table 40–1. **The underlying cause for respiratory alkalosis should be pursued.** Patients with psychogenic hyperventilation (anxiety) should be instructed to rebreathe air using a bag, which increases the systemic $PACO_2$; these measures raise the $PACO_2$ and pH, and also may help to reduce the pH in patients with mixed, severe life-threatening alkalosis (pH >7.70). The only acid-base disorder that can return back to a normal pH of 7.40 in the absence of a secondary acid-base disorder is chronic respiratory alkalosis.

Example 2: A 27-year-old woman presents with a 1-day history of severe anxiety and hysteria. She is being evaluated because of weakness and dizziness and an onset of paresthesias. She had a new onset of seizures that lasted 1 minute in which she had an episode of emesis. This led to her admission to the ICU for suspected aspiration pneumonia and treatment of possible rhabdomyolisis. Laboratory studies show serum sodium, 140 mEq/L; serum potassium, 5 mEq/L; serum chloride, 110 mEq/L, and serum bicarbonate of 21 mEq/L. Arterial blood gas studies on room air reveal pH, 7.54; $PACO_2$ 25 mm Hg, PAO_2 77 mm Hg on 40% FIO_2.

What is the acid–base abnormality?

- Is the patient acidemic or alkalemic? (pH = 7.54) **Alkalemic**
- Is the acid–base disorder primarily metabolic or respiratory? **Respiratory**
- What is the anion gap? 140 – (110 + 21) = **9**
- If a metabolic/respiratory acidosis exists, is there appropriate metabolic/respiratory compensation? **Yes.** The change from the normal $PACO_2$ of 40 mm Hg is 15 mm Hg so the expected compensation is 1.5 × 2 = 3 (normal HCO_3 24 mEq/L) 24 – 3 = 21. The measured HCO_3 is 21.

Answer: This patient has an acute respiratory alkalosis with metabolic compensation.

Patients with restrictive lung diseases can only increase minute ventilation by increasing the respiratory rate. Some of these conditions include CHF, pneumonia, pulmonary fibrosis, obesity, ascites, chest bellows restriction, chest wall abnormalities, chest pain, trauma, contusions.

CLINICAL CASE CORRELATION

- **See also Case 22 (Acute Liver Failure) and Case 24 (Acid–Base Abnormalities I).**

COMPREHENSION QUESTIONS

25.1 A 68-year-old man is brought to the ICU after being dyspneic and tachypneic for 5 days. Axial CT scan diagnosed a pulmonary embolism. On physical examination, the patient's temperature is 36.7°C (98°F), heart rate is 79 beats/minute, respiratory rate is 32 breaths/minute, and blood pressure is 156/80 mm Hg. He is lethargic and weak, in moderate respiratory distress, and oriented only to place and person. Laboratory studies revealed sodium 135 mEq/L, potassium 3.9 mEq/L, chloride 115 meEq/L, bicarbonate 11 mEq/L. Arterial blood gas studies (on room air) identified the following: pH 7.49, $PACO_2$ 15 mm Hg, and PAO_2 67 mm Hg. Which of the following best characterizes the patient's acid–base disorder?

A. Mixed anion gap metabolic acidosis and respiratory acidosis
B. Mixed anion gap metabolic acidosis and respiratory alkalosis
C. Mixed metabolic alkalosis and respiratory alkalosis
D. Mixed non–anion gap metabolic acidosis and respiratory alkalosis
E. Chronic respiratory alkalosis with appropriate compensation

25.2 A 55-year-old woman is admitted to the ICU with a urinary tract infection and septic shock. She is now intubated but is not on mechanical ventilation. Over the past 4 days, she has had increasing shortness of breath and fever. Her medications are limited to amlodipine and hydrochlorothiazide. On physical examination, her temperature is 38.8°C (101.8°F), heart rate is 110 beats/minute, respiration rate is 22 breaths/minute, and blood pressure is 85/50 mm Hg. Other than tachycardia, the cardiac examination is normal. On pulmonary examination, there are crackles over the bilateral lungs. Laboratory studies on admission: sodium 140 mEq/L, potassium 4.5 mEq/L, chloride 100 mEq/L, bicarbonate 14 mEq/L, ABG study (on 50% FIO_2) showed: pH 6.94, $PACO_2$ 80 mm Hg, PAO_2 58 mm Hg. Which of the following acid–base conditions is most likely present in this patient?

A. Anion gap metabolic acidosis
B. Mixed anion gap metabolic acidosis and respiratory acidosis
C. Mixed anion gap metabolic acidosis and respiratory alkalosis
D. Mixed non–anion gap metabolic acidosis and respiratory acidosis
E. Mixed non–anion gap metabolic acidosis and respiratory alkalosis

ANSWERS TO QUESTIONS

25.1 **E.** In a patient with a diagnosis of pulmonary emboli and a chronically high respiratory rate for 5 days, the presence of a chronic respiratory alkalosis is expected. This patient has a respiratory alkalosis with appropriate compensation. The presence of an alkaline pH with a decreased serum HCO_3 level suggests a respiratory alkalosis with ongoing renal compensation or a metabolic acidosis with a respiratory alkalosis. A mixed disorder should be raised in a patient whose pH is above normal in the presence of a metabolic acidosis. To confirm the suspicion of a mixed disorder, Winter formula can be used to estimate the expected P_{CO_2}: Expected $P_{CO_2} = 1.5 \times [HCO_3^-] + 8 \pm 2 = 24.5 \pm 2$ mm Hg. According to this formula, the expected P_{CO_2} is approximately 22.5 to 26.5 mm Hg, but the measured P_{CO_2} was 15 mm Hg, which confirms the presence of a respiratory alkalosis. The most likely cause of a mixed anion gap metabolic acidosis and respiratory alkalosis in this patient is salicylate toxicity.

25.2 **B.** A decrease in the pH and HCO_3 level is consistent with an anion gap metabolic acidosis. There is also a primary respiratory acidosis. This patient has a mixed anion gap metabolic acidosis and respiratory acidosis. The pH <7.38 indicates an acidosis. This anion gap metabolic acidosis is most likely due to septic shock–associated lactic acidosis. Winter formula can be used to estimate the expected P_{CO_2} for the degree of acidosis: Expected $P_{CO_2} = 1.5 \times [HCO_3^-] + 8 \pm 2 = 29 \pm 2$ mm Hg. According to this formula, this patient's P_{CO_2} is significantly increased above the expected level, which indicates the presence of carbon dioxide retention and respiratory acidosis. This is due to ventilatory failure secondary to the patient's respiratory distress, likely due to ARDS.

CLINICAL PEARLS

- ► The only acid–base disorder that returns to a normal pH without another acid–base cause being present is chronic respiratory alkalosis.
- ► The anion gap formula is $[Na+] - ([Cl^-] + [HCO_3^-])$. The normal value is 12 +/− 2 (with an albumin of 4 g/L). It is the albumin that represents the anion gap.
- ► Each gram of albumin is responsible for 3 points of the normal anion gap of 12 +/− 2. Adjust the normal range of the anion gap accordingly. (Eg, Albumin of 2 g = 6 ± 2)
- ► Changes in P_{ACO_2} and HCO_3 always move in the same direction.
- ► Acute respiratory alkalosis with significant elevation in pH can de-ionize calcium and induce a seizure via a relative hypocalcemia.

REFERENCES

American College of Physicians and the Clerkship Directors in Internal Medicine. *Internal Medicine Essentials for Clerkship Students*. Philadelphia: ACP Press; 2007-2008.

Loscalzo J. *Harrison's Pulmonary and Critical Care Medicine*, New York, NY: McGraw-Hill; 2011.

Toy EC, Simon B, Takenaka K, Liu T, Rosh A, *Case Files Emergency Medicine*. 2nd ed, New York, NY: Lange Medical Books/McGraw-Hill; 2009.

CASE 26

A 66-year-old man was hospitalized two days ago following an acute hemorrhagic stroke. His CT findings demonstrated a left intracerebral hemorrhage with subarachnoid hemorrhage. The patient's Glascow coma score (GCS) is 13. He was admitted to the ICU for monitoring and management of his hypertension. Today, on hospital day 2, you receive a call from the ICU nurse because the patient appears to be more somnolent. The examination reveals that the patient has the same right extremity weakness as before, no new focal neurological findings. He is lethargic, answers slowly to commands, and appears confused. A repeat brain CT demonstrates no changes from his initial CT. Laboratory findings reveal WBC 8000 cells/mm^3, hemoglobin/hematocrit 13.4 g/dL and 42%, sodium 124 mmol/L, serum osmolality 288 mOsm/kg (normal: 278-305 mOsm/kg).

- ▶ What is the most likely cause of the patient's mental status changes?
- ▶ What is the best treatment for this patient?

ANSWERS TO CASE 26: Fluid/Electrolyte Abnormalities

Summary: A 66-year-old man with intracerebral and subarachnoid hemorrhage develops hyponatremia and mental status changes 2 days after admission to the ICU.

- **Cause of mental status change:** Acute hyponatremia, most likely due to cerebral salt wasting.
- **Treatment:** Correct hyponatremia with normal saline infusion. Recheck serum electrolytes every 2 to 4 hours, and carefully monitor mental status and neurological examination.

ANALYSIS

Objectives

1. To learn to identify the patients "at-risk" for the development of fluid/electrolyte abnormalities.
2. To learn the detrimental effects of fluid and electrolyte abnormalities and replacement strategies.

Considerations

This patient was admitted to the ICU for management of hemorrhagic stroke and subarachnoid hemorrhage. Acute changes in mental status necessitate immediate repeat CT of the brain to rule out cerebral vasospasm as the etiology. In this case, the repeat head CT returned with no interval changes. However, laboratory testing reveals an electrolyte abnormality, namely hyponatremia, which may explain the newly altered mental status. Hyponatremia is a common problem in patients with CNS disease because the brain's ability to regulate sodium and water homeostasis is often altered. It is the most common electrolyte abnormality after an aneurysmal subarachnoid hemorrhage (SAH), occurring in 34% of patients after SAH. It usually occurs between the 2nd and 10th post-bleed day, closely paralleling the period of cerebral vasospasm. It is likely due to cerebral salt wasting, but the trigger is unknown. Natriuresis and volume depletion from cerebral salt wasting may contribute to severe vasospasm in SAH. The diagnosis and management of other fluid and electrolyte abnormalities is paramount.

APPROACH TO: Fluid/Electrolyte Abnormalities

DEFINITIONS

HYPONATREMIA: Serum sodium concentration <135 mmol/L. Hyponatremia is usually asymptomatic unless the absolute level is <120 mmol/L or the change in sodium concentration is very rapid (within hours).

TOTAL BODY WATER (TBW): The amount of water in the body, estimated as 60% of a person's weight for men, or 50% of a person's weight for women. One-third of the total body water is located in the extracellular fluid (ECF) compartment, whereas two-thirds of the total body water is located in the intracellular fluid (ICF) compartment.

OSMOLALITY: The concentration of solute particles in a solution is referred to as osmotic activity, expressed in osmoles (Osm). *Osmolality* is the osmotic activity *per volume of water* and is expressed in mOsm/kg H_2O.

PLASMA OSMOLALITY: The primary extracellular solutes are sodium and its anions, chloride and bicarbonate, glucose, and urea. Plasma osmolality can be calculated with the following formula:

$$\textbf{Serum osmolality} = [\text{Na}] \times 2 + [\text{glucose}]/18 + \text{BUN}/2.8.$$

TONICITY: A measure of the *relative* osmotic activity in 2 solutions separated by a membrane that is permeable to water but not solutes. Tonicity is also referred to as *effective osmolality*.

PLASMA TONICITY: The cell membrane is permeable to water, but solutes that are unable to move across the cell membrane passively are called "effective" solutes because they create osmotic gradients across cell membranes. These osmotic gradients affect water movement between the ICF and ECF compartments. Because water moves freely between the ICF and ECF, osmolality will always be equivalent in both of these compartments. The effective solutes in the ECF include sodium and its anions, as well as glucose. Urea is able to move freely through the cell membrane. However, it makes up a very small portion of the plasma osmolality. As such, the plasma osmolality can often be considered equivalent to the plasma tonicity, also known as the *effective plasma osmolality*.

CLINICAL APPROACH

Patients "at-risk" for the development fluid/electrolyte abnormalities include those with pulmonary or mediastinal disease and CNS diseases. Hyponatremia, which manifests as vague constitutional or mental status changes, can be found in up to 15% to 30% of hospitalized patients. Hyponatremia has the potential to cause substantial morbidity and mortality, and has been identified as an independent risk factor for mortality in hospitalized patients. Moreover, overly rapid correction of chronic hyponatremia can cause severe neurological deficits and death.

Sodium homeostasis: Abnormalities of plasma sodium concentration usually reflect an abnormality in total body water rather than a problem with sodium balance. Total body water and its composition are tightly regulated by both osmotic and nonosmotic processes. Under normal circumstances, plasma osmolality is the major determinant of water balance, where plasma osmolality is maintained at approximately 280 to 295 mOsm/kg by arginine vasopressin (AVP), otherwise known as antidiuretic hormone (ADH). Changes in plasma osmolality are monitored by the host by changes in the size of specialized neurons in the hypothalamus, called osmoreceptors. These changes in tonicity are relayed to the magnocellular neurons in the supraoptic and paraventricular nuclei of the hypothalamus, which synthesize AVP for subsequent storage and release. An increase in plasma osmolality triggers the release of AVP, which act on V2 receptors in the kidneys to increase water permeability in the distal tubule and collecting duct of the nephrons, resulting in water retention and a subsequent fall in the osmolality. At serum osmolarity levels >295 mOsm/kg, a person's thirst mechanism is also stimulated, triggering an increase in free-water consumption if the person is able to drink. On the contrary, a decrease in plasma osmolality of just 1% to 2% with water intake suppresses AVP secretion and leads to urinary excretion of excess water, thus raising the plasma osmolality back toward normal.

Plasma AVP is also regulated by *nonosmotic* factors, such as blood pressure and circulating blood volume. Arterial stretch baroreceptors are located in the carotid sinus, aortic arch, cardiac atria, and pulmonary venous system. With an 8% to 10% decrease in arterial pressure, the baroreceptors signal the hypothalamus to release AVP into the plasma. The circulating AVP acts on V2 receptors in the kidney, increasing free-water reabsorption. In addition, AVP acts on V1 receptors on blood vessels, causing an increase in vascular resistance and in blood pressure. When hyponatremia is with associated hypovolemia, the nonosmotic stimulation of AVP can cause an increase in water retention and worsening of hyponatremia, despite the presence of hypo-osmolality. During periods of low blood volume or blood pressure, baroreceptors in the cardiac atria stimulate the adrenal release of aldosterone, which contributes to sodium and water reabsorption via the proximal renal tubule.

Hyponatremia usually is a result of dysregulation of the tightly regulated process described earlier. As such, persons at risk of developing hyponatremia include those patients who are likely to have disrupted control over their water homeostasis. **Risk factors for the development of hyponatremia include head or other traumatic injury, subarachnoid hemorrhage (SAH), acute meningitis, transsphenoidal surgery, other general surgical operations, medications (ie, carbamazepine), and advancing age (due to a decline in blood flow to the kidney and GFR with age).**

Detrimental effects of fluid and electrolyte abnormalities and replacement strategies: The detrimental effects of fluid and electrolyte imbalance in the intensive care unit can evolve as the result of pathologic states or iatrogenically.

Symptomatic hyponatremia usually occurs with absolute sodium levels <120 mmol/L. However, symptoms may also arise secondary to very rapid changes in the serum sodium concentration. **Acute hyponatremia is classified as occurring within 48 hours**, whereas chronic hyponatremia takes >48 hours to develop. Initial symptoms associated with hyponatremia can be mild, including headache, nausea and vomiting, muscle cramps, aches, or generalized restlessness. With increasing severity, patients may become apathetic, lethargic, or acutely confused. If left undiagnosed and untreated, hyponatremia can progress to seizures, apnea, coma, and death. These symptoms are the manifestations of cerebral edema progression.

Hyponatremia in most cases reflects a state of relative intravascular and extravascular free-water excess, which causes water in the extracellular space to move across the cell membrane into the intracellular space, leading to cell swelling. Within the calvarium, because the skull provides a finite space for the brain to expand, cerebral edema that is left uncorrected can lead to the symptoms detailed earlier as well as eventual brain herniation and death.

Adaptive processes to cerebral edema in the brain include shifting of intracellular potassium to the extracellular fluid, thereby decreasing intracellular osmolality. As a result, brain cells lose water, and globally, the brain returns to normal volume within the skull. This occurs within hours of the onset of cerebral edema. The brain's acute adaptation helps explain why hyponatremia often remains asymptomatic except with rapid changes in sodium concentrations.

Though the brain has developed adaptive processes to deal with imbalances in body water and solute homeostasis, these adaptive processes occur at the expense of losing intracellular potassium and organic osmolytes in the brain. This becomes relevant during the treatment of hyponatremia, particularly chronic hyponatremia. Treatment for hypotonic hyponatremia causes a rise in the serum osmolality toward normal ranges, which draws water out of brain cells as the total body water equilibrates. **When the movement of water out of the neurons occurs too rapidly, brain cells that have previously adapted may not have enough time to re-accumulate the intracellular potassium and organic osmolytes that were lost.** Consequently, neurons may shrivel and become prone to **risk for osmotic demyelination**. For unknown reasons, the areas of the brain that are most sensitive to this process are near the **pons**. **Patients who are at high risk of osmotic demyelination after acutely correcting chronic hyponatremia include those with severe malnutrition, alcoholism, or advanced liver disease.**

Osmotic demyelination often presents after a period of initial improvement from the symptoms of severe hyponatremia. Several days after correction, new and progressive neurologic symptoms may develop, including spastic quadriparesis or quadriplegia, pseudobulbar palsy, and changes in levels of consciousness. This diagnosis can be established by brain MRI to assess for demyelinated regions in the brain.

Diagnosis and Management

Management of hyponatremia begins with a precise, often multistep, diagnostic algorithm that helps pinpoint the cause of hyponatremia to guide its treatment. This diagnostic process is multistep because hyponatremia can be categorized according to different etiologies that culminate in one similar clinical presentation. For example, unlike hypernatremia, which always is associated with hypertonicity, **hyponatremia can occur in the settings of hypotonicity, isotonicity, or hypertonicity. Thus, the first step in patient evaluation is to measure the serum osmolality.** *Hypertonic* hyponatremia occurs when effective solutes other than sodium, such as glucose or mannitol, accumulate in the ECF compartment. These solutes draw water from within cells into the extracellular space, resulting in a hypertonic hyponatremia as the sodium concentration is diluted. **A rise in the serum glucose of 100 mg/dL will cause a fall of ~1.6 mmol/L in serum sodium concentration.** *Isotonic* **hyponatremia, also called pseudohyponatremia, is usually produced by lab artifacts caused by severe hypertriglyceridemia, hypercholesterolemia, or paraproteinemia that causes measured serum sodium levels to be falsely low while serum osmolality remains normal.** Isotonic hyponatremia should trigger a search for an underlying cause of increased serum lipids or paraproteins. Treatment for hypertonic and isotonic hyponatremia centers on treating the underlying cause.

Hypotonic hyponatremia can be *dilutional* or *depletional*. Dilutional hyponatremia occurs when extracellular sodium concentrations are low *relative to* increases in total body water, and this can take place under 2 different scenarios: 1) The absolute sodium level may stay the same, but the total body water increases; and 2) the absolute sodium level increases, but not as much as the total body water, leading to a relative dilution of sodium concentration. Depletional hyponatremia develops when sodium loss outpaces water loss.

After establishing a patient's low serum osmolality, the diagnosis of hypotonic hyponatremia requires further investigation. The next step in diagnosis is to assess the patient's volume status. This is done using a combination of clinical and laboratory signs. Examination of the patient should include assessment of weight changes, orthostatic variations in vital signs, skin turgor (less useful in elderly patients), jugular venous pressure, central venous pressure if central access is available, and an echocardiogram to assess cardiac filling and inferior vena cava engorgement or compressibility. Laboratory measures of fluid status include hemo-concentration or -dilution and the BUN/Cr ratio. Evaluating volume status allows for the placement of a patient's hypotonic hyponatremia into 3 categories: hypovolemia, euvolemia, and hypervolemia.

Hypovolemic hyponatremia is depletional, and can be caused by either renal or extrarenal loss of sodium. Causes of renal sodium loss include diuretic use, cerebral salt wasting syndrome, mineralocorticoid deficiency, and salt-wasting nephropathy. Causes of extrarenal loss of sodium include gastrointestinal losses via vomiting or diarrhea, third space losses from bowel obstruction, pancreatitis, or burns, or sweat losses from endurance exercises. Differentiating between renal and extrarenal sodium loss is done by measuring urine sodium excretion. If the kidney is the site of sodium loss, a spot urine sodium concentration will be >20 mmol/L. On the contrary, a urine sodium concentration of <20 mmol/L points to an extrarenal etiology of sodium loss.

Euvolemic hyponatremia **has many causes, the most common being SIADH.** The diagnosis of SIADH remains a diagnosis of exclusion and requires a demonstration of (1) hyponatremia, (2) low serum osmolality, (3) inappropriately concentrated urine (U_{Osm} >100 mOsm/kg), (4) persistent urinary sodium excretion (U_{Na} >20 mmol/L), and (5) exclusion of hypothyroidism or hypoadrenalism. There must also be an absence of any stimuli that might explain an increased secretion of AVP, such as hypovolemia and hypotension. If a measure of the urine osmolality returns with appropriately dilute urine (U_{Osm} <100 mOsm/kg), the cause of hyponatremia can be explained by excessive water intake (primary polydipsia or beer potomania).

Hypervolemic hyponatremia is caused by clinical entities of volume overload, such as congestive heart failure (CHF), cirrhosis, nephrotic syndrome, and other renal failure.

Distinguishing between SIADH and cerebral salt wasting is important in the management of patients with CNS injury. The biggest distinction between the two pathological entities is that SIADH is a *volume-expanded state*, whereas cerebral salt wasting is a *volume-depleted state*. In SIADH, despite low serum osmolality, increased expression of AVP leads to an ongoing dilutional hyponatremia. However, patients are not clinically hypervolemic because only one-third of the total retained water remains in the extracellular space. Cerebral salt wasting, on the contrary, is a state characterized by hypovolemia secondary to primary natriuresis. As such, patients have a negative sodium balance. Though the pathogenesis of cerebral salt wasting is not definitive, it is theorized that impaired sodium reabsorption occurs in the proximal nephron. Reduced sympathetic tone may explain the failure of renin and aldosterone levels to rise despite volume depletion. Volume depletion will ultimately trigger AVP release despite the low serum osmolality, often causing confusion between a diagnosis of SIADH and CSW. However, CSW is always associated with an initial presentation of volume contraction and negative sodium balance.

The goals of treating hyponatremia are (1) to achieve euvolemia and (2) to correct low sodium levels to a *safe*, but not necessarily normal, range in a controlled manner to avoid the potential of osmotic demyelination. In the case of hypovolemic hypotonic hyponatremia, including cerebral salt wasting seen in SAH, volume replacement with normal saline (0.9% NaCl in water) to euvolemia generally is enough to correct the low sodium level. With volume expansion, the trigger for nonosmotic AVP release is taken away, and the kidneys will then excrete excess free water and correct the serum sodium concentration toward normal. For symptomatic hyponatremia in euvolemic or hypervolemic contexts, correction of sodium levels should take place with hypertonic saline (3% NaCl in water). Because of the risk of osmotic demyelination, this should happen in a controlled manner. **Osmotic demyelination can be avoided by limiting correction of hyponatremia to ≤10 to 12 mmol/L in 24 hours and to <18 mmol/L in 48 hours. Rate of correction should be even slower in patients with risk factors such as severe malnutrition, alcoholism, or advanced liver disease.** Acute treatment should be stopped once the patient's symptoms resolve, a safe serum sodium level (≥120 mmol/L) is achieved, or a total magnitude of correction of 18 mmol/L is achieved. During this acute treatment phase, serum sodium levels should be monitored at frequent intervals (every 2-4 hours).

How does one estimate the amount of infusion of hypertonic saline needed to stay within the safe rates of correction? Adrogué and Madias in 2000 published a seminal article on hyponatremia that included a formula that can be used to calculate the effect of 1 L of infusate on the serum sodium.

$$\textbf{Change in serum } Na^+ = (\textbf{Infusate } Na^+ - \textbf{serum } Na^+)/(\textbf{TBW} + 1)$$

Along with acute reversal of symptomatic hyponatremia, fluid restriction is warranted for euvolemic and hypervolemic hyponatremia. All fluids, not only water, need to be restricted. Nonfood fluids should be limited to 500 mL/d below the average daily urine volume. Several days of restriction are needed to make a significant change in the plasma osmolality. Alternative therapy in cases of SIADH includes demeclocycline, which induces a nephrogenic form of diabetes insipidus and excretion of excess free water.

Research is currently underway for new treatments for hyponatremia. The FDA has approved conivaptan, a nonselective vasopressin receptor antagonist, for 4-day IV use to treat euvolemic and hypervolemic hyponatremia. However, the use of this medication in patients with advanced cirrhosis is cautioned, as it also antagonizes

V1 receptors in the splanchnic region, thus increasing splanchnic flow and further elevating portal pressures in patients with liver disease; this predisposes to esophageal bleeding. Because of these concerns, selective V2 receptor antagonists are currently being tested in phase 3 clinical studies.

OTHER ELECTROLYTE ABNORMALITIES

Beyond disturbances in body water and sodium homeostasis, other electrolyte abnormalities in critically ill patients are also common and associated with poor patient outcomes. The following is a discussion on 3 electrolytes that are commonly measured daily in the intensive care unit: **potassium, magnesium**, and **phosphorus**. For a summary of causes of abnormalities in these 3 electrolytes, please refer to Table 26–1.

Potassium

Potassium is the body's predominant intracellular cation. The importance of potassium lies in the fact that **potassium is the primary determinant of a cell's resting membrane potential.** However, only 2% of the body's total potassium stores are found in the ECF, making plasma potassium concentration an insensitive marker of changes in the total body potassium level. Furthermore, the plasma potassium concentration is regulated by a variety of signals, including catecholamines, the renin-angiotensis-aldosterone system, glucose and insulin metabolism, and direct release from exercising or injured muscle. Nevertheless, because potassium is essential for cellular functions, it is important to maintain the potassium level in the normal range (3.5 to 5 mEq/L).

Hypokalemia: [K] <3.5 mEq/L can be caused by transcellular shifts or total body potassium depletion. Transcellular shifts occur when potassium moves between the ICF and the ECF. Despite the low measured serum potassium, these states do not represent true depletion. Factors that shift potassium into cells include β-agonists (such as albuterol), insulin, alkalosis, and hypothermia. Hypokalemia due to potassium depletion, on the other hand, represents a decrease in total body potassium stores and can be caused by either renal or extra-renal etiologies. For example, diuretics increase sodium delivery to the renal collecting ducts by blocking more proximal tubular sodium reabsorption; this produces a rise in electrochemical gradient in the collecting ducts favoring sodium reabsorption at the expense of potassium secretion. Hypokalemia can occur from extra-renal sources such as from gastrointestinal losses. In patient with excess GI secretion losses, the chloride loss activates the renin-angiotensin-aldosterone system, resulting in renal potassium wasting.

Hypokalemia is generally asymptomatic; however, **severe hypokalemia can present as diffuse muscle weakness, EKG changes (U waves, flat or inverted T waves, prolonged QT interval), ileus, and constipation.** Although hypokalemia usually does not produce serious arrhythmias, this condition can potentiate arrhythmias. The first goal of potassium replacement is to eliminate or treat the condition underlying a transcellular shift. The second goal is to replace the serum potassium to a concentration of 4 mEq/L, which can be accomplished with an IV or PO dose of potassium chloride. It should be noted that magnesium depletion impairs potassium reabsorption across the renal tubules, and hypomagnesemia (see the next section)

Table 26–1 • COMMON CAUSES OF ELECTROLYTE ABNORMALITIES IN THE ICU	
Electrolyte Abnormality	**Etiology**
Hypokalemia	*Transcellular Shift* • β-Adrenergic activity • Insulin • Alkalemia • Hypothermia *Increased Losses* • Extra-renal (diarrhea, enterocutaneous fistula, ostomies) • Renal (diuretics, renal tubal acidosis (RTA), metabolic alkalosis, hypomagnesemia) • Hyperaldosteronism *Decreased Intake* • Anorexia • Malnutrition/malabsorption
Hyperkalemia	• Acidosis (transcellular shift) • Renal insufficiency • Adrenal insufficiency • Rhabdomyolysis • Drugs (β-antagonists, ACE inhibitors, spironolactone, heparin, β-blockers, Bactrim, pentamidine) • Blood transfusions
Hypomagnesemia	*Renal Losses* • Diuretics • Volume expansion and increased tubular flow • Hyperaldosteronism *Extra-renal Losses* • Diarrhea • Malabsorption/malnutrition (short gut, alcoholism) • Inflammatory bowel disease • Gastric suction • Chronic pancreatitis • Burns
Hypophosphatemia	*Transcellular Shift* • Carbohydrate infusion/refeeding syndrome • Calcitonin • Catecholamines • Insulin and glucose loading • Respiratory alkalosis *Decreased Intake* • Dietary insufficiency • Malabsorption • Phosphate binders • Vitamin D deficiency *Increased Renal Excretion* • Diuretics • Hyperaldosteronism • SIADH • Glucocorticoid use • Metabolic acidosis • Hypercalcemia

can be a cause of refractory hypokalemia. As such, magnesium also must be replaced to a normal level when replacing serum potassium.

Hyperkalemia: [K] >5.5 mEq/L is often more clinically apparent in comparison to hypokalemia. It is **associated with slowing of cardiac electrical conduction and manifests with classic ECG findings.** These include peaked T waves, decreased amplitude of the P wave, increased PR interval, loss of P waves, and eventually QRS prolongation that can lead to asystole if left untreated. However, hyperkalemia can often be spurious due to traumatic venipuncture and subsequent potassium release, or specimen hemolysis. Thus, unexpected hyperkalemia should be validated with repeat blood draw if possible.

The causes of hyperkalemia can also be categorized as transcellular shifts versus impaired renal excretion. Impaired renal excretion in critical care patients is mostly due to renal insufficiency. Adrenal insufficiency can also be a cause of hyperkalemia, but this is not commonly seen in ICU patients. Furthermore, many drugs, such as sulfamethoxazole (Bactrim), subcutaneous heparin, and pentamidine can cause hyperkalemia by inhibiting the renin-angiotensin-aldosterone system. Lastly, blood transfusions can contribute to hyperkalemia, as the potassium in stored erythrocytes leaks out slowly. The accumulation of extracellular potassium in stored blood is usually cleared renally in patients receiving transfusions, but this may become a problem in patients with acute renal failure or hemodynamic shock.

There are 3 ways of managing hyperkalemia. First, to **inhibit the arrhythmogenic nature of hyperkalemia, calcium infusions are used to stabilize the myocardium.** These infusions are temporary, lasting 20 to 30 minutes, and will temporize the condition until the effects of definitive measures take place. Second, medications that **shift potassium from the ECF to the ICF are employed to temporarily decrease the plasma potassium concentrations.** These include insulin and glucose, albuterol, and bicarbonate. Note, however, that bicarbonate actually has little clinical value because it binds to calcium in the plasma, which would render our calcium infusion ineffective if given together. **Third, more definitive measures should be undertaken to remove excess potassium from the body.** These include sodium polystyrene (Kayexalate), a cation exchange resin, furosemide, a loop diuretic that enhances urinary potassium excretion, and dialysis, the most effective method in patients with acute renal failure.

Magnesium

As the body's second most abundant cation, magnesium serves as an important cofactor in a multitude of enzyme reactions. One such magnesium-dependent system is the membrane pump that generates a cell's resting membrane potential. Magnesium is also responsible for regulating calcium movement into smooth muscle cells. As such, it is essential in helping the body maintain cardiac contractility and peripheral vascular tone. These functions make it important for magnesium levels in the plasma to be maintained at normal values.

Hypomagnesemia, defined as a serum magnesium concentration <2 mEq/L, occurs in 20% of hospitalized patients and 65% of ICU patients. Diuretics can cause hypomagnesemia, as inhibition of sodium reabsorption interferes with magnesium reabsorption. The gastrointestinal tract can also be a direct source of magnesium depletion.

Diarrhea leads to a loss of magnesium; therefore, short gut syndrome and other malabsorptive states are associated with decreased magnesium absorption. Furthermore, in patients with chronic and heavy alcohol use, hypomagnesemia in the ICU may be exacerbated by depleted total body stores produced by chronic malnutrition, diarrhea, and thiamine deficiency associated with chronic alcohol abuse.

Similar to potassium, deficiencies in plasma magnesium are largely asymptomatic. However, when manifested, symptoms include weakness, tetany, and seizures. Beyond its essential role in many of the body's enzymatic reactions, magnesium replacement is important because hypomagnesemia is usually associated with other electrolyte abnormalities that will be refractory to treatment unless the magnesium level is normal. Magnesium replacement is accomplished with IV infusions of magnesium sulfate in normal saline.

Phosphorus

Phosphorus is an important electrolyte because of its participation in aerobic energy production. The presentation of phosphorus abnormalities is usually subclinical, though impaired cellular energy production may develop secondary to hypophosphatemia and can be detrimental to systemic oxygen delivery. Decreased energy production in the heart can cause decreased inotropy and cardiac output. Hypophosphatemia is also associated with reduced deformability of red blood cells, leading to hemolytic anemia. Lastly, low phosphate levels are associated with low levels of 2,3-DPG, which shifts the oxygen-hemoglobin dissociation curve to the left and reduces the release of oxygen to tissues.

Hypophosphatemia is defined as a plasma phosphate concentration of <2.5 mg/dL and can be caused by many factors. Glucose loads can decrease ECF phosphate as phosphate enters cells along with glucose. The use of phosphate binders, such as sucralfate, can iatrogenically lower the phosphate level in the serum. The reintroduction of nutrition in patients with prolonged periods of nonfeeding can cause low phosphate levels via the refeeding syndrome. Hypophosphatemia is also commonly seen in patients with respiratory alkalosis, sepsis, and DKA. Phosphate replacement is accomplished with IV or PO preparations of potassium phosphate or sodium phosphate.

CLINICAL CASE CORRELATION

- **See also case Case 23 (Acute Kidney Injury), Cases 24 and 25 (Acid–Base Abnormalities I and II), and Case 27 (Traumatic Brain Injury).**

COMPREHENSION QUESTIONS

26.1 A 53-year-old woman with a history of uncontrolled hypertension is admitted to the ICU with subarachnoid hemorrhage. She has had endovascular coiling of an anterior communicating artery aneurysm. On post-procedure day 4, she becomes acutely confused and lethargic. On evaluation of the patient, you find her vital signs to be the following: temperature 37.5°C, HR 110 beats/minute, BP 150/90 mm Hg, RR 16 breaths/min, O_2 saturation 98% on 2L/min oxygen by nasal cannula. She is somnolent, oriented only to person, and has a GCS of E3 V4 M6 (13). She has no focal neurologic deficits. Her mucous membranes are dry, her urine output has been 25 mL/h in the past 2 hours, and her CVP is 5. While awaiting a repeat CT scan of the head, laboratory values return and reveal serum sodium of 128 mmol/L and serum osmolarity of 260 mOsm/kg water. What is your next step in management of this patient?

A. Fluid bolus with 3% NS.

B. Fluid bolus with 0.9% NS.

C. Fluid restriction.

D. Give demeclocycline.

E. Give the patient salt tabs to take PO.

F. Urgent hemodialysis.

26.2 An otherwise healthy 40-year-old woman with a history of remote appendectomy is postoperative day 5 after an exploratory laparotomy and adhesiolysis for complete bowel obstruction. Yesterday, her nasogastric tube was removed and she was started on a clear liquid diet. You are notified by her nurse to evaluate her for altered mental status. Upon your evaluation, she is confused and agitated. Her vital signs are stable and normal. She is clinically euvolemic and weighs 60 kg. Laboratory testing reveals a serum sodium concentration of 122 mmol/L and serum osmolarity of 240 mOsm/kg water. You decide to correct her hyponatremia using 3% saline. At what rate will you run your infusion for the next 12 to 24 hours?

A. 33 mL/h.

B. 66 mL/h.

C. 100 mL/h.

D. Give the infusion as a bolus over 1 hour.

E. 133 mL/h.

26.3 An 18-year-old gentleman is intubated and sedated in your ICU following an exploratory laparotomy for multiple gunshot wounds to the abdomen. On postoperative day 1, morning labs reveal a serum potassium concentration of 6.2 mmol/L. Which of the following is the LEAST IMPORTANT part of your initial evaluation and management of this patient?

A. Repeat potassium measurement

B. 12-lead ECG

C. Infusion of calcium gluconate

D. Treatment with insulin and glucose

E. Fluid bolus with 0.9% saline

ANSWERS TO QUESTIONS

26.1 **B.** The patient in question has had coiling of an intracerebral aneurysm. She most likely presents with altered mental status due to hyponatremia secondary to cerebral salt wasting syndrome. Several clues in the vignette help you decide that she is clinically hypovolemic (mild tachycardia, low urine output, dry mucous membranes, and low CVP). The first goal of treating symptomatic hyponatremia is to achieve euvolemia. As such, this woman should be fluid bolused with an isotonic solution, such as normal saline. Once euvolemia is achieved, the impetus for nonosmotic AVP release is resolved. If the patient still remains symptomatic at that time, considerations should then be made for correction with hypertonic saline.

26.2 **A.** The patient in question weighs 60 kg, and as such, her TBW is estimated at 30 L (0.5×60). Using the equation from Adrogue et al, infusion of a liter of 3% saline will change the serum concentration by 12.7 mmol. The calculation is done below:

$$\text{3\% Saline} = 513 \text{ mmol/L of sodium}$$
$$\text{Patient's serum sodium} = 122 \text{ mmol/L}$$
$$\text{TBW} = 30$$
$$\text{Change in serum [Na]} = (513 - 122)/(30 + 1) = 12.7 \text{ mmol}$$

A safe target for correction of serum sodium is 10 mmol in 24 hours. For this patient, a correction of 10 mmol would take 790 mL ($10/12.7 = .79$). To infuse 790 mL over 24 hours would take a rate of 33 mL/h.

26.3 **E.** The evaluation and treatment of hyperkalemia involves all of the aforementioned answers except for fluid boluses. Repeat measurements should be pursued to confirm a true hyperkalemia. An ECG should be performed to assess for myocardial instability. A calcium infusion should be given to stabilize the myocardium. Temporary correction of hyperkalemia can be done with albuterol or insulin. More definitive treatment includes giving polystyrene (Kayexalate), furosemide, or undergoing hemodialysis if the patient is in acute renal failure. There is no role for fluid boluses in the management of hyperkalemia.

CLINICAL PEARLS

- High-risk patients for osmotic demyelination after acutely correcting chronic hyponatremia include those with severe malnutrition, alcoholism, or advanced liver disease.
- Osmotic demyelination associated with hyponatremia treatment can be avoided by limiting correction of hyponatremia to ≤10 to 12 mmol/L in 24 hours and to <18 mmol/L in 48 hours.
- Treatment of hyperkalemia include several categories: **temporary** – insulin + glucose, sodium bicarbonate; **membrane stabilization** – calcium infusion; **elimination (definitive)** – sodium polysty – rene (Kayexelate), loop diuretics, and hemodyalsis.

REFERENCES

Adrogué HJ, Madias NE. Hyponatremia. *N Engl J Med*. 2000;342:1581-1589.

Diringer MN, Zazulia AR. Hyponatremia in neurologic patients: consequences and approaches to treatment. *The Neurologist*. 2006;12(3):117-126.

Kapoor M, Chan GZ. Fluid and electrolyte abnormalities. *Crit Care Clin*. 2001;17(3):503-529.

Marino PL. *The ICU Book*. 3rd ed. Philadelphia, PA: Lippincott, Williams & Wilkins: 2007.

Rabinstein AA, Wijdicks EFM. Hyponatremia in critically ill neurological patients. *Neurologist*. 2003;9(6):290-300.

Schrier RW, Bansal S. Diagnosis and management of hyponatremia in acute illness. *Curr Opin Crit Care*. 2008;14:627-634.

Tisdall M, Crocker M, Watkiss J, Smith M. Disturbances in sodium in critically ill adult neurologic patients: a clinical review. *J Neurosurg Anesthesiol*. 2006;18:57-63.

Topf JM, Rankin S, Murray P. Electrolyte disorders in critical care. In: Hall JB, Schmidt GA, Lawrence DH, eds. *Principles Critical Care*. New York, NY: McGraw-Hill; 2005: Chapter 76.

Verbalis JG, et al. Hyponatremia treatment guidelines 2007: expert panel recommendations. *Am J Med*. 2007;120(11A):S1-S21.

CASE 27

An 18-year-old man had an unintentional fall from a second story balcony. He had a Glasgow coma scale (GCS) of 5 (E1, V1, M3), normal blood pressure, and normal pulse rate in the emergency department. The patient was immediately intubated, and a brain CT scan revealed linear skull fractures, bilateral frontal lobe contusions, intraparenchymal hematoma, and diffuse cerebral swelling. The neurosurgeon determined that these injuries do not warrant surgical treatment at this time. A ventriculostomy drain was placed in the ICU for monitoring and revealed intracranial pressure (ICP) of 26 mm Hg.

- ▶ What is the primary goal in the management of this patient?
- ▶ What are appropriate management steps?

ANSWERS TO CASE 27:

Traumatic Brain Injury

Summary: An 18-year-old man has fallen from 20 ft and has a traumatic brain injury. His CT scan shows intraparenchymal hemorrhage and diffuse swelling. Placement of the ventriculostomy shows that he has intracranial hypertension.

- **Primary goal in the management:** The primary goal in the treatment of this patient is to decrease the amount of secondary brain injury.
- **Appropriate management steps:** This patient has a traumatic brain injury (TBI) and an elevated ICP. The next steps need to include measures to reduce the ICP and maintain the cerebral perfusion pressure (CPP). These measures include the use of mannitol, vasopressors, brief hyperventilation, elevation of the head of bed (if possible), and maintaining the head in midline position. If these measures do not work, surgical intervention may be necessary.

ANALYSIS

Objectives

1. To learn the prognostic factors for traumatic brain injuries.
2. To learn the optimal supportive strategies (ventilation, fluid/electrolyte, and hemodynamic strategies) for patients with severe brain injuries and intracranial hypertension.
3. To learn the factors that contribute to secondary brain injury.

Considerations

This patient suffered a significant fall and presented with a GCS that is indicative of severe intracranial injury. His CT scan has shown that he has skull fractures and severe injury to the brain. The ability to minimize swelling and maintain adequate perfusion to the brain is of the utmost importance, as secondary injury to the brain significantly worsens the outcome. Special attention needs to be paid to ensure that there are no episodes of hypotension or hypoxia. A ventriculostomy is helpful in the diagnosis and treatment of traumatic brain injury. This device can be used not only for ICP measurements, but it can be used to remove cerebrospinal fluid (CSF) for temporary relief of intractable intracranial hypertension.

APPROACH TO:
Traumatic Brain Injury

DEFINITIONS

TRAUMATIC BRAIN INJURY: Injury to the brain as a result of an external force leading to disruption of brain tissue and blood vessels. The injury can consist of skull fractures, intracranial bleeding (subdural, epidural, intraparenchymal), and diffuse axonal injury.

MONRO-KELLIE DOCTRINE: Doctrine that describes cerebral compliance. Within the skull, there is brain tissue, cerebrospinal fluid, and intracranial blood. As the volume of one of these increases, the skull does not allow for expansion, so there is a mandatory increase in ICP. Only with the reduction of one of these (skull restrictions, tissue, fluid, or blood) can there be a reduction in ICP.

CEREBRAL PERFUSION PRESSURE (CPP) = MAP – ICP. Under normal circumstances, the cerebral blood flow remains constant over a wide range of cerebral perfusion pressure. This is often referred to as the zone of autoregulation. Normally, CPP below 50 mm Hg causes ischemic damage, while CPP above 150 can cause hyperperfusion injury. Acute disease processes can alter the range of the zone of autoregulation, leading to increased risk of cerebral damage.

CLINICAL APPROACH

Prognostic Factors for Traumatic Brain Injuries

Traumatic brain injury remains one of the major causes of morbidity and mortality. In the United States, brain injury was only recently surpassed by gunshot wounds as the number 1 cause of death in trauma patients. There is a significant amount of post-injury care needed in this population, since many patients require rehabilitation or suffer from posttraumatic stress disorder (PTSD). **The goal in treating patients with TBI is to minimize the risk for developing secondary brain injury.** Identifying those factors which tend toward a worse prognosis is not as clear, however. The prognosis for TBI is dependent on a multitude of factors including the type and severity of the injury, the time before initiation of treatment, and physiologic occurrences after the injury. There have been models based on large numbers of retrospective analysis that have identified some prognostic factors for TBI.

The most commonly identified factors in almost all models that identify risk factors for poor outcomes are **age**, **initial motor score in the GCS**, and **pupillary reactivity** at admission. Additional prognostic information is provided by the initial CT scan. The inclusion of other clinical information such as secondary insults (hypotension and hypoxia), and laboratory parameters (glucose and hemoglobin) appears to strengthen the prognostic indication.

The GCS (Table 27–1) was introduced to help improve uniformity, reproducibility, and communication of patients' neurological conditions between different care providers. The routine use of the GCS allows stratification of patients for initial therapy. The GCS measures the patient's consciousness in 3 separate components.

Table 27–1 • GLASCOW COMA SCALE SCORE

Motor Response		Verbal Response		Eye-Opening Response	
Obeys commands	6	Oriented	5	Opens spontaneously	4
Localizes to pain	5	Confused	4	Opens to speech	3
Withdraws from pain	4	Inappropriate words	3	Opens to pain	2
Flexor posturing	3	Unintelligible sounds	2	No eye opening	1
Extensor posturing	2	No sounds	1		
No movement	1				

They are scored for their eye-opening response, their verbal response, and their motor response with a minimum score of 3 and maximum of 15. The patient is awarded the best score possible for each category. For example, a patient who is a new paraplegic, but can follow commands with their arms is given a score of 6 on the motor scale (not a 1 because he does not move his legs). A low score for the motor component of the GCS has been identified as the most important predictor of poor outcome.

The pupillary examination is an essential component of the initial examination **for all trauma patients. Detection of a pupil asymmetry, dilation or loss of light reflex in an unconscious patient is concerning for ipsilateral intracranial pressure increase.** The mass effect of intracranial injuries increases the intracranial pressure and this is reflected by compression of the cranial nerves and pupillary changes. Patients who have concerns for intracranial injury and have unequal or nonreactive pupils should have rapid lowering of their ICP.

The type of injury seen on the CT scan appears to indicate the likelihood of poor outcome. Direct lacerations of epidural arteries produce epidural hematomas, while it is the disruption of bridging subdural veins that causes subdural hematomas. Intracerebral contusions are most likely the result of tissue disruption from the direct force of the injury. Contra-coup injuries are common and can be on the more severely injured side. **A subarachnoid hemorrhage has been stated to double the mortality.** Conversely, an epidural hematoma was associated with a better outcome, possibly due to the ability to emergently evacuate the hematoma. The brain damage caused by an epidural hematoma is secondary to compression, instead of intrinsic brain injury. Relief of this pressure likely results in full recovery.

Diffuse axonal injury (DAI) may not be seen on initial CT scan, but often results in poor long-term outcome. Small punctate lesions seen on initial CT scan may hint toward DAI, but MRI is the definitive imaging for diagnosis. The MRI for diagnosis of DAI does not need to be done in the early treatment stages. CT findings can also correlate with increased intracranial pressures. The loss or compression of the basilar cisterns is an indication of elevated ICP and predictor of poor outcome. With improved transport times and rapid access to CT scans, there is new risk for underestimating early intracranial injuries seen on the initial CT scan. Therefore, any patient with TBI who has intracranial pathology should have an early follow-up CT image.

Supportive strategies for severe brain injuries and intracranial hypertension: Aggressive restoration of intravascular volume, maintenance of adequate cerebral perfusion pressure, and avoidance of hypoxia are the primary endpoints in the supportive therapy for patients with intracranial hypertension. There are several different therapies and maneuvers that can be utilized to achieve these goals. Cerebrospinal fluid drainage, controlled hyperventilation, mannitol, and barbiturates are among the most commonly used therapies to alleviate intracranial hypertension. Maneuvers directed at improving cerebral perfusion require that patients have appropriate continuous monitoring with intracranial pressure monitors, central venous catheters, and arterial lines. Patients with increased intracranial pressures should be positioned to optimize venous drainage from the brain, and this can be accomplished with elevation of the head of the bed and positioning the head in a neutral, midline position.

The monitoring of ICP is essential for all patients with severe head injury. The concern for herniation from elevated ICP is the impetus for placement of ICP monitoring. The range for when to treat elevated ICP is not as clear, but is usually recommended at ICP >20 to 25 mm Hg. Increased intracranial pressure may have a direct injurious effect on the brain tissue, but the greatest harm associated with increased ICP is the increase in resistance to cerebral blood flow, which produces additional secondary brain injury.

Maintaining adequate blood flow to the brain is important treatment therapy, but it is not as easy as it would seem. Under normal circumstances, cerebral pressure autoregulation maintains CBF stable over a wide range of CPP (approximately 50-150 mm Hg). However, this zone of autoregulation is disrupted in patients with traumatic brain injuries, resulting in an increased reliance on raised MAP for brain perfusion. Previously, a CPP of >70 mm Hg was the goal for treating patients with TBI. However, data from the National Institutes of Health (NIH)-funded North American Brain Injury Study on Hypothermia suggested that transient decreases in CPP ≤60 mm Hg were not associated with worse outcome than CPP >60 mm Hg. The recent data seem to question the utility of maintaining the MAP artificially high to improve CPP, and this practice in fact may increase the duration of intracranial hypertension. It appears that attention to CPP is important; however, the best strategy for management is not clear. However, it is accepted that routinely elevating CPP to values above 60 mm Hg is not associated with improved outcome.

Brain cell metabolism is more important than total blood flow; thus, methods have been devised to try and monitor cerebral cellular metabolism. Two methods involve measuring 1) the oxygen saturation in the internal jugular vein ($JVSo_2$), and 2) the tissue oxygen tension in the brain ($Ptio_2$). These methods have obvious limitations. The $JVSo_2$ is a measurement of entire brain oxygen utilization which may not help when there is a focal lesion. Conversely, the brain tissue oxygenation measures only a focal area of tissue and may not be representative of other areas of injury. Currently no device can be singled out as an ideal monitor.

Avoidance of hypotensive episodes is important and is accomplished by use of plasma expansion (crystalloids, colloids, blood products) and vasopressors. It is important to recognize that while patients with TBI may have hypotension as a result of their TBI, this is an uncommon occurrence, so any hypotension in a patient with a TBI should be considered to be hypovolemic in nature. The achievement of euvolemia is necessary prior to the addition of vasopressors, as the constriction of cerebral blood vessels in a hypovolemic patient can contribute to worsening ischemia. Crystalloid administration is best accomplished by use of normal saline. This is different from patients who need volume resuscitation as the result of hemorrhage. The normal saline can aid in expanding the intravascular volume and may aid in decreasing brain tissue swelling. For similar reason, fluids containing dextrose and water should not be given to patients with TBI, as the free water may infuse into the brain tissue and thereby increase brain swelling. Vasopressor use usually involves an α-agonist that has focused activity on vasculature. Treatment of hypertension is rarely indicated in the patient with head injury. There is no evidence that hypertension promotes continued intracranial hemorrhage.

Patients with severe brain injury (GCS ≤8) require early intubation for protection of their airway. This also allows for the provision of increased oxygen administration to reduce hypoxia. Additionally, the minute ventilation can be controlled, and the patient can be **hyperventilated** to decrease the Pa_{CO_2} and thus cause vasoconstriction. This will decrease both the cerebral blood flow and cerebral blood volume. The decrease in blood volume can aid in the acute decrease in elevated ICP. Potential benefits of controlled hyperventilation are probably most prominent in the first 24 to 48 hours after injury, so hyperventilation to decrease ICP should be used with extreme caution and only for short periods of time. Thereafter, if intracranial hypertension persists, controlled hyperventilation to Pa_{CO_2} values of 30 to 35 mm Hg may be considered, but again for only short time periods. For the majority of individuals, controlled ventilation to maintain Pa_{CO_2} between 35 and 40 mm Hg is optimal.

Cerebral edema in patients with TBI can result from direct cellular injuries from the traumatic event or later from vasogenic edema during the recovery phase. Currently, the strategies for removing cerebral edema are limited to osmotic agents, usually mannitol or hypertonic saline. **Mannitol increases the osmotic gradient and by Starling forces, draws fluid from the interstitial compartment of the brain into the plasma, thereby decreasing the brain volume and ICP.** Mannitol can have adverse consequences as it is a potent diuretic and can significantly decrease the intravascular volume and, consequently, decrease the CBF. As such, it should only be given to patients who have documented euvolemia and ongoing continuous monitoring to avoid treatment-related hypotension. Hypertonic saline has been implemented more recently in the treatment of patients with TBI. The same mechanism of action to reduce ICP is hypothesized for hypertonic saline, but there is currently no data to support its efficacy.

Painful and noxious stimuli in patients with TBI can contribute to increase in ICP. Adequate pain control and sedation is critical when caring for these patients. However, the use of such agents can limit the neurologic examination; therefore, short-acting agents are preferred. Barbiturate comas have also been utilized to aid in the decrease of cerebral metabolism, but this intervention should be limited to situations where sedation alone is insufficient to maintain patient comfort. Neuromuscular blockade may be added if further ICP control is needed, but again, it interferes with the ability for neurological examination.

Factors Contributing to Secondary Brain Injury

Secondary brain injury refers to the injurious events that occur after the initial injury. Other than public safety intervention measures (ie, requirement of helmet wearing, etc), there is little that can be done to prevent the primary injury. It is the severity of the secondary insult that often determines the overall outcome of patients with TBI and as such, it has become the major goal in the treatment of patients with TBI. The 2 factors that are most injurious are hypotension and hypoxia. Another significant factor that can contribute to secondary brain injury is secondary hemorrhage, often referred to as "blossoming" of the initial hemorrhage.

The pathophysiology behind secondary injury involves biochemical processes and injury to the "supporting cells" in the brain including microglia, astrocytes, oligodendrocytes, and endothelial cells; these are critical to the survival of neurons. Numerous clinical trials of patients with brain trauma have investigated of use of various pharmacologic agents to mitigate secondary injury. However, to date, there has been limited success demonstrated in these investigations.

Since there are no real pharmacologic interventions that can prevent or reverse secondary injury, the primary management is to minimize hypotension and hypoxia. **A single episode of systolic blood pressure of ≤90 mm Hg that occurs during the period from injury through resuscitation doubles the mortality and significantly increases the morbidity of any given brain injury.** This reinforces the priority of avoiding hypovolemia and early consideration for vasopressor initiation when hypotension is refractory to fluid management.

Hypoxia is also known as a significant contributor to poor outcome in patients with TBI. The incidence of hypoxic episodes has decreased with the practice of early intubation and mechanical ventilator support. The avoidance of decreased oxygen-carrying capacity (anemia) is often cited in the literature as a need to maintain a hematocrit of above 30%. Currently, this level of hematocrit is not substantiated by the literature, and the adverse effects of blood transfusions are well known. However, it is generally accepted that patients with TBI should avoid significant anemia and the need for transfusion is left to the judgment of individual physicians.

Secondary brain hemorrhage is certainly one of the most devastating forms of secondary injury. The additional blood volume increases the mass effect and ICP, limiting the ability to maintain adequate CBF. Additionally, the increased bleeding initiates oxidative stress, inflammation, and edema, which all can result in cell death. Reducing secondary hemorrhage after CNS trauma may have profound effects on overall outcome. Monitoring the patient's coagulation status, especially those who have undergone significant blood transfusions is critical, as coagulopathies will contribute to further bleeding and increased mass effects.

Another important source of secondary injury is continued fever. It is not clear as to how or why continued fever increases secondary brain injury, but it is thought that the increased metabolic requirement of the cells is the cause. Patients with severe brain injuries and fevers should be treated aggressively with medications and mechanical cooling devices to reduce their core temperatures.

CLINICAL CASE CORRELATION

- **See Case 7 (Ethics in Critical Care), Case 28 (Blunt Trauma), and Case 30 (Altered Mental Status).**

COMPREHENSION QUESTIONS

27.1 An 18-year-old man is riding his motorcycle when he crashed into a light pole. On presentation to the trauma bay, his eyes open to pain, he his mumbling, and he has flexor posturing. What is his GCS?

A. 6

B. 7

C. 8

D. 9

E. 10

27.2 A 35-year-old woman is the passenger in a car that is involved in rollover. When she arrives at the trauma bay, her GCS is 5 (E1 V1 M3), and she is intubated. She is hypotensive with a systolic blood pressure of 80 mm Hg that is not responsive to fluid resuscitation. Her FAST shows free fluid in the abdomen. The initial management should be:

A. Immediately place a ventriculostomy in the trauma bay.

B. Take the patient to the CT scanner to image their brain and cervical spine.

C. Take the patient immediately to the operating room.

D. Admit to the ICU, start fluid boluses and blood transfusions.

E. Take patient to the angiography suite for aortic angiography and embolization.

27.3 A 21-year-old man had a bicycle crash with subsequent intracerebral hemorrhage and ventriculostomy placement. Later that day, his ICP rises to 35 mm Hg and he is given 100 g of mannitol. Over the next hour, his blood pressure decreases from 120/80 to 90/60 mm Hg. The most likely cause of his hypotension is:

A. Increased intracerebral pressure

B. New intracranial bleeding

C. Spinal shock

D. Decreased intravascular volume

E. Myocardial depression

27.4 A 19-year-old man is hit in the head with a baseball bat and is brought to the hospital by his friends 5 minutes after being assaulted. His GCS is 10 and his blood pressure is 150/90 mm Hg. He has a CT scan of his brain that shows a small area with intraparenchymal hemorrhage (~3 cm in diameter). He is taken to the ICU for monitoring. His treatment should include which of the following:

A. Mannitol administration, repetition of CT scan in 24 to 48 hours, and monitoring in the ward

B. Ventriculostomy placement and admission to the ICU for monitoring

C. Intubation, fluid administration, vasopressors, and repetition of CT in 6 hours

D. Admission to the ICU for monitoring and repetition of CT in 6 hours

E. Emergent craniectomy and evacuation of the intracerebral hematoma

ANSWERS TO QUESTIONS

27.1 **B.** His GCS is 7. Using this value, he receives 2 points for opening his eyes to pain, 2 points for incoherent speech, and 3 points for flexor posturing.

27.2 **C.** This patient was involved in a significant trauma and presents to the trauma bay with a decreased GCS. She is intubated for airway protection. She is receiving fluid for her hypotension, but it does not respond to fluid administration and her FAST examination shows that there is free fluid in the abdomen. The 2 most injurious events in a patient with a TBI is hypotension and hypoxia. It appears that the patient has continued bleeding in her abdomen as seen by free fluid there and a blood pressure that does not respond to fluids. Controlling the bleeding in the operating room is the best method to decrease the likelihood of hypotensive episodes.

27.3 **D.** Mannitol works to decrease cerebral edema by increasing the osmotic gradient from brain tissue to the plasma, thereby drawing the fluid out of the brain tissue. However, mannitol also acts as a significant diuretic and can deplete the total intravascular volume. This can lead to hypotension and increase the risk of secondary brain injury. It should only be used in patients who are known to be euvolemic.

27.4 **D.** This patient has a moderate head injury as indicated by his GCS. He has a small intraparenchymal bleed, but because of his rapid presentation to the emergency department, this bleed may "blossom" later. His injury is not severe enough at the moment to warrant intubation, ventriculostomy placement, vasopressors, or surgical decompression. However, because of the risk of increased bleeding, he does need to be monitored in the ICU with frequent neurologic examinations and a repeat head CT in about 6 hours.

CLINICAL PEARLS

- Early supportive therapy in patients with TBI includes restoration of intravascular volume, maintenance of adequate cerebral perfusion pressure, and avoidance of hypoxia.
- Hypotension in a patient with TBI should be considered to be hypovolemic first, and efforts should be concentrated on identifying and correcting the source of hypovolemia.
- Reducing the ICP can be accomplished with elevation of the head of bed, neutral head position, osmotic diuresis, and brief hyperventilation.
- Reduction of secondary brain injury is the primary goal in treating patients with TBI.

REFERENCES

Chang CWJ. Neurologic injury: prevention and initial care. In: Gabrielli A, Layon AJ, Yu M, eds. *Civetta, Taylor, & Kirby's Critical Care*. 4th ed. Philadelphia, PA: Lippincott Williams & Wilkins; 2009:1245-1260.

Clifton GL, Drever P, Valadka A, Zygun D, Okonkwo D. Multicenter trial of early hypothermia in severe brain injury. *J Neurotrauma*. 2009 Mar;26(3):393-397.

Nortje J, Menon DK. Traumatic brain injury: physiology, mechanisms, and outcome. *Curr Opin Neurol*. 2004 Dec;17(6):711-718.

Winter CD, Adamides AA, Lewis PM, Rosenfeld JV. A review of the current management of severe traumatic brain injury. *Surgeon*. 2005;3:329-337.

CASE 28

A 48-year-old man was an unrestrained driver who fell asleep at the wheel while driving on a highway. His car struck the highway divider resulting in a vehicle rollover, and he was ejected from the vehicle. He was evaluated in the emergency department (ED), and the following injuries were identified by CT imaging: bi-frontal cerebral contusions, facial fractures, left-sided rib fractures, a left pulmonary contusion, a nondisplaced bilateral pubic rami fracture, a left mid-shaft femur fracture, and a grade 2 splenic laceration. In the ED, the patient received 2 L of crystalloid and had a blood pressure of 100/80 mm Hg, pulse of 98 beats/minute, respiratory rate of 24 breaths/minute, and GCS of 13. He is transferred to the ICU for monitoring and further care.

- How should this patient be monitored?
- What are the priorities in the management of this patient?

ANSWERS TO CASE 28:

Blunt Trauma

Summary: A 48-year-old man has been in a high-speed motor vehicle collision sustaining blunt mechanism polytrauma. His injuries include: brain injury, pulmonary contusion with multiple rib fractures, pelvic fracture, grade 2 splenic laceration, and a femur fracture. He is hemodynamically stable with a GCS of 13 and is now in the ICU.

- **Monitoring:** This patient will need to be monitored for signs of deterioration in his pulmonary status, hemodynamic status, and neurological status. **Pulse oximetry** will be helpful for continuous monitoring of oxygenation. **Respiratory rate and respiratory efforts** are important to monitor given his pulmonary contusion and chest wall injuries. **Hemodynamic monitoring with CVP catheters and/or intra-arterial pressure monitors** should be considered for close monitoring for possible continued blood loss from his multiple injured sources. Close follow-up of his neurological functions with **serial GCS** evaluation will be important to monitor his intracranial injury. Often a repeat brain CT 8 to 12 hours following the initial CT can be helpful.
- **Priority in management:** 1) Breathing concerns (chest wall and lungs) first, 2) bleeding sources (spleen and pelvis) are next, followed by 3) brain injury, and lastly 4) non-life-threatening orthopedic injuries.

ANALYSIS

Objectives

1. To learn common injuries produced by blunt trauma.
2. To learn to prioritize and coordinate the management of patients with multiple injuries including intra-abdominal injuries, blunt chest injuries, orthopedic injuries, and brain injuries.
3. To learn the criteria for the selection of nonoperative management of solid organ intra-abdominal injuries.

Considerations

The patient is a 48-year-old man who has been in a high-energy mechanism motor vehicle crash. This represents significant mechanism for major injuries. He has undergone radiographic imaging and his identified injuries include a brain injury, thoracic injuries, pelvic fracture, splenic laceration and a femur fracture. He is currently in the ICU for observation of his head injury, optimization of his pulmonary status, and for monitoring of potential bleeding from his splenic laceration and pelvic fracture. He is at risk for deterioration of his mental status secondary to his brain injury or from developing shock due to splenic or pelvic hemorrhage. Additionally, his respiratory status may deteriorate requiring potential intubation to maintain adequate oxygenation and ventilation. Two factors have been consistently identified as leading to worse outcomes in head-injured patients: hypotension, and hypoxemia. These complications should be prevented and/or addressed aggressively in this patient.

APPROACH TO: Blunt Trauma

CLINICAL APPROACH

Common Injuries Produced by Blunt Injury

Blunt trauma is the most common mechanism causing injury in trauma patients. However, different types of blunt mechanisms produce different types of injuries. For example high-speed motor vehicle crash, fall from a roof, and fall from standing all produce different injury patterns. Blunt trauma patients are often quite challenging to treat due to the fact that with a severe mechanism multiple organ systems may be involved. In these patients, the prioritization of care is important to optimize outcomes.

Commonly affected organ systems include the central nervous system (skull, brain, and spine), respiratory system (chest wall and lung), solid intra-abdominal organs (liver and spleen), gastrointestinal system (intestines and the mesentery), urologic system (kidneys and bladder), and musculoskeletal system (long bone and pelvis fractures).

Central nervous system injuries will include skull fractures and brain injuries. The main issue with skull fractures is that there is often underlying associated brain injury. Brain injuries include cerebral contusions, epidural hematoma, subdural hematoma, and subarachnoid hemorrhage. These injuries are clinically manifested as altered mental status, or depressed level of consciousness as reflected in a decreased Glasgow coma scale score. A brain injury or skull fracture mandates neurosurgical consultation, although the majority of these injuries are treated by observation and serial neurological examinations.

Respiratory system injuries include rib fractures, pulmonary contusion, pneumothorax, and hemothorax. Rib fractures contribute to significant morbidity and even mortality particularly in patients over the age of 45. Rib fractures cause significant pain which can lead to splinted respiration and poor inspiratory effort. The sequelae of this may be pneumonia and respiratory failure requiring mechanical ventilatory support, which carries its own set of complications. Pulmonary contusions are believed to be due to direct impact of pulmonary parenchyma against the chest wall as a result of significant deceleration force. Clinically, they result in decreased oxygenation as there is a physiologic shunt of damaged lung which may not exchange gas effectively while being perfused. **Unfortunately, pulmonary contusions often worsen post injury as intravenous fluids may sequester within the injured lung parenchyma.**

Pneumothorax may occur as a result of a bone fragment from a broken rib lacerating the pulmonary parenchyma, causing air to accumulate in the pleural space. At its extreme it may lead to enough air occupying the thorax to cause the mediastinum to shift and impede venous return to the heart. This may result in circulatory collapse and is termed **tension pneumothorax**. Prompt recognition and treatment with tube thoracostomy is a life-saving procedure in these patients. Hemothorax is the result of bleeding into the pleural space, most often from the thoracic cage. Besides the risk of exsanguination, accumulated blood in the thorax may lead to infection, resulting in an empyema and sepsis. This would require operative drainage.

Solid abdominal organ injury (liver and spleen) manifests as hemorrhage during the initial hours or 1 to 2 days following injuries. Intervention in the form of operation or angiography/embolization may be necessary to control hemorrhage. Most clinically significant bleeding will be manifested as drop in blood pressure or hemoglobin and hematocrit within the first 24 hours following the injury. Patients with severe liver injuries may develop bile leaks; these patients may present with bile peritonitis. Treatment options include nonoperative methods such as CTguided drain placement and biliary decompression by ERCP with endoscopic stent placement.

Hollow viscus injury may result in the development of peritonitis if enteric contents irritate the peritoneal cavity. Clinically, the patients will often exhibit a hyperdynamic picture associated with leukocytosis. This will result in a profound inflammatory/septic response and requires operation and possible bowel resection for therapy. Mesenteric injuries may result in exsanguinating hemorrhage or bowel ischemia with delayed presentation of peritonitis. These injuries are best treated operatively.

Renal injuries from a blunt mechanism may result in parenchymal laceration or in renovascular injuries. Renal lacerations result in hemorrhage and perinephric hematoma. In extremely rare circumstances, particularly if the renal pelvis is involved, these injuries may result in the development of a urinoma and sepsis which would require drainage either operatively or percutaneously. Renovascular injuries occur as a result of the kidney's retroperitoneal location. The forces involved in a high-energy mechanism in effect cause a "stretch" of the renal artery from its origin at the aorta. This causes an intimal injury to the renal artery which will lead to renal artery thrombosis and renal ischemia. Unfortunately, success with revascularization of the kidney following blunt traumatic injury has been dismal. An ischemic kidney may result in the development of persistent hypertension or chronic flank pain requiring nephrectomy.

Pelvic fractures can result in life-threatening hemorrhage. The pelvis can be thought of as a "ring." When this ring is disrupted by fracture, two potential problems may develop: bleeding and internal injury. The pelvis is well vascularized so hemorrhage from veins and arteries may develop. Additionally, the disrupted "ring" leads to an expanded pelvic volume. As a consequence, greater blood loss occurs due to the larger capacity, and absence of tamponade effect which normally would exerted from an intact pelvic bony ring. Additionally, bone fragments from the pelvis may lacerate pelvic organs such as the rectum, the vagina, and the urethra. Pelvic fractures in and of themselves may be fatal, and unfortunately they are frequently associated with other life-threatening injuries.

Prioritizing and Coordinating the Blunt Trauma Management

Patients often have multiple injuries such as involving intra-abdominal, chest, orthopedic, and brain structures.

Mortality from trauma demonstrates a temporal relationship. Immediate deaths occur from devastating brain injury or massive exsanguination on scene from aortic ruptures. Fatality that occurs in minutes may be a result of airway issues, overwhelming brain injury, or hemorrhage. Fatality that occurs from a few hours up to the first 2 days after injury is often caused by hemorrhage or injury to the brain. Mortality that occurs subsequent to this time period is usually due to multi-system organ dysfunction or sepsis/infection. As a result, the key to triaging injury is recognizing this temporal pattern of mortality. These principles guide the Advanced Trauma Life Support guidelines for resuscitation. In brief, these principles are:

A-Airway

B-Breathing

C-Circulation

D-Disability

E-Exposure/Environment

Inability to maintain an airway leads to the rapid demise of the patient. Airway problems are most often due to the patient's inability to protect his airway secondary to diminished level of consciousness caused by brain injury or shock. **If a patient is not alert or responsive, it is critical that the airway is secured, ideally via orotracheal intubation.** This is the first priority in trauma patients with a blunt mechanism. In the scenario described, the patient has a GCS of 13 which implies adequate mentation/sensorium to protect his airway. As a result, he does not require emergent intubation in the ER or in the ICU. If, however his condition deteriorates, there should be no hesitation in establishing a definitive airway. **A GCS of 8 or less is defined as coma and would mandate intubation for securing airway.**

With a GCS of 13, it would be appropriate to monitor this patient in the ICU with frequent neuro/mental status checks. If the patient's mental status degrades as represented by a decrease in GCS, it would be appropriate to notify the neurosurgical consultant and obtain a repeat head CT to evaluate for progression of head injury. Additionally, if the GCS drops significantly, it would be prudent to intubate the patient urgently in order to prevent hypoxia from an inability to maintain an airway secondary to diminished consciousness.

If, on presentation, the patient's GCS was 8 or less, a Level II recommendation from the American Association of Neurological Surgeons suggests that intracranial pressure monitoring is warranted. This requires an invasive procedure performed by a neurosurgeon but may be done at the patient's bedside (Figure 28–1).

Patients with multiple rib fractures and pulmonary contusion need to undergo close observation, preferably with cardiac monitoring and pulse oximetry. Management of patients with significant pulmonary contusion and other hemorrhagic injuries is challenging; the fluid and blood products used to resuscitate the patient from hemorrhagic shock can aggravate the pulmonary contusion-related oxygenation defects. The process can be even further complicated if the patient also has a severe brain injury, because any further hypoxic and hypotensive insult will cause secondary brain injuries and worsen the neurologic outcome.

Grade	Hematoma	Laceration
I	Subcapsular; <10% area	Capsular tear; <1 cm, nonbleeding
II	Subcapsular; 10% to 50% area	Intraparenchymal; 1-3 cm in diameter
III	Subcapsular; >50% area, >3 cm or involving trabecular vessels	Intraparenchymal >2 cm
IV	Ruptured hematoma with active bleeding	Segmental or hilar vessel involvement with >25% spleen devascularized
V	Completely shattered	Hilar vessel involvement with complete vascularization

Splenic injuries cause concerns for further bleeding. A computed tomography (CT) scan for grading splenic injuries has been developed:

The majority of splenic injuries may be observed. Those that are prone to failure of nonoperative management include:

1. Lower hematocrit at admission
2. Lower blood pressure at admission
3. Higher CT grade of injury
4. Higher Injury Severity Score
5. Lower Glasgow coma scale
6. Larger volume of hemoperitoneum

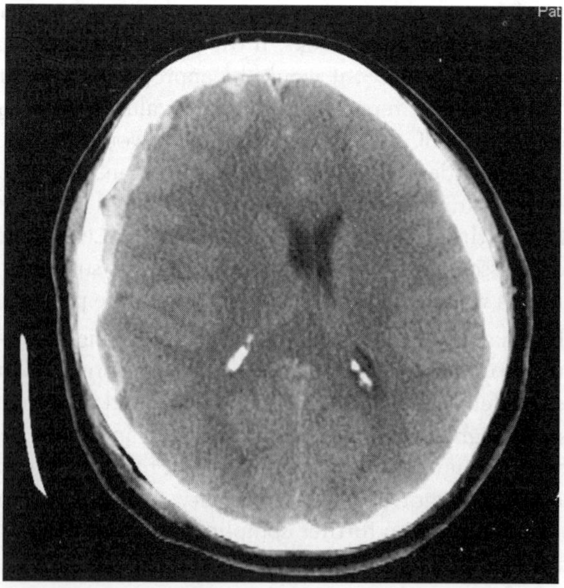

Figure 28–1. This brain CT demonstrates a subdural hemorrhage of the right side with midline shift. Hemorrhage on a noncontrast head CT is demonstrated by white density. (Courtesy of J Sadjadi, MD.)

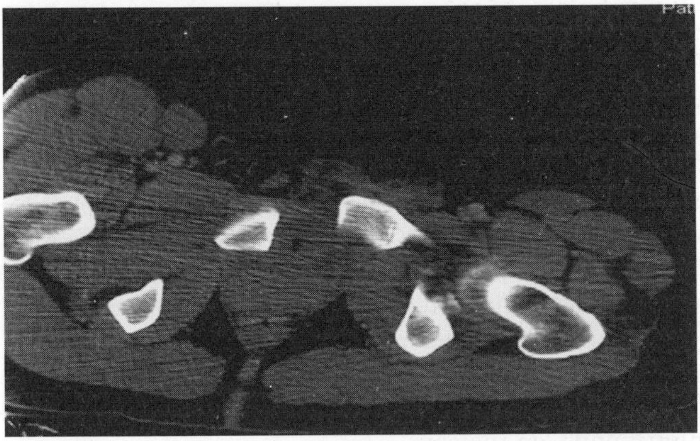

Figure 28–2. The image demonstrates an "open book" pelvic fracture with disruption of the pubic symphysis. This injury is prone to bleeding and requires a binder to be placed. (Courtesy of J Sadjadi, MD.)

Data from retrospective reviews has suggested that the addition of angioembolization may lead to increased rates of successful nonoperative management of spleen injuries.

Pelvic fractures may also lead to clinically significant hemorrhage. The disruption of the bony ring causes injury to the venous plexus of pelvis and also to branches of the internal iliac artery. Additionally, bleeding from the fractured bone edges themselves occurs. Bleeding is most pronounced in pubic rami and symphysis fractures. Acetabular and iliac wing fractures tend not to bleed, but may result in early onset osteoarthritis. Pelvic hemorrhage can often be controlled by placing a pelvic binder, which reduces the potential volume of hemorrhage and can assist in tamponade of pelvic bleeding. If a binder does not control the hemorrhage, angiography with embolization or preperitoneal pelvic packing performed in the operating room are options (Figure 28–2).

Femur fractures may result in bleeding of up to 1 L within the thigh. However, it may be unwise to perform definitive operative fixation of this patient's femur at this time as it is unclear whether this patient's head injury or splenic injury is going to progress. An operation for his femur at the time of admission may mask worsening of his other injuries while he is under general anesthesia for his orthopedic injury. This has lead to the development of the concept of damage control orthopedic surgery. It is possible to realign this patient's femur and control hemorrhage and potentially reduce pulmonary complications by placing a Steinman pin at the bedside. This weighted traction would reduce his femur fracture to length until his physiologic status is optimized prior to undergoing definitive operative femur fixation.

In summary, patients with multiple blunt traumatic injuries from high-energy mechanisms are best managed by being monitored in the ICU. Prioritization of the management of the various injuries is essential to optimize outcome. The intensive care provider must communicate and coordinate care for these patients to optimize outcome.

Criteria for the Selection of Nonoperative Management of Solid Organ Intra-abdominal Injuries

The management of spleen and liver injuries in blunt trauma patients has shifted toward a nonoperative paradigm. The Focused Abdominal Sonogram for Trauma (FAST) has changed the method of diagnosis of intraperitoneal hemorrhage following blunt trauma. Traditionally, physical examination and the invasive adjunct of diagnostic peritoneal lavage were the main tools used to diagnose intra-abdominal hemorrhage. However, the FAST examination is noninvasive and rapid and can readily identify intra-abdominal free fluid which in a hemodynamically unstable patient is presumed to be blood and mandates an operative exploration.

However, if the patient is hemodynamically stable, the next step even with a positive FAST examination is CT of the abdomen/pelvis. This allows the physician to identify injuries and plan therapy.

A large multicenter database review identified several risk factors for failed nonoperative spleen injury management. These risk factors were:

1. Increased age
2. Increased injury severity score
3. Decreased hematocrit
4. Increased grade of injury
5. Increased amount of hemoperitoneum

Additionally, the study delineated the percentage chance of splenectomy by grade of injury:

Grade	% Requiring Splenectomy
I	4.8
II	9.5
III	19.6
IV	33.7
V	75

Any development of hemodynamic instability mandates exploration and likely splenectomy.

Liver lacerations behave somewhat differently then spleen lacerations. Patients who present with a blunt hepatic injury but are hemodynamically stable and undergo a CT scan rarely require operation. The necessity of operation for blunt liver injury is dictated by clinical findings, not radiographic findings (Figure 28–3).

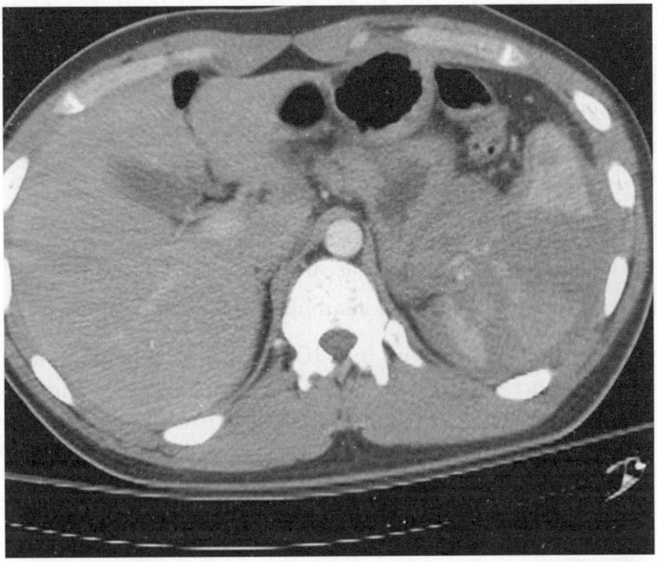

Figure 28–3. The image demonstrates a Grade IV spleen injury with 2 large fractures affecting the splenic hilum with a small vascular blush and some hemoperitoneum. This patient was successfully treated nonoperatively with angioembolization. (Courtesy of J Sadjadi, MD.)

CLINICAL CASE CORRELATION

- **See also Case 27 (Traumatic Brain Injury), Case 33 (Multiorgan Dysfunction), and Case 34 (Endocrinopathies).**

COMPREHENSION QUESTIONS

28.1 Which of the following patients may benefit from placement of an intracranial pressure monitor?

A. A 24year-old man who fell from 10 ft and presented with a GCS of 7 but a normal head CT scan.

B. A 28-year-old man involved in a high-speed motor vehicle collision with a GCS of 8 who is receiving propofol and has a right-sided subdural hematoma.

C. A 19-year-old woman who has fallen from standing and has a witnessed seizure but has a GCS of 9 and a small subarachnoid hemorrhage.

D. An 82-year-old man who fell from his bed, is confused, and cannot move his left side.

E. A 17-year-old man with an epidural hematoma based on CT and GCS of 15.

28.2 A 35-year-old woman is in a high-speed motor vehicle crash. On presentation, she is complaining of abdominal pain. Her pulse is 136, blood pressure is 76/40, and she is confused. A FAST examination is positive for fluid. The best next step is:

A. Intubation
B. CT scan of the abdomen/pelvis
C. Exploratory laparotomy
D. Admission to the intensive care unit
E. Mesenteric angiography and embolization of bleeding vessels

28.3 A 23-year-old man is involved in a 10-ft fall from a ladder. He complains of pelvic pain. On arrival his heart rate is 120 beats/minute and his blood pressure is 90/65 mm Hg. On examination he has ecchymoses of his buttocks. X-rays identify pelvic fracture with a widened pubic symphysis. FAST examination is normal. The best next step is:

A. Placement of pelvic binder in emergency room
B. Angiography
C. Exploratory laparotomy
D. CT of the abdomen/pelvis
E. Open reduction and internal fixation of the pelvis

ANSWERS TO QUESTIONS

28.1 **B.** Although there are insufficient data to make Level I recommendations, patient B does fulfill the criteria of the American Association of Neurological Surgeons for possible intracranial pressure monitoring. These criteria are: CT confirmed intracranial hemorrhage, GCS of 8 or less, and receiving sedation.

28.2 **C.** This scenario describes a patient who was involved in a high-speed motor vehicle collision and is hemodynamically unstable. Her FAST examination is positive suggesting intra-abdominal hemorrhage. She requires exploratory laparotomy. Bleeding takes priority in this instance, since without control of hemorrhage she is likely to die; she is already hemodynamically unstable, suggesting that she is in Class IV shock. Angiography and embolization are options for relatively stable patients with solid organ injuries, and reasoning behind embolization is that early embolization can help avoid surgical interventions in some of the patients. If this patient stabilizes with resuscitation and a CT demonstrates such injuries, then angiography and embolization can be viable options.

28.3 **A.** This patient has a pelvic fracture with a pattern known to result in bleeding. Additionally, he is hemodynamically unstable. A normal FAST examination has ruled out intra-abdominal hemorrhage. It must be assumed that his hemodynamic instability is secondary to bleeding from his pelvic fracture. The first step is to place a pelvic binder to reduce the potential pelvic space where bleeding can occur. If his hemodynamic status improves, he would not need angiography. If he continues to deteriorate despite placement of the binder and transfusion, he would require angiography and possible embolization of branches of the internal iliac artery which may be bleeding.

CLINICAL PEARLS

- Patients who have suffered blunt polytrauma can have multiple potentially lethal injuries. It is the physician's responsibility to triage the patient's injuries.
- The great majority of mild head injuries (GCS 13-15) can be monitored and do not require intervention.
- A positive FAST examination in a hypotensive patient mandates exploration.
- Several radiographic findings can help predict success of nonoperative management of spleen injuries.
- Liver injury management (operative vs nonoperative) is dictated by the patient's clinical status.

REFERENCES

Bratton SL, Carney NA. Guidelines for the management of severe traumatic brain injury. VI. Indications for intracranial pressure monitoring. *J Neurotrauma*. 2007;24(Suppl 1):S37-S44.

Moore EE, Cogbill TH, Jurkovich GJ, et al. Organ injury scaling: spleen and liver (1994 revision). *J Trauma*. 1995;38:323-324.

Peitzman AB, Heil B, Rivera L, et al. Blunt splenic injury in adults: multi-institutional study of the Eastern Association for the Surgery of Trauma. *J Trauma*. 2000;49:177-189.

CASE 29

A 30-year-old man is admitted to the ICU. The patient is a fire fighter who was inside a burning building when the floor of the room collapsed, causing him to fall 3 floors into the basement. The patient was trapped under a large amount of debris and was rescued after approximately 35 minutes. On examination at the scene, he had a pulse of 112 beats/minute, a blood pressure of 90/70 mm Hg, and bilateral thigh deformities with accompanying soft tissue swelling. He had burn wounds involving the entire anterior chest and abdomen and circumferential burns involving both upper arms. The wounds on his legs appear to extend into the muscles. His GCS in the emergency center was 10, and the patient was intubated. His carboxyhemoglobin level was 27%. Dark, tea-colored urine returned after the insertion of the urinary catheter. A CT scan of the abdomen and pelvis was done and revealed a laceration of the liver with minimal amount of free fluid in the abdomen. A fracture of the right iliac crest was also noted.

- ▶ What are your priorities for this patient's care in the ICU?
- ▶ How do you manage his fluid resuscitation?
- ▶ What are the measures that you would take to prevent organ injuries that may develop as results of his burns?

ANSWERS TO CASE 29:
Trauma and Burns

Summary: This patient is a 30-year-old man with severe burns on his trunk and upper extremities in association with multiple other traumatic injuries. His presentation to the emergency department is consistent with shock and inhalation injury.

- **Priorities:** Orotracheal intubation to secure the airway. Place the patient on 100% oxygen to minimize injuries from his carbon monoxide inhalation. Large-bore secured intravenous access should be placed for ongoing fluid resuscitation and for central venous pressure monitoring. His thigh deformities likely indicate femur fractures that should be verified by x-rays, followed by reduction and stabilization. The burn wounds should be gently cleaned and covered with silver sulfadiazine and gauze dressing.
- **Fluid resuscitation:** Initial fluid resuscitation can begin using either the Parkland formula or the modified Brooke formula. Endpoint of resuscitation to follow include urine output >0.5 to 1.0 mL/kg/h and adequate central venous pressures. The initial fluid administration may need to be greater in this patient because of the other associated injuries (liver, pelvis, and long bones) and his myoglobinuria. Similarly, because of these potential bleeding sources, the patient's hemoglobin, hematocrit, coagulation profile, and platelet counts need to be closely monitored during the early resuscitation period.
- **Measures to prevent organ injuries:** Large burns produce cardiac depression from circulating systemic inflammatory mediators. Pulmonary injuries may result from direct burn effects or acute lung injury (ALI), and acute kidney injury may develop as the result of insufficient fluid resuscitation and myoglobin-induced injuries. Primary prevention begins with timely and appropriate fluid resuscitation based on hemodynamic monitoring and responses to resuscitation (urine output, lactate, and base deficits). Early and timely wound management is also important in the prevention of distant organ dysfunction. For example, early burn wound excision has been demonstrated to produce fewer burn wound–associated septic complications and improved survival.

ANALYSIS

Objectives

1. To learn the management of thermal injuries (inhalation injuries, infections, acute kidney injuries, pain management, metabolic and nutritional support).
2. To learn to recognize and prioritize the care of burn patients with other associated injuries.

Considerations

This firefighter suffered severe burn injuries as evident by the extent of his wounds, which involve the entire circumference of his trunk and upper extremities.

Because he was trapped in a burning building for quite some time, he was exposed to the by-products of fire, mainly carbon monoxide and cyanide. Inhalation of these toxins along with direct heat and the steam of the flames can cause edema and severe damage to the airway. Hence, early intubation is warranted. The patient's carboxyhemoglobin of 27% is concerning and indicates significant carbon monoxide (CO) inhalation; COHgb levels of 30% are often associated with permanent central nervous system dysfunction, and COHgb levels greater than 60% commonly produce coma and death. Carbon monoxide has a 240-fold greater affinity for hemoglobin than oxygen; therefore, the half-life of CO in blood in room air is 250 minutes. The half-life of COHgb can be reduced to 40 to 60 minutes by placing the patient on 100% O_2. This patient's history of having fallen several stories to the basement resulting in severe bony injuries and subsequent immobility are concerning for the occurrence of muscle degradation and rhabdomyolysis; therefore, precautions should be taken to identify and treat this potential complication. This patient's associated injuries of pelvic fracture, bilateral femur abnormalities, and a liver laceration are worrisome. This patient needs diagnostic studies to ensure that there is no active retroperitoneal bleeding (ie, angiography or CT angiography). Additionally, urgent orthopedic consultation is necessary for early skeletal stabilization. The grade of the liver laceration can be determined based on the CT findings, and serial hemoglobin and hematocrit levels can be helpful to determine if operative or angiographic interventions are needed.

APPROACH TO:
Burns and Trauma

CLINICAL APPROACH

Management of Thermal Injuries

Burns are a major cause of trauma in the United States, as over 1 million cases occur annually. Burn injuries can be produced by heat, chemicals, electricity, or radiation, with thermal injuries being the most common. Thermal injuries are a significant cause of morbidity and mortality because of the profound inflammatory response generated both locally and systemically.

Skin Biology and Pathophysiology

The epidermis and dermis are 2 distinct layers which make up the skin. The epidermis is the outermost layer and has the unique responsibility of protecting the host from infection, fluid loss, and ultraviolet light. It is also the site of vitamin D absorption and provides much of our thermal regulation. It is derived from ectoderm and hence is capable of regeneration. In contrast, the dermis lies underneath the epidermis and provides the structural framework of skin. Collagen is the principal structural molecule found in this layer. It is the dermis that gives skin its durability and elasticity.

Burns can cause significant damage to the structure and function of the skin. Jackson's classification of the burn wound outlines the pathophysiology of thermal injury. There are **3 zones of tissue injury resulting from a burn: the zone of coagulation, the zone of stasis, and the zone of hyperemia**. The zone of coagulation is in the center and constitutes the most severely injured tissue. The cells in this zone are coagulated and necrotic. The zone of stasis is immediately beyond the zone of coagulation and is characterized by ischemia and vasoconstriction. The zone of stasis is important as it oftentimes is initially viable but can progress to the zone of coagulation when exposed to severe edema and/or hypoperfusion (consequences of inappropriate initial fluid management). Beyond the zone of stasis is the zone of hyperemia. In this zone the tissue is viable but often involved in profound inflammatory changes from surrounding cells.

Clinical Assessment

A burn patient should be treated similar to any other trauma patient, meaning the initial assessment should focus on the patient's airway, breathing, and circulatory systems. Assessment of the extent of the burns and other major injuries should also take place at this time. Inspection of the airway includes evaluation of the mouth, nose, oropharynx, and trachea. Facial burns, cinched nose hairs, the presence of soot, foamy oral secretions, and mucosal edema should alarm the provider of possible inhalation injury, and early intubation should take place. Additionally, labored breathing with shallow breaths, use of accessory muscles, stridor, or diminished neurologic function also warrant intubation. **A significant portion of initial deaths from fires occur secondary to hypoxia from oxygen deprivation or toxin inhalation.**

Perhaps one of the biggest advances in managing severely burned patients is the use of early aggressive fluid resuscitation. The Parkland formula, named after the hospital in Dallas, Texas, is a guide to volume repletion. For adults with affected TBSA% >15 or children with affected TBSA% >10, it is recommended that supportive care, continued monitoring, and aggressive fluid resuscitation be given. The Parkland formula calculates the amount of volume that should be given in a 24-hour period by measuring the (affected TBSA%) x (4 mL of lactated Ringer solution) x (weight of the patient in kg). Half of the calculated amount should be given in the first 8 hours following the injury, and the second half should be given in the subsequent 16 hours. This is only a guide for resuscitation and should be used in conjunction with other information (eg, urine output, central venous pressure, etc) to determine volume status. The modified Brooke formula is an alternative resuscitation approach using lactated Ringer solution at 2 mL/kg per% TBSA, with one-half of the fluid administered in the first 2 hours and the remaining half in the subsequent 16 hours; during second 24 hours, colloid is given at (0.3 to 0.5 mL/kg)/% TBSA burn + D_5W to maintain urine output of at least 0.5 mL/kg/h.

Calculating TBSA can be tricky. Usually only second- and third-degree burns are included in estimating TBSA. Wallace rule of nines is a way of estimating the extent of burn injury in adults. The body is divided into sections and given a percentage (a fraction or multiple of 9) of body surface area. In this schema the anterior chest, posterior chest, abdomen, buttocks, unilateral anterior lower extremities, unilateral posterior extremities, circumferential unilateral arm, and circumferential head each equal 9%. The perineum equals 1%. In total, the entire body is 100% (Figure 29–1).

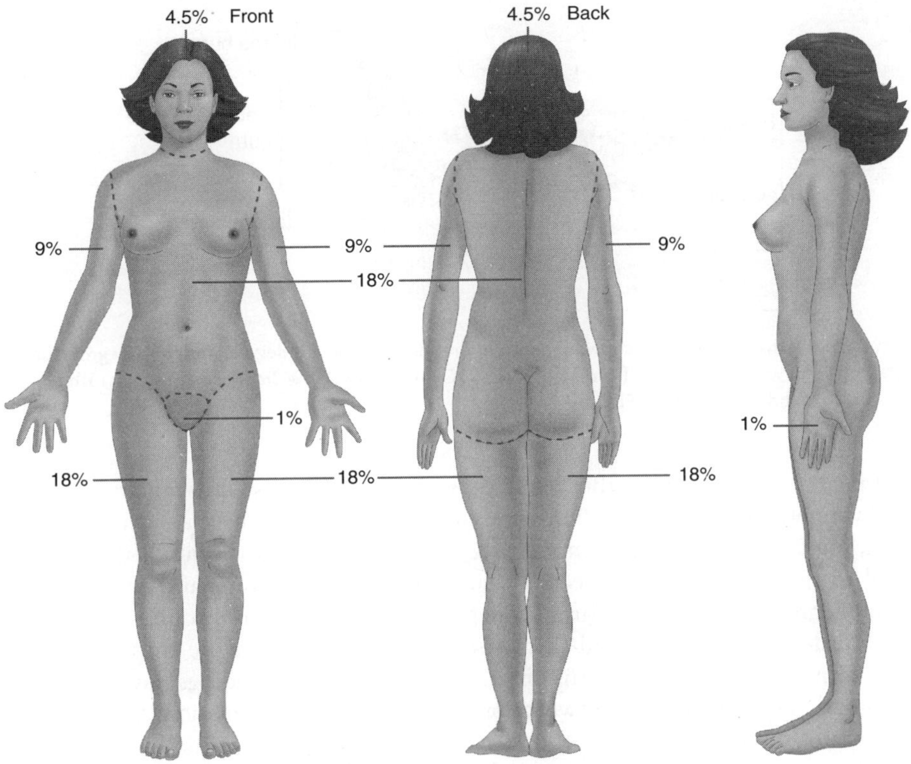

Figure 29–1. Rule of nines to estimate patient's burn size by dividing the body into regions in which the body total surface area can be calculated by multiples of nine. (Reproduced, with permission, from Brunicardi FC, Andersen DK, Billiar TR, et al. *Schwartz's Principles of Surgery*. 9th ed. New York, NY: McGraw-Hill Education; 2010. Figure 8-1.)

The rule of nines does not apply to children as they are proportionately different from adults. Hence, an adaptation of the rule of nines estimates a larger surface area for the circumferential head and less for the extremities (Figure 29–1). In our patient, the calculated TBSA equals 36%.

Management of Burn Wounds

Determining the depth of the burn wound can provide some insight into the direction of management (see Figure 29–2). First-degree burns are superficial and only involve the epidermis. They appear erythematous in color and do not have any blisters. Healing usually occurs within a few days but can take up to 2 weeks. Treatment usually consists of applying a topical cream for symptom relief and serve as a barrier against infection.

Partial-thickness burns (formerly known as second-degree burns) extend beyond the epidermis and are further classified as superficial or deep. Superficial partial-thickness burns are characterized by painful blisters that are usually pink in color. Topical agents such as silver sulfadiazine can be used for management of these burns, which usually heal within 2 weeks without much residual impairment and with

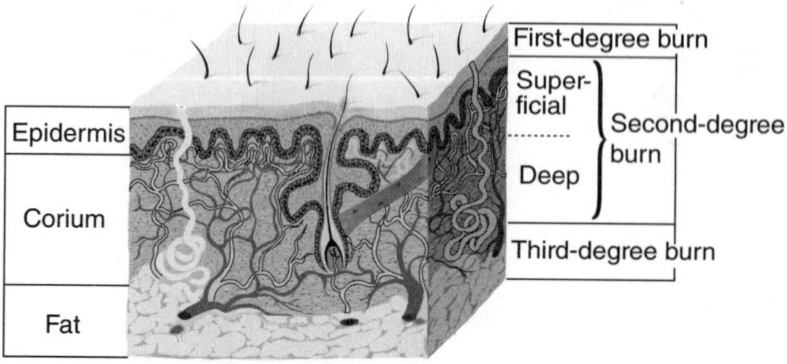

Figure 29–2. Layers of the skin showing depth of first-degree, second-degree, and third-degree burns. (Reproduced, with permission, from Doherty GM. *Current Diagnosis & Treatment: Surgery*. 13th ed, McGraw-Hill Education, 2010. Figure 14-1.)

minimal scarring. On the other hand, deep partial-thickness burns are dry, mottled, and variably painful. Silver sulfadiazine can also be used in their management; however, surgical excision and skin grafting may be necessary for wounds that do not heal within 3 weeks. Severe scarring, subsequent functional impairment, and contracture are associated with chronic deep partial-thickness burn wounds.

Third-degree burns are full-thickness burns, which involve the entire epidermis and dermis. Usually, these burns are painless as the nerve endings have also been damaged. These burns appear white or black with eschar formation. Spontaneous healing of these wounds can only take place by contraction, since the precursors for skin regeneration have been damaged. Similarly, deep partial-thickness burns have limited regenerative capacity, in which spontaneous regeneration is usually prolonged. Therefore, full-thickness and deep partial-thickness burns usually benefit from operative interventions with surgical excision and skin grafting for optimal functional outcomes. Early excision of devitalized tissue also reduces the local and systemic effects of inflammatory mediators.

Multiple Organ Dysfunction Syndrome After Burns

Due to the profound local and systemic inflammatory response from thermal injury, nearly every organ system has the potential to be compromised following a severe burn. **In the immediate post-injury period, the neurologic, pulmonary, and cardiovascular systems are most commonly affected.** Neurologically, burn victims can have a decline in their level of alertness for a number of reasons including hypoxia, inhalation of toxins, and associated traumatic head injuries. Supplemental oxygen should be given immediately. A low GCS warrants endotracheal intubation and mechanical ventilation. In patients who are alert, it is important to be aware that superficial and partial-thickness burns can cause excruciating pain and warrant careful and continuous dosing of analgesics.

A substantial percentage of patients who suffer severe burns have **inhalation injury**. Direct heat and steam can cause damage to the upper and lower airways and cause significant swelling leading to airway obstruction. **Carbon monoxide and hydrogen cyanide** are the byproducts of fires, and these toxins lead to inflammation and pulmonary edema that prevent adequate gas exchange. Hence, early intubation and mechanical ventilation should be considered. In the ICU, regular tracheobronchial care (ie, deep suctioning, therapeutic bronchoscopy, use of adjuvant pharmacologic agents such as bronchodilators or *N*-acetylcysteine) should be provided.

Cardiovascular collapse following severe burn injury is usually caused by volume depletion from fluid loss after skin disruption and vasodilation from local and systemic inflammatory mediator releases. To combat hypovolemia, **aggressive fluid resuscitation** should be initiated in the emergency department and continued in the ICU. The Parkland formula provides an initial guideline for fluid resuscitation (4 mL of lactated Ringer solution × %TBSA × weight in kg with one-half given in the first 8 hours and the second half given in the subsequent 16 hours). In the ICU, continued measurements of urine output and central venous pressure should be used to determine the patient's response to fluid management. Often, the initial fluid resuscitation plans need to be adjusted to minimize the effects of under- or over-resuscitation.

One of the most devastating conditions associated with extensive burns is burn **wound sepsis**. Burn injuries disrupt the skin's protective barrier which, in turn, renders the host susceptible to burn wound infections. Severe thermal injuries induce a relative immunocompromised state which can lead to sepsis. Initially, burn wounds are sterile but quickly become colonized with indigenous skin flora such as *Staphylococcus*. The wounds can become subsequently colonized with gram-positive and gram-negative organisms, as well as yeast from the host's oral-digestive flora and contaminants from health-care workers and the hospital environment. ***Pseudomonas aueroginosa* is a common organism found in burn wounds** in many US hospitals. The application of digestive tract decontamination reduces hosts' GI tract colonization and has been shown to reduce the occurrence of burn wound sepsis in the ICU setting.

The metabolic demands are significantly increased after thermal injury. For severe burn patients (>20% TBSA injured), **early nutritional support is critical**, with the nitrogen repletion and the maintenance of nitrogen balance being the most critical aspect of therapy. Early enteral nutritional support in this patient population is associated with improved maintenance of gastrointestinal tract, physiological and immunological functions, decreased burn wound sepsis, and decreased hospital length of stay. Nutritional goals should include a high protein diet with considerations for supplemental glutamine. Daily protein intake should be in the range of 1.5 to 2.0 g/kg/d. Avoidance of hyperglycemia is critical for minimizing infectious complications. Daily weight measurements with weekly assessment of pre-albumin levels are helpful for the determination of response and for guiding nutritional planning. Nutritional strategies are optimal when a multidisciplinary team approach is taken, including inputs from nutritionists.

MANAGING ASSOCIATED INJURIES

Burn victims often have associated traumatic injuries which can be life-threatening or compromise functional outcomes if not identified and treated in a timely manner. Burn victims should be treated as any other trauma patient. The initial assessment should begin with the ABCs of trauma but should be followed by a comprehensive secondary survey to identify other potential injuries. Radiographic imaging, such as, x-rays, CT scans, and ultrasound examinations are useful diagnostic tools.

Severe thermal injuries are often associated with immobility and subsequent muscle degradation. In addition to hypovolemia from capillary leak as a result of a profound systemic inflammatory response, the renal system can be affected secondary to rhabdomyolysis. Urine output measurements are important in the monitoring of volume status. Serial laboratory measurements of blood urinary nitrogen, creatinine, and CPK are useful in the management of rhabdomylosis and the prevention of acute kidney injuries.

LONG-TERM CONSEQUENCES

Should a patient survive a severe thermal injury, there are still several long-term consequences of burns. Psychiatric issues may develop as the result of prolonged hospitalization, multiple surgical procedures, severe skin scarring, contracture, and/or impaired function. Long-term rehabilitation and counseling are important to improve functional recovery. Additionally, the severely injured burn patient has an increased risk of developing skin cancer. A *Marjolin ulcer* is a squamous cell carcinoma that arises from a burn scar. Any changes in a burn scar should prompt further investigation via tissue biopsy to rule out malignancy.

CLINICAL CASE CORRELATION

- **See also Case 4 (Hemodynamic Monitoring), Case 5 (Vasoactive Drugs), Case 8 (Airway Management), Case 28 (Blunt Trauma), and Case 33 (Multiorgan Dysfunction).**

COMPREHENSION QUESTIONS

29.1 A patient has deep partial burn wounds involving the entire anterior chest and abdomen, and circumferential burns involving both upper arms. His estimated weight is 75 kg. Based on the Parkland formula, how much IV fluid should he receive in the first 8 hours following his injury?

A. 2000-4000 mL LR

B. 4000-6000 mL LR

C. 8000-12,000 mL LR

D. 10,000-12,000 mL albumin

E. 4000-8000 mL albumin

29.2 A 45-year-old woman suffered a thermal injury to her dominant arm 2 years ago. It took 6 months of aggressive wound care for the initial injury to heal. She presents to her physician with itching at the scar, which is irregularly bordered and has changed in shape over the past few months. Her PMD calls you to discuss the case since you cared for the patient in the ICU during her hospitalization. Which of the following is the best next step in management?

A. Observe the wound as it does not appear to be infected.

B. Prescribe an antibiotic as it may be infected.

C. Prescribe hydrocortisone cream which the patient should apply daily.

D. Take a tissue biopsy of the wound to rule out malignant transformation.

E. Refer the patient to a dermatologist.

ANSWERS TO QUESTIONS

29.1 **B.** This patient has burns to the anterior chest and abdomen and both arms, so the total body surface area involvement can be estimated at 18% (abdomen and chest) + 9% × 2 (both arms) = 36%. Based on the Parkland formula that provides 4 mL/kg × percent BSA, the calculation would be 4 × 75 × 36 = 10,800 mL over 24 hours. During the first 8 hours, half of the calculated volume will be given, which is approximately 5400 mL.

29.2 **D.** Patients with chronic wounds including burn scars are at risk of developing malignance transformation in the chronic wounds. Squamous cell carcinoma has been known to develop, and a history of shape change or growth would mandate tissue biopsy.

CLINICAL PEARLS

- A burn patient is a trauma patient. Therefore, initial assessment should begin with the ABCs of trauma with assessment of the severity of burn wounds and other traumatic injuries.
- Every major organ system can be compromised following severe burns.
- Early intubation, mechanical ventilation, aggressive fluid resuscitation, infection control, and enteral nutrition will reduce morbidity and mortality in the severely burned patient.
- Tissue biopsy is necessary for all changes in burn wound scars to rule out malignancy.

REFERENCES

Chipp E, Milner C, Blackburn A. Sepsis in burns: a review of current practice and future therapies. *Ann Plastic Surg*. 2010;65:228-236.

Church D, Elsayed S, Reid O, Winston B, Lindsay R. Burn Wound Infections. *Clin Microbiol Rev*. 2006 Apr;19(2):403-434.

Enkhbaatar P, Traber DL. Pathophysiology of acute lung injury in combined burn and smoke inhalation injury. *Clin Sci (Lond)*. 2004 Aug;107(2):137-143.

Evers L, Bhavsar D, Mailander P. The biology of burn injury. *Experimental Dermatol*. 2010;19:777-783.

CASE 30

A 60-year-old man was admitted to the ICU because of changes in his mental status after 2 short tonic-clonic seizures lasting <1 minute each. He had suffered a bout of seizures 5 years previously, and none since that time. The patient has a heavy alcohol history, averaging a 6-pack of beer a day for the past 20 years. He presented with confusion and dehydration, and it has been 4 days since his last drink. He is unable to respond coherently to questions and rambles with an unclear flow of ideas. His family members admitted that his mental status has deteriorated quickly over several weeks, at first with inattention and slight forgetfulness, and then later progressing to confusion and lethargy. He was given thiamine in the ED. IV fluids are being aggressively administered in the ICU. His vitals include a temperature of 101°F, a BP of 170/90 mm Hg, a regular heart rate of 135 beats/minute, and an oxygen saturation of 95% on room air. A CT of the brain without contrast revealed no acute changes, only slight brain atrophy compatible with his age. On physical examination, the pupils demonstrate equal size and reactivity and react to light and accommodation. The rest of the neurological examination was within normal limits.

- What is the most likely diagnosis?
- What are the initial steps in the management of this patient?

ANSWERS TO CASE 30: Altered Mental Status

Summary: A 60-year-old man is admitted to the ICU for an altered mental status. The patient has a long history of alcohol use and is confused. His BP is elevated, and he is febrile.

- **Most likely diagnosis:** Alcohol withdrawal with delirium tremens.
- **Initial management steps:** Secure the patient safety by stabilizing his clinical status with a rapid evaluation for the most common treatable and reversible causes of altered mental status (AMS).

ANALYSIS

Objectives

1. To list the common causes of alterations in mental status.
2. To understand the methods used to evaluate alterations in mental status.
3. To understand the possible choices in the treatment of patients in delirium.

Considerations

This 60-year-old man has a long history of alcohol use and has been noted by his family members to have a deterioration of his mental capabilities over several weeks. The patient's last drink was 4 days previously, and he is having alcohol withdrawal, that has progressed to delirium tremens (DT). The first priority is to stabilize the patient by controlling the seizures and withdrawal symptoms with benzodiazepines. Thiamine, folic acid, vitamin B_{12}, and other vitamins should be administered and aggressive hydration should be initiated. Glucose should be avoided until thiamine is given. Although this patient's findings are likely to be due to alcoholism and the complications of alcohol, a careful differential diagnosis for neurological problems should be undertaken to assess for conditions such as meningitis, drug toxicity, electrolyte abnormalities, and stroke.

APPROACH TO: Altered Mental Status

DEFINITIONS

DELIRIUM: It is an acute state of confusion.

COMA: It is a sleeplike state in which the eyes are closed and the patient is unarousable even when vigorously stimulated.

CLINICAL APPROACH

In the ICU, evaluating and monitoring the mental status of patients with multiple serious disease processes is a daunting task. It is estimated that **half the patients admitted to a hospital in an acute condition will undergo some form of delirium during their admission.** Half of these cases of delirium go undiagnosed. In normal consciousness, there is a state of awareness of self and the environment and the ability of the patient to interact with the activities of daily living (ADL); an intact and functioning brain stem and reticular activating system and its cortical projections are required for normal consciousness. Alterations in mental status (AMS) may range from an agitated, confused state (delirium) to an unarousable, unresponsive state (coma). Whether it is delirium, coma, or some state in between, each category represents a stage of the same disease process and is investigated in the same manner. The potential causes are broad and diverse; major causes include metabolic derangement, exposure to toxins, structural lesions, vascular insult, seizure, infection, and substance abuse.

Differential Diagnosis of AMS

Metabolic derangements may include disorders of temperature control, electrolyte balance, glucose or hormone levels, or vitamin insufficiency. Both hyperthermia and hypothermia can cause alterations in mental status. Electrolyte disorders include hypernatremia, hyponatremia, hyper and hypoglycemia, and hypercalcemia. Hypoglycemia occurs commonly in the treatment of diabetes mellitus and is life-threatening. Severe untreated hypothyroidism can result in a myxedema-derived coma. Thyrotoxic crisis, or "thyroid storm," is a life-threatening complication of hyperthyroidism characterized by marked agitation, restlessness, delirium, or coma. AMS is a broad term that can encompass anything from sudden confusion and agitation to impaired awareness and profound unresponsiveness, even coma. A patient's mental status is assessed by the level of consciousness (ie, attentiveness) via the reticular system, while cognition (ie, thought process) happens via the cortical projections. **Delirium is an acute altered level of consciousness described as waxing and waning with fluctuating inattentiveness and perceptual disturbances.** A patient in delirium will present in a confused and agitated state, unaware of his/her surroundings. It is common to see delirium superimposed on dementia in the elderly in up to 80% of cases.

A **patient in a comatose state is considered a medical emergency and must be assessed immediately for underlying, reversible causes**. The most common causes of coma are cerebrovascular disease or hypoxic injury, electrolyte disorders, encephalopathies, and drug toxicity. The longer the coma state lasts, the less likelihood there is of recovery. Hepatic encephalopathy needs to be investigated immediately as a possible cause of coma. The administration of $D_{50}W$ is standard in patients found in a comatose state since reversing hypoglycemia, if present, can be lifesaving. Coma without focal signs but with meningismus, with or without fever, suggests meningitis, meningoencephalitis, or subarachnoid hemorrhage. Coma with focal signs implies a structural lesion such as stroke, hemorrhage, tumor, or abscess formation.

Acute pituitary gland hemorrhage or infarction can lead to pituitary apoplexy. Lastly, thiamine deficiency in alcoholics or the malnourished may lead to Wernicke encephalopathy when glucose-containing fluids are administered. Toxins can arise from exogenous or endogenous sources. Exogenous sources include illicit and prescription drugs, alcohol, and noxious fumes. Endogenous sources can arise from organ system failure. Examples include liver failure (hepatic encephalopathy), kidney failure (uremic encephalopathy), and cardiopulmonary insufficiency (hypoxia and/or hypercapnia). Structural lesions can cause coma through diffuse insult to the cerebral hemispheres, damage to the reticular activating system in the brainstem, or interruption of the connections between the two. Massive hemispheric lesions result in coma either by expanding across the midline laterally to compromise both cerebral hemispheres (lateral herniation) or by impinging on the brain stem to compress the rostral reticular formation (transtentorial herniation). Mass lesions of the brain stem produce coma by directly affecting reticular formation. Because the pathways for lateral eye movements traverse the reticular activating system, impaired eye movements (doll's eye) are often an element of diagnosis.

Space-occupying lesions include neoplasms (primary or metastatic), intracranial hemorrhage, and infection. Vascular insults include hemorrhagic or ischemic phenomena, inflammation, and hypertension. Subarachnoid hemorrhage and hemorrhagic stroke cause intracerebral hemorrhage, and cerebral ischemia can result from thrombotic or embolic occlusion of a major vessel. Unilateral hemispheric lesions from stroke can blunt awareness, but do not result in coma unless edema and mass effect cause compression of the other hemisphere. Global cerebral ischemia, usually resulting from cardiac arrest or ventricular fibrillation, may cause anoxic encephalopathy and coma. Vasculitis of the central nervous system may also cause AMS, as well as other systemic signs and symptoms.

Malignant hypertension can lead to a stroke or hypertensive encephalopathy. Central nervous system infections also adversely affect mental status. Examples of these include meningitis, encephalitis, and subdural empyema. Infection may also travel from a distant site to cause AMS, such as the development of septic emboli from endocarditis. Infection or fever from any source can cause delirium in the elderly. Delirium tremens is characterized by hallucinations, disorientation, tachycardia, hypertension, low-grade fever, agitation, and diaphoresis. **Most commonly, altered mental status is caused by metabolic derangements, toxin exposure, structural lesions, vascular insults, seizures, infections, and withdrawal syndromes. A mnemonic used to remember the most common causes of altered mental status is: WITCH HAT—*w*ithdrawal, *i*nfection, *t*oxins/drugs, CNS pathology, *h*ypoxia, *h*eavy metals, *a*cute vascular insult, and *t*rauma.**

Evaluation

Rapid identification of the cause of AMS is required to treat the patient effectively. The etiologies of AMS are various and multifactorial in most instances. Patient safety is foremost, and the ABCs of resuscitation and adequate hydration must be prioritized. Vital signs, O_2 sat levels, glucose, electrolytes, CBC, and urine analysis should be evaluated. The patient should be screened for illicit drugs and possible toxic levels of prescribed medications. Potential interactions of medications should not be ignored. When possible, a history obtained from family members can help pinpoint the cause of AMS. Pertinent details of the patient's history, including the use of prescribed or over-the-counter medications, vitamin supplements, and drug abuse will aid the correct diagnosis and treatment.

The laboratory evaluation should include an arterial blood gas, complete metabolic panel, CBC with differential, ammonia, and liver enzyme level. Focused testing for ASA, acetaminophen, and tricyclic antidepressants depends upon the history and clinical suspicion. The physical examination should address 3 main questions: (1) does the patient have meningitis? (2) are signs of a mass lesion present? and (3) is this a diffuse syndrome of exogenous or endogenous metabolic origin?

The neurological examination should focus on whether there are lateralizing signs suggesting a focal lesion or signs of meningismus and fever that would suggest an infection. The key features to be noted during the physical examination are pupil size and reactivity, ocular motility, motor activity (including posturing), and certain respiratory patterns. Coma without focal signs, fever, or meningismus suggests a diffuse insult such as hypoxia or a metabolic, drug-induced toxicity, an infectious or postictal state. In the case of coma after cardiac arrest, patients who lack pupillary and corneal reflexes at 24 hours and lack motor responses at 72 hours have a poor chance of meaningful recovery.

Patients with focal findings on examination or who exhibit unexplained coma should undergo emergent imaging to exclude hemorrhage or mass lesion. Lumbar puncture is indicated when meningitis or subarachnoid hemorrhage is suspected and when neuroimaging is normal. The possibility of nonconvulsive status epilepticus should be evaluated by emergent electroencephalogram. Delirium may predispose patients to prolonged hospitalization, frequent impairment of physical function, and increased rates of institutionalization. Therefore, rapid detection, evaluation, and intervention are essential. Diagnosis of delirium is based upon clinical information. The **confusion assessment method (CAM) algorithm** is a useful tool in diagnosing delirium. Physical examination is useful in determining the etiology of AMS. Assessing for neurologic causes may help determine the severity of damage to the CNS. Focal neurologic signs should be assessed, and a CT scan should be performed to evaluate intracranial pathology. It is important to remember that before performing a lumbar puncture in the case of suspected meningitis, CT imaging of the brain should be performed first. This will detect any structural abnormalities and possibly avoid herniation from a lumbar puncture.

Diagnosis of Delirium

It is critical to diagnose and determine the cause of delirium. To diagnose delirium, a patient must have an acute change in mental status that is fluctuating between altered levels of consciousness. Laboratory testing and physical examination can shed light on the source of the delirium. The confusion assessment method (CAM) is the most accurate tool available to diagnose delirium. Table 30–1 outlines the CAM method allowing clinicians to evaluate delirium and to present focused questions that expedite the correct diagnosis of the delirium.

There are no laboratory tests, imaging studies, or other tests that can provide greater accuracy than the CAM algorithm (sensitivity 94%-100%; specificity, 90%-95%). Some clues that can help in identifying the etiology of the AMS include: the time course of mental status changes, the association of those changes with other events (eg, medication changes or development of physical symptoms), the presence of sensory deprivation (absence of glasses or hearing aids), and the

Table 30–1 • CONFUSION ASSESSMENT METHOD FOR THE DIAGNOSIS OF DELIRIUM

Feature	Comment
1. Acute onset and fluctuating course	Usually obtained from a family member or nurse and shown by positive responses to the questions, "Is there evidence of an acute change in mental status from the patient's baseline? Does the abnormal behavior fluctuate during the day, that is, tend to come and go, or increase or decrease in severity?"
2. Inattention	Shown by a positive response to the following: "Did the patient have difficulty focusing or concentrating? For example, being easily distracted or having difficulty keeping track of what was being said?"
3. Disorganized thinking	Shown by positive response to the following: "Was the patient's thinking disorganized or incoherent, such as rambling or irrelevant conversation, unclear or illogical flow of ideas, or unpredictable switching from subject to subject?"
4. Altered level of consciousness	Shown by any answer other than "alert" to the following: "Overall, how would you say what the level of consciousness of the patient is?" Normal = alert; Hyperalert = vigilant; Drowsy, easily aroused = lethargy; Difficult to arouse = stupor; Unarousable = coma Diagnosis of delirium requires the presence of the features of 1 and 2 plus either 3 or 4

presence of uncontrolled pain. A medication history with particular attention to sedative hypnotics, barbiturates, alcohol, antidepressants, anticholinergics, opioid analgesics, antipsychotics, anticonvulsants, antihistamines, and medications for Parkinson disease is very useful in including or excluding these in the list of possible etiologies of the patient's AMS. The more medications the patient is taking, the greater the likelihood that a medication is causing or contributing to the delirium. Patients and caretakers must be aware that medications include any over-the-counter medications, vitamins, supplements, elixirs, and creams.

Performance of a complete neurological and medical examination is critical in determining the patient's mental status. One should seek for signs of infection, heart failure, myocardial ischemia, dehydration, malnutrition, urinary retention, and fecal impaction. The laboratory evaluation should be tailored to the specific clinical situation. Cerebral imaging, although commonly used, is usually not helpful in the diagnosis of delirium unless there is a history of a fall or evidence of focal neurologic impairment. Targeting intervention to the individual's risk factors, such as cognitive impairment, sleep deprivation, immobility, visual and hearing impairment, and dehydration may reduce the incidence of delirium. Delirium often results from a combination of underlying vulnerability and acute precipitating factors (Table 30–2).

Amelioration of underlying vulnerability and prevention of acute precipitants will reduce the incidence of delirium. The use of **physical restraints** is generally **avoided** because they can increase agitation and the risk for patient injury. However, if other measures to control a patient's behavior are ineffective and it seems likely that the patient, if unrestrained, may cause personal injury or injury to others, restraints can be used with caution. The use of sedating agents may exacerbate or

Table 30–2 • COMMON CAUSES OF DELIRIUM	
Category	**Diseases**
Autoimmune	• CNS vasculitis • Lupus cerebritis
Neoplastic	• Diffuse brain metastases • Brain tumors
Hospitalization	• ICU psychosis
Toxins	• Prescription medications (narcotics, anticholinergics, benzodiazepines) • Drugs of abuse (alcohol, illicit drugs) • Poisons (carbon monoxide, pesticides)
Metabolic	• Electrolyte abnormalities • Hypothermia and hyperthermia • Vital organ failure (liver failure, renal failure, cardiac failure) • Vitamin deficiency (B_{12}, thiamine, folate) • Severe anemia • Severe malnutrition
Infectious	• Systemic infections • CNS infections
Endocrine	• Thyroid (hyper or hypo) • Hyperparathyroidism • Adrenal insufficiency
Cerebrovascular	• Hypoperfusion • Hypertensive encephalopathy • Focal ischemic strokes and hemorrhages

prolong delirium. **Antipsychotics or anxiolytics** should only be used in life-threatening circumstances such as in the ICU or when behavioral measures have been ineffective. Low-dose haloperidol, risperidone, and olanzapine are equally effective in treating agitation associated with delirium. These are associated with little respiratory depressive effect, a feature much desired in the respiratory compromised patient. One should attempt to use the lowest dose of the least toxic agent that successfully controls the agitation. Lorazepam used along with antipsychotics agents is complementary without adding undesirable side effects.

Treatment

The treatment of AMS depends upon its etiology. A significant part of the treatment of delirium is to institute preventive measures. In prevention of relapses of DTs, precipitating factors such as lack of sleep and dehydration should be addressed. Vitamin B_{12} and folic acid should also be administered and patients be hydrated adequately. A quiet, lowly lit environment during the day and an even darker environment during the evening and sleeping hours should be maintained. The patient should be advised to avoid reversing the normal rest and sleeping pattern.

Medications

Neuroleptics should be used with caution to avoid possible undesirable side effects. Newer neuroleptics such as risperidone, olanzapine, and quetiapine have fewer adverse effects than haloperidol. The lowest effective dose should be used, and therapy should be tapered downward ASAP, especially in the elderly. Low-dose haloperidol causes less sedation and is highly effective in treating delirium, especially when used in combination with lorazepam. The combination of 5 mg of haloperidol with 1 mg of lorazepam is effective in the treatment of delirium. The use of risperidone has fewer side effects than haloperidol and should be substituted for the latter when possible. Sedatives such as lorazepam are the drugs of choice when treating delirium due to alcohol withdrawal. These agents are also useful in decreasing anxiety. Respiratory depression can be minimized by careful monitoring, especially in the elderly.

Flumazenil can be used for benzodiazepine intoxication. This can lead to rapid withdrawal symptoms including seizures, which now may be untreatable with benzodiazepines since flumazenil will block its effect. Dexmedetomidine is also a sedative that does not cause respiratory depression. Naloxone and naltrexone should also be kept in mind with narcotic drug overdose, especially opioid intoxication where they competitively inhibit opioid-binding sites and are therefore useful in any opioid intoxication. Proper nutrition and removal of precipitating factors are essential in preventing a relapse. Weeks of treatment are needed to recover from delirium and the patient should be monitored continuously.

CLINICAL CASE CORRELATION

- **See also Case 3 (Scoring Systems and Patient Prognosis), Case 27 (Traumatic Brain Injury), Case 32 (Stroke), and Case 37 (Poisoning).**

COMPREHENSION QUESTIONS

30.1 A 78-year-old woman who has acute respiratory distress syndrome and was admitted to the ICU for mechanical ventilation (MV) 2 days ago is being evaluated for disorientation. Prior to hospitalization, she lived alone and functioned well independently. The patient is receiving MV. She received lorazepam over the past 48 hours for periods of agitation. The nurse indicates that the patient recently became disoriented and is not interacting as clearly with her family as she had done previously. Her mental status has fluctuated over the past 24 hours. On physical examination, her vital signs were normal except for a sinus tachycardia of 110 beats/minute. She is awake but does not follow directions. Neurologic examination shows no focal abnormalities and the cranial nerve examination is normal. Which of the following is the most likely cause of her current symptoms?

A. Cerebrovascular accident

B. Delirium

C. Dementia

D. Paranoid psychosis

E. Transient ischemic attack

30.2 A 19-year-old man is admitted to the ICU after presenting to the ED 6 hours ago with a drug overdose. His friends brought him to the ED after he collapsed at a party. They admitted to mixing codeine and oxycodone with alcohol and ingesting multiple drinks throughout the night. The patient is intubated for airway control and MV. His vital signs are stable. Upon physical examination, the patient's pupils are constricted and the mucous membranes appear dry. The patient is unresponsive except to deep stimuli. What is the next best step in the management of this patient?

A. Benzodiazepines intravenously
B. Haloperidol and psychiatry consult
C. Flumazenil intravenously
D. Nalaxone or naltrexone intravenously
E. Thiamine intravenous infusion

ANSWERS TO QUESTIONS

30.1 **B.** This patient has several causes for delirium: advanced age, intubation, and mechanical ventilation, unfamiliar surroundings, and underlying significant medical problems like ARDS. Protection of the patient to avoid self-harm and self-removal of the ventilation tubing and lines is the first consideration. The early treatment should involve the use of haloperidol and lorazepam to control the agitation and delirium. Propofol may be also used here to control agitation and to improve the coordination between the patient and the MV. Avoid the "sundown syndrome" by increasing the patient's awareness of her surroundings. The TV should be on. Frequent communication with the patient explaining her condition, intended therapy, and why low level lighting and control of sunlight entering the room are the key first steps in easing the patient's anxiety. Controlling the ambient lighting will assist the patient to discern the difference between day and night. Close attention to hydration and potential electrolyte disorders and the immediate correction of any such abnormalities is important in improving the underlying medical conditions.

30.2 **D.** Reversal of the narcotic overdose, which is the source of the respiratory depression and coma, is accomplished by giving nalxoxone expeditiously. This reversal is usually rapid but may be blunted since it was accompanied by alcohol. By reversing the narcotic quickly, the patient may awaken in an aggressive state. Ethanol and acetaminophen levels should be evaluated. Oxycodone and codeine are frequently available in combination with acetaminophen. Acetaminophen overdose should also be considered. If acetaminophen levels are elevated, acetyl cysteine should be administered to avoid irreversible hepatic damage. Codeine and oxycodone are not water soluble but acetaminophen is, so abusers frequently dissolve the combined medications in water and filter out the acetaminophen leaving the narcotic compound free of acetaminophen. The patient's airway should be controlled via ETI. MV is advised to control hypoventilation and hypercapnia induced by the narcotic overdose. Elevating the head of the bed to 45 degrees should be done to avoid aspiration. Narcotic overdose can cause ARDS and a chest x-ray and blood gases should be evaluated. If an osmolal gap between measured and calculated osmolality of >10 mOm/kg water exists in the presence of a positive gap metabolic acidosis, ethylene glycol and methyl alcohol should be considered as the cause of the coma. Isopropyl alcohol causes an osmolal gap but not acidosis.

CLINICAL PEARLS

- AMS is an acute change in consciousness and cognition and considered a medical emergency that must be diagnosed early and treated immediately to reach the best outcome.
- The most common causes for AMS are (WITCH HAT); **W**ithdrawal, **I**nfection, **T**oxins/drugs, **C**NS pathology, **H**ypoxia, **H**eavy metal, **A**cute vascular insult, **T**rauma.
- CAM assessment of delirium is the most accurate test available for diagnosing delirium.
- Differentiate dementia from delirium in the elderly as the 2 may superimpose each other.
- Haloperidol, risperidone, and olanzapine are all effective in treating agitation with delirium.
- Delirium is a disturbance of consciousness and cognition over a short period of time, and is associated with increased morbidity and mortality no matter the cause.

REFERENCES

Clifford S, Deutschman MS. *Evidence Based Practice of Critical Care. Saunders*; 2010.

Loscalzo J. *Harrison's Pulmonary and Critical Care Medicine*. McGraw-Hill; 2010.

Toy E, Simon B, Takenaka K, Liu T, Rosh A. *Case Files Emergency Medicine*, 2nd ed McGraw-Hill, Lange, 2009.

CASE 31

A 68-year-old white woman is hospitalized in the coronary care unit and has suffered 3 continuous tonic-clonic seizures within the past 45 minutes, each lasting about 5 minutes. She is 2 days postoperative from a repaired ascending aortic aneurysm. She never recovered wakefulness in the postoperative period. There are multiple hypodense embolic strokes revealed on a CT scan of the brain performed the day after her surgery. Her electroencephalogram (EEG) shows bursts of active seizure activity. Her respiratory rate is 18 breaths/minute, blood pressure is 160/90 mm Hg, heart rate is 150 beats/minute, and temperature is 99.9°F. She weighs 60 kg.

- ▶ What is the most likely diagnosis?
- ▶ What is the most likely mechanism responsible for the patient's condition?
- ▶ What is the best immediate treatment?

ANSWERS TO CASE 31:
Status Epilepticus

Summary: This 68-year-old patient has undergone multiple embolic strokes following aortic bypass surgery for the repair of an ascending aortic aneurysm. She has had 3 seizures within 45 minutes and had decreased sensorium since surgery.

- **Most likely siagnosis:** Status epilepticus.
- **Mechanism**: Multiple embolic strokes after aortic bypass surgery, leading to a decreased seizure threshold.
- **Best immediate treatment:** Intravenous benzodiazepines followed by an antiepileptic such as phenytoin. If needed, general anesthesia with midazolam or propofol can be used to assist in seizure control.

ANALYSIS

Objectives

1. To understand the most common causes for seizures.
2. To discuss the diagnosis and treatment of status epilepticus.
3. To understand the role of medications and toxins in causing seizures.

Considerations

This 68-year-old patient has undergone an aortic bypass surgery for the repair of an ascending aortic aneurysm. She has been in coma since surgery, and the brain imaging reveals multiple embolic strokes. She has had 3 seizures within 45 minutes each lasting 5 minutes, which is consistent with **status epilepticus.** The most likely mechanism for the multiple seizures are the multiple embolic strokes after aortic bypass surgery leading to decreased seizure threshold in the region of the cerebrovascular accidents (CVAs). The most management important steps are to maintain oxygenation, suction oral secretions to prevent aspiration, and control the seizures. The best immediate treatment includes **intravenous benzodiazepines, followed by an antiepileptic such as phenytoin.** As a last resort, general anesthesia with IV midazolam or propofol can be used to assist in seizure control. Associated complications include aspiration of gastric secretions (airway control, elevation of head of bed to 45 degrees), trauma from seizure activity (bed padding), and elevated creatine phosphokinase (CPK) levels with rhabdomyolisis and renal toxicity (hydration).

APPROACH TO:
Status Epilepticus

Status epilepticus (SE) is defined as a condition in which continuous or rapidly repeated seizures occur without regaining consciousness between seizures. The pathophysiology of status epilepticus is incompletely understood. Up to 30% of adult

Table 31–1 • DEFINITIONS OF SEIZURE DISORDERS

Definitions	Comments
Status epilepticus (SE)	>30 minutes of continuous seizure activity or >2 or more seizures without full recovery of previous baseline mental status
Epilepsy	When 2 or more seizures occur more than 24 hours apart or become recurrent
Seizure	Any event causing a change in behavior associated with alteration and erratic brain function

patients with a new diagnosis of epilepsy present as SE. The frequency of cases in the United States is approximately 150,000 per year, with 55,000 deaths annually. The mortality rate of status epilepticus is high, especially if treatment is not initiated quickly.

SE is a life-threatening condition requiring prompt management. SE with seizures lasting longer than 30 minutes or failure to regain consciousness between seizures carries a poor prognosis. **SE is considered a medical emergency**. An ambulance should be called for seizures lasting longer than 5 minutes. Approximately 2 million persons in the United States have epilepsy, making the prevalence of this disorder similar to that of type 1 diabetes mellitus. Annually, 100,000 new cases of epilepsy are diagnosed in the United States. Among the elderly epilepsy is dramatically higher (see Table 31–1).

MANAGEMENT

Control of the airway and effective ventilation are imperative. Hyperventilation and hypocapnia help offset the SE associated metabolic acidosis which results from the increased muscle metabolism and lactic acidosis. Once the seizures cease, this acidosis rapidly reverses if adequate perfusion returns the skeletal muscle. The use of intravenous bicarbonate should be avoided except in the most severe cases of acidosis. The patient must remain in a controlled environment to avoid bodily trauma. Periods of hypoventilation, cyanosis, and high mechanical ventilator (MV) pressures during active seizures should be anticipated. This may require paralysis of the patient if mechanical ventilation cannot be undertaken because of the high MV pressures. The patient should not be overly restrained while in an active state of seizure to avoid fractures and dislocations.

SE most commonly manifests itself as a series of tonic-clonic seizures. Tonic-clonic SE is managed by a regimen of intravenous diazepam or lorazepam plus intravenous phenytoin or fosphenytoin. If this fails to control the seizures, the patient is at risk for prolonged seizures and brain damage. Some patients with SE are unresponsive and may have myoclonus or focal motor activity. A characteristic series of electroencephalographic changes accompanies status epilepticus, and **an electroencephalogram (EEG) must be obtained to confirm the diagnosis**. SE is still a dangerous condition that is difficult to treat.

Benzodiazepines are the drugs of choice for the acute control of SE. Subsequent medications should include phenytoin or fosphenytoin in a continuous fashion to maintain therapeutic blood levels. If SE persists after the use of benzodiazepines and phenytoin compounds, drugs such as phenobarbital to induce coma should be

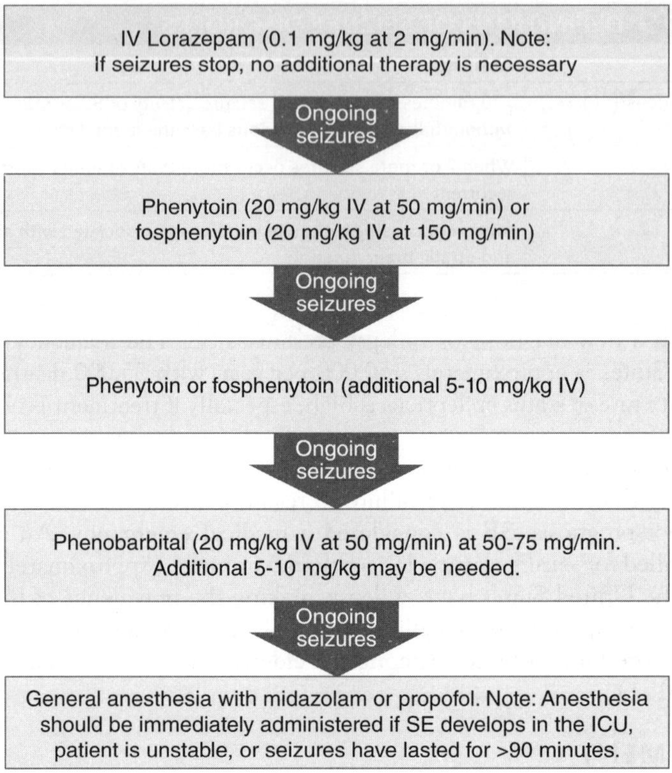

Figure 31–1. Algorithm for the treatment of status epilepticus.

considered. Failure to stop the convulsions with the regimen above requires anesthesia with midazolam or propofol as the next step in management. SE or seizures that have continued for more than 60 to 90 minutes while in the ICU tend to have severe systemic disturbances (eg, extreme hyperthermia, acidosis). Figure 31–1 indicates the approach to a stepwise treatment and the preferred dosages of antiepileptic medications, respectively.

Neurological Consultation

Neurological consultation should be undertaken in the evaluation of SE, especially if the diagnosis is uncertain, 2 or more antiepileptic drugs have failed to control the seizures, the patient is considering becoming pregnant, or the patient has a form of epilepsy that is particularly difficult to treat.

CAUSES OF SEIZURES

Drug-Induced seizures

The most common reason for seizures is noncompliance with antiepileptic drug therapy, most commonly phenytoin. **Many medications are known to decrease the seizure threshold** and cause seizures in otherwise healthy patients. Table 31–2 summarizes these drugs by class. Special attention must be paid to patients in renal

Table 31–2 • MEDICATIONS KNOWN TO LOWER THE SEIZURE THRESHOLD	
Medication Class	**Medications Known to Lower Seizure Threshold**
Antimicrobials	Imipenem, penicillin (high dose), cefazolin, cefmetazole, fluoroquinolones, metronidazole, isoniazid, aztreonam
Psychiatric drugs	Bupropion, lithium, clozapine, flumazenil, phenothiazines
Anesthetics	Lidocaine, bupivacaine
Miscellaneous	Theophylline, cyclosporine, metrizamide (IV contrast)

insufficiency or with CNS comorbidity when determining the preferred dosage of any of these antiepileptic drugs. Phenytoin itself can induce a positive antinuclear antibody (ANA) test, a lupus-like syndrome, drug fever, and even Stevens-Johnson syndrome. The ANA in drug-induced cases is of RNA origin; ANA of DNA origin is seen in SLE.

Infectious Causes

Infections are an important cause of seizures. Infections of the CNS and other sites produce acute seizures and can lead to chronic epilepsy. Direct infection of CNS tissues as in bacterial meningitis, viral encephalitis, neurosyphilis, cerebral malaria, and disseminated Lyme disease can all cause seizures. Systemic infections, such as bacterial endocarditis, include vegetations that embolize to the brain which can lead to a seizure. HIV/AIDS are also associated with several pathogens that can lead to convulsive states, including *Toxoplasma* and *Polyomavirus*, the agent of progressive multifocal encephalopathy (PME). Cryptococcal meningitis may also induce epilepsy. Among the childhood exanthems, measles can give rise to subacute sclerosing panencephalitis (SSPE) years after the infection, leading to a state of chronic recurrent seizures. Neurocysticercosis, caused by infection with *Taenia solium* (the pork tapeworm), is the most common parasitic pathogen of the CNS, which can lead to SE and is the most common cause of acquired epilepsy in developing countries.

Ethanol

Ethanol, through its effects on the GABA neurotransmitter, produces seizures both in instances of acute intoxication and in withdrawal situations (delirium tremens, DT). Complications of alcohol abuse such as head trauma, subdural hematomas, and stroke may lead to seizures. **Alcohol withdrawal seizures carry a 5% risk of progressing to DT**, a severe state of alcohol withdrawal associated with a hypermetabolic state and a high mortality. The treatment of seizures related to alcohol involves long-acting benzodiazepines (lorazepam, diazepam, or chlordiazepoxide). Chronic phenytoin therapy is not effective and should not be used.

Pseudoseizures

Psychogenic nonepileptic seizures (PNES), or pseudoseizures, must be distinguished from SE or any other true epileptic condition. Iatrogenic complications may ensue from improper treatment with anticonvulsants. Features that should raise suspicion of pseudoseizures are psychiatric comorbidities, gradual onset of the seizures, motor activity characterized by pelvic thrusting or head rolling, and vocalization such as crying and shouting in the middle of the seizure. Physical examination often reveals geotropic eye movements or eyes moving away from the examiner, and briskly reactive pupils. The absence of cyanosis and seizure activity that intensifies when the patient is restrained are also consistent with pseudoseizures. **The gold standard for diagnosis of PNES is video electroencephalography**, in which no encephalographic changes would be expected while the patient was observed to have a seizure. Management of PNES must also concentrate on treating any underlying psychiatric comorbidity.

Electroencephalographic Studies

Approximately 50% of epileptic patients will have no abnormality on a single EEG. The EEG provides confirmation of abnormal electrical activity, the type of seizure, and its location. EEG results shortly after a seizure may be misleading; therefore, EEG studies should be performed 48 hours or more after a suspected seizure. The EEG should include recordings with provocation such as with sleep deprivation, photic stimulation, and hyperventilation.

Neuroleptic Malignant Syndrome

Neuroleptic malignant syndrome (NMS) is a life-threatening neurological disorder caused by an adverse reaction to *neuroleptic or antipsychotic drugs* (haloperidol). NMS presents with muscle rigidity, *fever*, autonomic instability, and *delirium*. NMS elevates CPK and causes renal failure. Antipsychotics users should be monitored for this side effect. Treatment includes removal of the drug, aggressive hydration, and dantrolene therapy.

CLINICAL CASE CORRELATION

- **See also Case 27 (Traumatic Brain Injury), Case 30 (Altered Mental Status), and Case 32 (Stroke).**

COMPREHENSION QUESTIONS

31.1 A 25-year-old insulin-dependent diabetic was found unconscious in bed. His mother stated that he had taken his morning insulin but had not eaten breakfast. She heard noises and saw the patient having a tonic-clonic seizure in his bedroom. He is now arousable but in a postictal state. What is the most likely cause of the seizure in this case?

A. Head trauma with cerebral bleeding

B. Neutropenia

C. New onset of seizure disorder

D. Nutritional deficiency

E. Occult alcohol use

31.2 A patient with SE refractory to benzodiazepines and phenytoin treatment is intubated for control of the airway. The patient has been seizing for the past 2 hours while in the ICU. What is the next best step in this patient's management?

A. Call neurosurgery for operative intervention.

B. Get an MRI.

C. Consider general anesthesia and or propofol.

D. Administer magnesium intravenous bolus followed by continuous drip.

E. Consider phenobarbital orally or IM.

ANSWERS TO QUESTIONS

31.1 **D.** The most likely cause for the seizure on this diabetic patient is hypoglycemia, especially with the omission of breakfast. Rapid reversal of hypoglycemia is the key to recovery. The use of intramuscular glucagon is indicated and avoids the risk of aspiration when oral glucose is given. If oral glucose must be used, powdered sugar is preferred over liquid forms to prevent aspiration. The longer the CNS is depleted of glucose and oxygen the greater the likelihood of a neurological insult, and of the affected brain tissue being predisposed to seizure activity.

31.2 **C.** Once the main resources to stop seizures have been exhausted, general anesthesia with midazolam or propofol must be considered. In the treatment cascade, phenobarbital may follow benzodiazepines and phenytoin. This patient has been in SE for more than 90 minutes. Management of intractable SE includes general anesthesia as a final resort to reduce mortality from SE.

CLINICAL PEARLS

- Early control of seizures reduces the risk of chronic neurological damage.
- The first drugs of choice for the control of tonic-clonic seizures are the benzodiazepines.
- Consider neuroleptic malignant syndrome as a cause of SE in cases where fever is present and there is a known use of haloperidol and/or succinylcholine.
- Patients with SE may have rhabdomyolysis and acidosis, which is treated with hydration and urinary alkalinization.
- Consider general anesthesia for cases of intractable SE.
- Endotracheal intubation may be needed for airway control.
- There is a 30% chance of seizures in a patient with a subdural hematoma.
- Commonly used drugs can decrease the seizure threshold, causing seizures in normal individuals.
- SE patients should be adequately hydrated, and CPK, electrolytes, BUN, and creatinine levels should be followed.
- Infections in the CNS and external to the CNS can cause acute as well as chronic seizure states.

REFERENCES

Browne T, Holmes G. Review article. Primary care, epilepsy. *N Engl J Med.* 2001;344:1145-1151.

Clifford S, Deutschman MS. *Evidence Based Practice of Critical Care*. Philadelphia: Saunders; 2010.

Loscalzo J. *Harrison's Pulmonary and Critical Care Medicine*. McGraw-Hill; 2010.

CASE 32

A 52-year-old man presents to the ED with a complaint of mild left-sided weakness that began approximately 2 hours ago while he was performing yard work. The patient has a history of COPD and still smokes 1 pack of cigarettes per day. While in the emergency department, he complains of a severe headache associated with emesis. His BP is 190/100 mm Hg; pulse is 76 beats/minute and regular. Neurologic examination shows no papilledema, dysarthria, or facial drooping. The patient then receives intravenous recombinant tissue plasminogen activator (rTPA) therapy and shortly thereafter develops acute weakness of the left arm and leg along with slurred speech. An emergent repeat CT scan is performed (Figure 32–1).

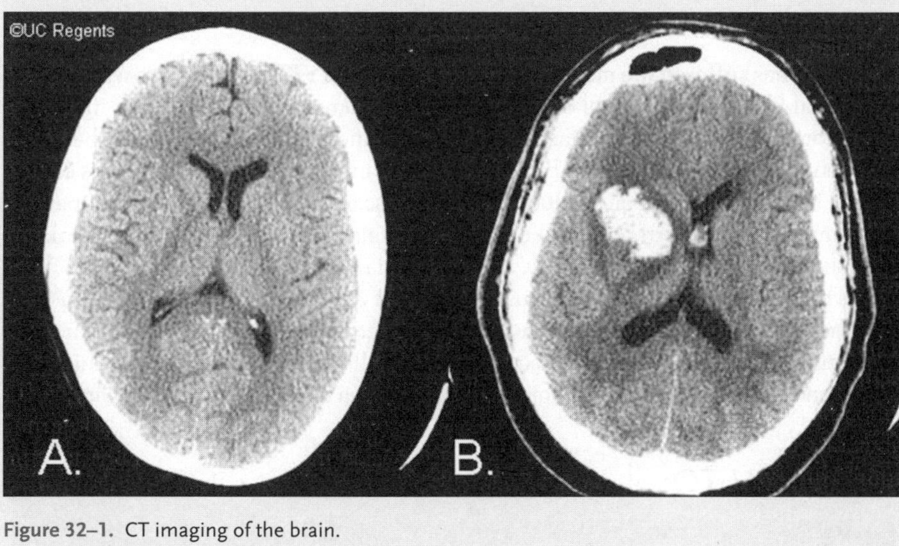

Figure 32–1. CT imaging of the brain.

- ▶ What is the most likely diagnosis?
- ▶ What is the next step in the treatment of this patient?

ANSWERS TO CASE 32:
Stroke

Summary: This 52-year-old man with COPD is seen in the ED for left-sided weakness. He receives rTPA therapy, and then develops marked left-sided weakness. A CT scan is performed.

- **Most likely diagnosis:** Initially TIA versus stroke, then hemorrhagic complication of rTPA.
- **Next step:** All anticoagulation therapy should be stopped, hypertension should be controlled, and any coagulopathy should be corrected.

ANALYSIS

Objectives

1. To understand the causes of cerebral vascular atherosclerosis and disease.
2. To understand the treatment of ongoing stroke.
3. To understand the common complications of stroke therapies.
4. To understand the medications for the prophylaxis of stroke.

Considerations

The patient has suffered the most feared complication of rTPA treatment, which is an intracranial bleed. The internal capsule is the most common area for strokes in hypertensive patients. Once intracranial bleeding is identified, all anticoagulation therapies are discontinued. Controlling the BP and reversing any clotting abnormalities is essential. The initial workup should include CT or MRI scans of the brain for determination of ischemic versus hemorrhagic stroke, while maintaining control of the BP. I think an extra space needs to be here? Initially, the patient has an acute nonhemorrhagic CVA. CVA is the second most common cause of death of adults in the United States. After rTPA therapy for his stroke, despite meeting all the criteria for administration of a clot-dissolving drug rTPA, the patient succumbed to a well-identified side effect of this class of drugs and developed a hemorrhagic bleed in the area of the right internal capsule.

APPROACH TO:
Stroke

Stroke and CVA rank second after ischemic heart disease (CAD) as a cause of life years lost to disability and death worldwide. The incidence of stroke varies among countries and increases exponentially with age. In Western societies, 80% of strokes are caused by focal cerebral ischemia due to arterial occlusion, and 20% are caused by hemorrhage. Ischemic brain injury culminates in anoxic cell death. Initially after arterial occlusion, an area of edema with structural integrity surrounds a central core of tissue death. This is the area that can recover from the first minutes to hours of the insult. No clinical deficits and findings necessarily reflect irreversible damage. Depending on the duration and severity of the ischemia, the edematous area may be incorporated into the infarct or normal tissue.

Thirty-day mortality rates are in the range of 10% to 17%. Older patients do worse after stroke; poor prognosis is also noted with the coexistence of ischemic heart disease and diabetes mellitus (DM). Mortality is related to the size of the infarct; the risk of death is as low as 2.5% with lacunar infarcts and as high as 78% with space-occupying hemispheric infarcts.

TREATMENT

The dictum is "time is brain tissue." Hence, as soon as a patient is diagnosed with possible stroke, acute imaging should be performed to rule out a hemorrhagic process and the patient screened for possible thrombolytic therapy. The treatment with intravenous rTPA (alteplase) or IV thrombolytics when started within 3 hours after the onset of symptoms are effective in limiting the severity of stroke. The recommended rTPA dose is 0.9 mg/kg with a maximum of 90 mg, with the first 10% being given IV over a period of 1 minute, and the remaining 90% given within 1 hour. Treatment leads to a 31% to 50% favorable neurologic or functional outcome at 3 months. Symptomatic intracranial hemorrhage occurred in 6.4% of the rTPA group versus 0.6% in controls. Trials of IV rTPA therapy failed to find a benefit when thrombolytics were given within 6 hours after the onset of symptoms. The benefit of rTPA is greater the sooner the treatment is started.

Intracranial hemorrhage after thrombolysis is higher in patients with more severe, larger strokes and with older patients. Concerns of hemorrhage, the efficacy and safety of rTPA in patients with early ischemic changes on CT still exist. In the first 3 hours after the onset of symptoms, the appearance of ischemic changes on CT was not associated with increased risk of symptomatic intracranial hemorrhage or other bleeding outcomes after rTPA treatment. IV thrombolysis with rTPA can be used in the community setting with efficacy and safety.

Anticoagulation

Ischemic stroke occurs because of a thrombus or narrowing of the arteries. ASA dosing (160 or 300 mg/d) initiated within 48 hours after the onset of stroke and continued for 2 weeks leads to better survival and function by reducing risk of recurrent ischemic stroke. Routine use of ASA is recommended for secondary prevention of stroke after the first few weeks. ASA is inexpensive, has a good safety profile, and is effective in patients with ischemic stroke; however, it should be withheld for 24 hours in patients treated with the use of IV thrombolytics to decrease the risk of bleeding. Dipyridamole or clopidogrel therapy in the acute phase of ischemic stroke has not been tested in randomized trials. The incidence of ischemic stroke has declined in the middle and elderly age groups but has increased in younger patients, likely due to obesity and hypertension being the contributing factors. Providers should be aware of the rising risk of stroke in younger people. The incidence of acute ischemic stroke has dramatically increased in people under age 35 in both sexes, but is still greater in males. Better detection of ischemic stroke with MRI may expose obesity and hypertension as the underlying cause. **The use of unfractionated heparin, low-molecular-weight heparins, heparinoids, thrombin inhibitors, or oral anticoagulants in the acute phase of stroke improves functional outcomes.**

Management of Cardiovascular Risk Factors

Aspirin (ASA) should be started after 24 hours (300 mg daily for the first 2 weeks) and extended release dipyridamole for secondary prevention. Aggressive management of cardiovascular risk factors including smoking cessation, treatment of hypertension, and initiating statin therapy is also recommended. **Atrial fibrillation (AF) is a common arrhythmia that increases the risk of stroke.** Warfarin (Coumadin) therapy (and now oral apixaban in nonvalvular AF) to keep the international normalized ratio (INR) between 2 and 3 is the accepted therapy. Apixaban, a direct antithrombin inhibitor, does not require monitoring of the INR. These agents have been more effective than ASA for the prevention of stroke in patients with AF. A narrow therapeutic window and the need for lifelong coagulation monitoring limits the use of warfarin (Coumadin). When warfarin (Coumadin) is used, maintenance of the INR in the therapeutic range is challenging and is achieved less than 60% of the time; suboptimal anticoagulation can lead to recurrent stoke. At least a third of patients with AF who are at risk for stroke are either not started on oral anticoagulant therapy or are not compliant with therapy. ASA reduces the risk of stroke in patients with AF by about 20% and is used to treat patients with atrial fibrillation for whom vitamin K antagonist therapy is contraindicated. Addition of clopidogrel to an ASA regimen in patients for whom vitamin K antagonist therapy is contraindicated further reduces the risk of stroke by 28%, but the combination increases the risk of major hemorrhage. A number of small molecular weight inhibitors of Factor Xa are currently available and can be delivered orally. Among these are rivaroxaban, apixaban, betrixaban, YM150, and DU-176b. Apixaban is a direct and competitive inhibitor of Factor Xa.

Prevention and Management of Complications

Patients with an acute stroke are at an increased risk for deep venous thrombosis (DVT) and pulmonary embolism (PE). This risk for DVT and PE increases with increasing age and stroke severity scores. Anticoagulant therapy does not improve the overall functional outcome, but subcutaneously administered low-dose unfractionated heparin (UFH) or low-molecular-weight heparin (LMWH) are recommended for patients at high risk for DVT and PE, and for those with immobility. Large supratentorial infarcts and space-occupying edema of the brain may lead to transtentorial or uncal herniation, usually between the second and fifth day after the onset of stroke. Intensive care units with these cases have reported early fatality rates of up to 78%. Medical therapy has proved ineffective in these cases of large space-occupying lesions. Compared to medical therapy, surgery (hemicraniectomy, duraplasty, a dural patch to enlarge the intradural space) in the first 48 hours of the onset of stroke reduced the case fatality rate (22% vs 71%). Surgery appeared to be less beneficial for patients with aphasia, patients older than 50 years of age, and patients in whom surgery was performed on the second day versus the first day after stroke onset. Patients who received care in a stroke unit were more likely to survive, regain independence, and return home than those who do not receive such specialized care.

Hypercoagulable States

Hypercoagulable conditions can lead to strokes. The most common conditions in this group include oral contraceptive use, pregnancy, Factor V Leiden deficiency, protein C and S deficiencies, antithrombin III deficiency, and lupus anticoagulant. Patients with these conditions usually present with some form of deep venous thrombosis. Procoagulant states should be suspected especially when recurrent episodes of deep venous thrombosis are diagnosed. Arterial thrombosis should definitely increase awareness of the presence of one of these conditions. Clots can travel from the venous circulation through the heart via an atrial or ventricular septal defect to the left side of the heart and to the arterial circulation leading to the brain (paradoxical emboli). Lupus anticoagulant is a specific immunoglobulin against phospholipids that prolongs the clotting time; it does not produce bleeding but instead a paradoxical procoagulant condition. It is seen in 25% of people with SLE, but is also seen in otherwise normal healthy subjects. In some people it is associated with an increased risk of blood clots and may be the cause of recurrent spontaneous abortions. Risk factors are SLE and a recent use of phenothiazine medication. Specialized clotting studies and levels of the factors involved are required to make an accurate diagnosis.

Prevention of Stroke

Secondary prevention of stroke and other cardiovascular complications is important. Prevention consists primarily of low-dose ASA and dipyridamole in patients with ischemic stroke, oral anticoagulation in patients with cardiac embolism, treatment of hypertension, statin therapy, and glucose control in patients with diabetes. Cessation of smoking and carotid endarterectomy in patients with ipsilateral carotid stenosis has been shown to be effective.

Even in the United States, only a minority of patients with acute ischemic stroke receive intravenous rTPA. The **use of intravenous rTPA is currently restricted to a 3-hour time window after the onset of symptoms with a potential benefit when used up to 6 hours after the onset of a stroke.** Later use was improved by quantification of the ischemic penumbra with perfusion MRI/CT. The intent of thrombolysis is to recanalize occluded arteries. **Complete recanalization of an occluded middle cerebral artery 2 hours after the start of thrombolysis was achieved in one-third of patients.** In some cases, continuous 2-MHz transcranial Doppler ultrasonography applied for 2 hours simultaneous with rTPA augmented the rate of arterial recanalization. The addition of intravenous galactose-based micro bubbles may also increase rates of recanalization along with Doppler therapy. Compared with intravenous thrombolysis, intra-arterial thrombolysis may increase the likelihood of recanalization. The administration of both intra-arterial recombinant pro-urokinase and intravenous heparin, compared with intravenous heparin alone, within 6 hours after the onset of stroke resulted in a higher rate of recanalization of the middle cerebral artery (66% vs 18%) and a higher rate of a favorable functional outcome at 3 months (40% vs 25%, $P = 0.04$).

Procedures required to deliver intra-arterial thrombolytic agents to the site of vascular occlusion involve more time than intravenous therapy. Thrombolytic therapy in which intravenous thrombolysis is followed by intra-arterial thrombolysis, may permit more rapid treatment and improved rates of recanalization. Mechanical thrombectomy in patients with acute intracranial occlusion of the intracranial carotid artery has resulted in a higher rate of recanalization.

Elevated blood pressure, hyperglycemia, and fever in the first hours to days after ischemic stroke have all been associated with poor long-term outcomes. Antihypertensive therapy during the acute phase of stroke is held unless the diastolic blood pressure exceeds 120 mm Hg or the systolic blood pressure exceeds 220 mm Hg in patients who do not receive rTPA. Monitoring blood pressure is recommended before, during, and after rTPA therapy. Intravenous antihypertensive therapy to maintain the systolic blood pressure <185 mm Hg and the diastolic blood pressure below 110 mm Hg is recommended. Hypothermia has also improved functional outcomes in trials involving patients with global cerebral ischemia after cardiac arrest and traumatic spinal cord injury, but the improvement was not consistent among those with traumatic brain injury.

Conclusions

Patients with signs and symptoms of CVA strongly suggestive of stroke should undergo prompt brain imaging (CT or MRI). MRI is more sensitive for early ischemic changes, but either method can fully rule out hemorrhage. In the absence of bleeding or other contraindications to thrombolysis such as spontaneous, complete clearing of the deficits, increase in BP to or >185/110 mm Hg, or presentation >3 hours (possibly 6 hours) after the onset of symptoms, the patient should receive therapy with intravenous rTPA. Cardiovascular risk factors should be addressed, and anticoagulation should be initiated when atrial fibrillation is present.

RECENT IMPORTANT DISCOVERIES

Compared to ASA, apixaban had superior efficacy in reducing the risk for embolic events in patients with AF. It has a 50% level of bioavailability, and is partially excreted by the kidneys. Apixaban, at a dose of 2.5 mg twice daily is effective and safe for the prevention of DVT after elective orthopedic surgery. **The direct thrombin inhibitor dabigatran gained a Class I recommendation as a useful alternative to warfarin (Coumadin) for the prevention of stroke and systemic thromboembolism in patients with paroxysmal to permanent AF.** Risk factors for stroke or systemic embolization are increased in patients with prosthetic heart valves, hemodynamically significant valvular disease, renal failure (creatinine clearance <15 mL/min), and advanced liver disease (impaired baseline clotting function).

Routinely switching patients to dabigatran who are already successfully taking warfarin is not recommended and remains an individual decision. Dabigatran requires a twice daily dosing and greater risk of nonhemorrhagic side effects; thus, patients already taking warfarin with excellent INR control have little to gain by changing to dabigatran. The patient's compliance with a twice-daily dosing is a real issue. Management to sustain monitoring of INR is needed with warfarin also adds to cost and compliance. Most studies demonstrate a benefit to routine blood-pressure lowering treatment in the acute phase of stroke.

Selective serotonin reuptake inhibitors (SSRI) are effective after ischemic stroke. Some SSRIs improved motor recovery after stroke but this has not been universally confirmed. Fewer fluoxetine recipients than placebo recipients had depression and treatment with thrombolytic agents did not alter the findings. The SSRIs are therapeutic treatment of stroke and should be considered as an adjunct to physiotherapy in the rehabilitation of motor deficits in moderate-to-severe stroke. Reports of a decreased effect of clopidogrel in patients taking proton pump inhibitors (PPI) did not conclude that there was an increase in the risk for a recurrence of stroke in clopidogrel/PPI users. Vitamin supplementation did not prevent major CV events in patients with previous myocardial infarction, unstable angina, or stroke.

CLINICAL CASE CORRELATION

- **See also Case 3 (Scoring Systems and Patient Prognosis), Case 27 (Traumatic Brain Injury), Case 30 (Altered Mental Status), and Case 31 (Status Epilepticus).**

COMPREHENSION QUESTIONS

32.1 A 38-year-old man who presented to the ED with right leg weakness and right hand numbness is admitted to the ICU. He states that his symptoms started shortly after the completion of a workout. The patient is a recent college graduate with no past medical history, an occasional cigarette smoker, and a social drinker. Upon examination the patient has a weakness in the right lower extremity and equal bilateral handgrip. The patient's vital signs illustrate tachycardia and blood pressure 140/90 mm Hg. He is alert, awake, with no visible signs of facial drooping or slurred speech. An ECG on arrival to the ICU shows normal sinus rhythm compared to an irregular rhythm without discernable P waves with multiple PVCs on arrival to the ED. The brain CT scan was negative. What is the most likely diagnosis responsible for this patient's neurological symptoms?

A. Ischemic stroke with atrial fibrillation

B. Hemorrhagic stroke

C. Exercise-induced hypertension

D. New-onset atrial flutter

E. Endocarditis

32.2 A 35-year-old woman presents to the emergency room with the complaint of having fallen down several steps at a movie theater. The patient is tachycardic and normotensive with muscle strength 2 over 5 of the left upper extremity compared to the right extremity. Doppler ultrasound of the left lower extremity detected a deep venous thrombosis. The CT of the brain revealed a small hypodense lesion in the area of the right internal capsule. Clotting studies are pending. What is the likely cause of this patient's neurological symptoms?

A. Intracranial bleed

B. Ischemic stroke secondary to a paradoxical emboli

C. Multiple sclerosis

D. Amyotrophic lateral sclerosis

E. Amniotic fluid embolism syndrome

ANSWERS TO QUESTIONS

32.1 **A.** This 35-year-old male patient has experienced exercise-induced AF, and likely passed blood clots from the heart to the brain. The change in heart rhythm from AF back to normal sinus rhythm (NSR) produced and released a clot, provoking the neurological symptoms. This clot could have been generated either in the left atrium or the right atrium (atrial septal defect, ASD) reaching the arterial circulation. This patient experienced paroxysmal AF, when he developed a blood clot, likely in the atrial appendage, which was pumped out of the heart and reached his cerebral circulation. Should the patient's neurological symptoms resolve, this patient is classified as a transient ischemic attack (TIA) in which blood flow to a certain area of the brain was intermittently decreased. If neurological deficits persist, a stroke is diagnosed, and a repeat CT of the brain at 48 hours should reveal a hypodense area in the part of the brain involved. The patient will need a 24-hour Holter monitor to document the atrial fibrillation. Paroxysmal AF is the most dangerous arrhythmia because of the constant transition from arrhythmia to NSR, which increases the risk of stroke by placing blood clots into the circulatory system. This patient will initially need 3 to 6 months of anticoagulation therapy along with medication to control his heart rhythm. Evaluation for AF in a young patient should be undertaken (hyperthyroidism, drugs). Examining the need for long-term anticoagulation therapy in the context of benefits versus risk of paroxysmal atrial AF associated with the formation of blood clots is indicated. Maintaining NSR and preventing spontaneous, infrequent AF is foremost in this patient.

32.2 **B.** The patient has developed multiple thrombi and blood clots secondary to a hypercoagulable condition. Some potential causes include Factor V Leiden disorder, pregnancy, and lupus anticoagulant. Many undiagnosed blood disorders are discovered during pregnancy. One clue that this patient has a hypercoagulable condition is that she has had 2 previous miscarriages. The higher than normal estrogen state of pregnancy triggers hypercoagulability risk factors in patients with clotting disorders like Factor V Leiden, protein C and S, and antithrombin III. This patient developed a DVT while sitting for a prolonged period of time at the movie theater. The patient's neurological symptoms are caused by her hypercoagulable state which contributes to the development of thrombi and emboli that have entered into the microcirculation of the cerebral vasculature. Admission to the ICU and complete hematological panel to determine the diagnosis of her blood clotting disorder is indicated. A hematology and obstetrical consultation is also warranted. The immediate therapy is anticoagulation with heparin or enoxaparin (Lovenox, an injectable Xa inhibitor). The use of warfarin (Coumadin) is contraindicated in pregnancy, as it is teratogenic. Long-term anticoagulation is needed. Lupus anticoagulant usually presents as prolonged prothrombin time (PTT) without evidence of bleeding, in which case, the PTT gets further prolonged when mixed with half-normal plasma confirms the presence of a factor antibody (antiphospholipid). A factor deficiency causing the PTT prolongation would correct when mixed with normal plasma.

REFERENCES

Foster C, Mistry N, Peddi PF, Sharma S. *The Washington Manual of Medical Therapeutics*. 33th ed. Philadephia: Lippincott Williams & Wilkins, 2010.

Van der Worp HB, Acute ischemic stroke. *N Engl J Med*. 2007;357:2203-2204.

Van der Worp HB, Raaijmakers TW, Kappelle LJ. Early complications of ischemic stroke. *Curr Treat Options Neurol*. 2008;10:440-449.

CASE 33

A 63-year-old man underwent a surgical appendectomy and colostomy formation for a ruptured appendicitis with abscess and devitalized cecum. At the time of the operation, he was noted to have necrosis and perforation of the cecum with fecal peritonitis. On postoperative day 8, the patient remains on the ventilator with $PAO_2/FIO_2 = 260$. Over the past 48 hours, he has developed worsening oliguria with urine output of <300 mL over the past 18 hours. The patient is becoming visibly jaundiced. A CT scan of the abdomen reveals no intrahepatic ductal dilatation, moderate amount of postoperative inflammatory changes throughout the peritoneal cavity, and no signs of active intrabdominal infections.

- What is the most likely diagnosis?
- What are the causes of the patient's current condition?
- How would you monitor and quantify the patient's organ dysfunction?
- What are your therapeutic strategies and goals for this patient?

ANSWERS TO CASE 33: Multiorgan Dysfunction

Summary: This is a 63-year-man who had an operation for a ruptured appendicitis, and his course was complicated by colonic perforation and fecal peritonitis. The patient is now developing organ dysfunction despite adequate source control. He is showing signs of pulmonary dysfunction with compromised oxygenation (P/F ratio = 260). In addition, he has new-onset compromised renal and hepatic functions as seen by his decreased urine output and visible jaundice. There is no evidence of continued intra-abdominal pathology.

- **Causes of the patient's current condition:** The patient's initial peritonitis and subsequent inflammatory response has resulted in organ dysfunction in multiple systems.
- **Monitoring and quantifying the organ dysfunction:** Continuous monitoring of his organ functions via standard measures (urine output, MAP, oxygen saturation, etc) is mandatory, and the level of dysfunction is quantified using the multiple organ dysfunction scale.
- **Therapeutic strategies and goals for this patient:** The therapy for multiple organ dysfunction is mainly supportive, addressing each organ system that is injured. The underlying cause should be treated. Mechanical support may be necessary, such as ventilatory support for pulmonary failure and hemodialysis for renal failure.

ANALYSIS

Objectives

1. To learn to identify, quantify, and manage multiple organ dysfunctions associated with critical illnesses.
2. To learn the factors that may contribute to the development of multiple organ dysfunction syndrome (MODS).
3. To learn the supportive care for patients with MODS.

Considerations

This patient presented with a single identifiable cause for his illness—appendicitis, cecal perforation with fecal peritonitis. His illness has not resolved with the removal of his diseased colon, irrigation of the peritoneal cavity, and antibiotic administration. Instead, despite appropriate treatment of his peritonitis, his overall status is continuing to deteriorate. His pulmonary function has declined with a P/F ratio that is indicative of acute lung injury. Likewise, he has acute kidney injury demonstrated by his progressive oliguria. His hepatic function has also deteriorated as evidenced by his visible jaundice. These organs become dysfunctional days following the inciting event and continue despite the resolution of his initial illness. These are indicative of secondary MODS.

APPROACH TO:
Multiple Organ Dysfunction Syndrome

DEFINITIONS

MULTIPLE ORGAN DYSFUNCTION SYNDROME: The continued dysfunction of two or more organ systems that occurs as a result of a disruption in homeostasis. The organ dysfunction may continue despite the resolution of the initial event.

SYSTEMIC INFLAMMATORY RESPONSE SYNDROME: Occurs when 2 of the following are present:

1. Body temperature <36°C or >38°C
2. Heart rate >90 beats/minute
3. Respiratory rate >20 breaths/minute
4. White blood cell count <4000 cells/mm^3 or >12,000 cells/mm^3 **or** the presence of >10% immature neutrophils (band forms)

ACUTE KIDNEY INJURY (AKI): AKI was formerly referred to as acute renal failure (ARF). AKI is defined by a rapid decline in renal function (<48 hours). The decrease in renal function is determined using urine output and/or serum creatinine levels. An absolute increase in serum creatinine of ≥0.3 mg/dL **or** a percentage increase in serum creatinine of ≥50% is indicative of AKI. Also, a reduction in urine output, defined as <0.5 mL/kg/h for more than 6 hours is also AKI.

ACUTE LUNG INJURY/ACUTE RESPIRATORY DISTRESS SYNDROME: Hypoxemic respiratory failure, of which the most severe form is acute respiratory distress syndrome (ARDS). Acute lung injury is defined as a P/F ratio of 200 to 300. ARDS is hypoxemic failure with a P/F ratio of <200, bilateral fluffy infiltrates on chest x-ray, and no evidence of congestive heart failure.

P/F RATIO: (PAO_2/FIO_2) × 100. This is used to identify the degree of pulmonary failure.

CLINICAL APPROACH

MODS is a clinical syndrome that has its origins in the ICU. MODS did not exist prior to the ability to keep patients alive who would have otherwise died from their disease processes. Once the ICU care began to evolve and became successful at sustaining patients after life-threatening illnesses, we began to see patients develop remote organ dysfunction despite resolution of their initial insults. Patients who develop MODS have increased length of ICU stays and a 20-fold increase in mortality rate when compared to those patients without MODS.

Pathophysiology

There are multiple factors that may contribute to the development of MODS. Originally, it was thought that MODS only occurred in patients who had severe sepsis. Although sepsis is responsible for almost three-fourths of MODS cases, any clinical scenario that leads to significant inflammation or host injury responses can cascade into MODS. The beginning of MODS starts with the normal, appropriate physiologic response to a single inciting event, such as pneumonia, pancreatitis, or a gunshot wound to the abdomen. This initial insult activates macrophages, which in turn release pro-inflammatory mediators, as well activate coagulation factors. The pro-inflammatory mediators interact with white blood cells resulting in their recruitment and activation. The inflammatory mediators also cause microvascular thromboses, apoptosis derangements, and increased capillary permeability. The procoagulant effects act in conjunction with the previously activated coagulation system, and serves to act as a local protective mechanism against injury. Once the original injury is treated, the inflammatory mediators and coagulation factors return to normal and healing is achieved.

However, occasionally, despite the resolution of the inciting event, the normal physiologic response acts as a positive feedback loop, leading to **overamplification of the immune response.** The activation of the white blood cells can also release pro-inflammatory mediators that activate more monocytes/macrophages, which in turn releases additional pro-inflammatory mediators. This continued inflammation and coagulation cause cellular damage, which in turn activates more inflammatory mediators. More cellular damage occurs with subsequent organ failure. Once this initial organ system fails, inflammatory mediators continue to be released, acting on other organ systems, until there is multiorgan dysfunction.

Once patients have been treated for their original injury and continue to have clinical deterioration, MODS should be considered as the diagnosis. Although the pulmonary system is often noted to be the first organ system to fail, there is no standard progression of organ failure. The degree of organ dysfunction is often graded by the multiple organ dysfunction syndrome score (see Table 33–1). **There is no single therapy for MODS and the treatment is largely supportive.** The goal of therapy is to decrease the continued cellular injury in each organ so that the positive feedback loop can be interrupted with an aim toward return of normal homeostasis.

The best treatment of MODS is to identify the patients at greatest risk for MODS and begin preemptive therapy to limit its progression. This is best accomplished by optimizing cardiac and pulmonary performance early in the disease process,

Table 33–1 • MULTIPLE ORGAN DYSFUNCTION SCORE (MODS)

	SCORE				
Organ System	0	1	2	3	4
Respiratory (P/F)	>300	226-300	151-225	76-150	<75
Renal (serum Cr) (μmol/L)	<100	101-200	201-350	351-500	>500
Hepatic (serum bilirubin) (μmol/L)	<20	21-60	61-120	121-240	>240
Cardiovascular (PAR)	<10	10.1-15	15.1-20	>20.1-30	>30
Hematologic (platelet count)	>120	81-120	51-80	21-50	<20
Neurologic (GCS)	15	13-14	10-12	7-9	<6

Table 33–2 • AVERAGE ICU STAY (DAYS)

MOD Score (Points)	ICU Mortality	Hospital Mortality	ICU Stay (days)
0	0%	0%	2
1-4	1%-2%	7%	3
5-8	3%-5%	16%	6
9-12	25%	50%	10
13-16	50%	70%	17
17-20	75%	82%	21
21-24	100%	100%	–

Data from: Marshall JC, Cook DJ, Christou NV, et al. Multiple organ dysfunction score: a reliable descriptor of a complex clinical outcome. *Crit Care Med.* 1995 Oct;23(10):1638-1652.

providing early and adequate nutritional support, giving appropriate antibiotics to decrease the risk of resistant "super" infections, and minimizing the use of blood transfusions.

The identification of organ failure in patients with MODS necessitates continuous monitoring and supportive therapy for that organ. Increased vigilance should also be used to monitor and detect new organ failure during treatment. Mortality in the ICU is related to the number of organs and the severity of organ injury. Prognosis depends on the MOD score (Table 33–2).

The **pulmonary system is frequently the earliest organ system to fail.** Patients who develop MODS are often already intubated and are unable to be weaned off the ventilator despite treatment of their original illness. Acute lung injury (ALI) is an umbrella term for hypoxemic respiratory failure. The most severe form of ALI is ARDS. In acute lung injury, there is a failure of normal gas exchange. The inflammation affects oxygen uptake more than carbon dioxide elimination. This occurs early because of atelectasis and intravascular thrombosis. As the inflammatory process progresses, there is an increase in capillary permeability, leading to increase in alveolar fluid that increases the distance for oxygen diffusion to occur.

Identification of a P/F ratio of <300 indicates that the patient has acute lung injury. A P/F ratio of <200 is a risk factor for having ARDS. The definition of ARDS is having a P/F ratio <200 with bilateral fluffy infiltrates without evidence of congestive heart failure. Once acute lung injury or ARDS is diagnosed, lung-protective ventilation should be initiated. The goal for treatment of these patients is to continue to provide adequate oxygenation without further damage to the alveoli. This is best accomplished with low tidal volumes, increased positive end expiratory pressure (PEEP), and limiting peak plateau pressures. This lung-protective ventilation strategy decreases the incidence of volutrauma and barotrauma, and also decreases the levels of inflammatory mediators.

The **biggest risk factor for developing MODS is circulatory failure within the first 24 hours of admission.** This is why early management of resuscitation is extremely important in critically ill patients. The cause of circulatory failure during MODS is multifactorial. During the initial phase of inflammation, TNF and reactive oxygen species inhibit cardiac contractility. Additionally, the early cytokines released result in increased vascular permeability and vasodilation. This combination results in loss of effective preload, contractility, and afterload. The treatment for circulatory failure is fluid resuscitation. However, this treatment may contribute to the worsening of the system, as the fluids administered may not stay intravascular because of the increased vascular permeability. This contributes to the increase in organ failure and the cycle continues. The use of pressors is advocated only once it is determined that the intravascular volume has been repleted. Likewise, the blood and blood products can be used to increase intravascular volume, but are associated with complications. The injudicious use of vasopressors and blood transfusions is known to increase morbidity and mortality. The use of $ScVO_2$ (central venous oxygen saturation obtained via central venous catheter), lactate, and base excess can help guide the initial resuscitation. The $ScVO_2$ reflects the upper body/head extraction of oxygen and is usually higher than the mixed venous O_2 in situations of shock.

Acute kidney injury (AKI), formerly referred to as acute renal failure (ARF) is a decline in renal function as determined by either a rise in serum creatinine levels or a decrease in urine output. Serum creatinine levels that increase by 0.3 mg/dL or by 50% from baseline is AKI. Urine output that is ≤0.5 mL/kg/h for more than 6 hours is also AKI. In MODS, the causes of AKI are both intrinsic and pre-renal. Early in the course of MODS, hypotension can lead to early AKI, while examples of late causes are nephrotoxic drugs and contrast-induced nephropathy. Hypoxemia can lead to cellular destruction and altered renal function. Renal replacement therapy (dialysis) may be necessary to support a patient with MODS and AKI.

Patients with MODS can develop hepatic dysfunction as identified by cholestasis and jaundice. Bilirubin levels are used to determine the severity of dysfunction on the MODS-scoring system. The elevation of bilirubin is most likely a result of leakage of bile from hepatic canaliculi that have been damaged by cytotoxins and inflammatory mediators. The elevation of acute-phase reactants, such as C-reactive protein and α_1 antitrypsin, is common during the inflammatory stages of MODS. The hepatic dysfunction identified in MODS is usually not life threatening. There is no specific supportive therapy aimed directly at the liver, so continued support of the other systems is all that is necessary.

CLINICAL CASE CORRELATION

- **See also Case 1 (Early Awareness of Critical Illness), Case 3 (Scoring Systems and Patient Prognosis), Case 22 (Acute Liver Failure), and Case 23 (Acute Kidney Injury).**

COMPREHENSION QUESTIONS

33.1 A 63-year-old, otherwise healthy man is admitted to the ICU with sepsis and right lower lobe pneumonia. He is started on broad-spectrum antibiotics and is being mechanically ventilated. The ventilator settings are assist-control ventilation, tidal volume of 9 mL/kg, oxygen concentration of 60%, and a PEEP of 8. Two days later, his chest x-ray shows bilateral fluffy infiltrates and a PAO_2/FIO_2 ratio of 195. His oxygen saturations are 85%. The best treatment for this patient is:

A. Increase the tidal volume on the ventilator.

B. Decrease the amount of PEEP.

C. Add additional antibiotic coverage.

D. Increase the PEEP and decrease the tidal volume.

E. Perform bronchoscopy to rule out atypical pneumonia.

33.2 A 35-year-old man with a history of chronic alcohol abuse is admitted with severe pancreatitis that does not appear to be necrotic on CT scan. He is admitted to the ICU with respiratory failure and low urine output. His bilirubin is 3.8 mg/dL. He has no history of cholelithiasis and ultrasound shows normal ductal anatomy. The most likely cause of his multiorgan failure is:

A. Release of pancreatic enzymes into the circulation, degrading level of serum proteins

B. Infection of the pancreas

C. Blockage of the biliary system

D. Malnutrition from chronic alcoholism

E. Release of inflammatory cytokines from monocytes

33.3 A 21-year-old man sustained a gunshot wound to the abdomen. He had multiple small bowel enterotomies repaired and a short segment of bowel was resected. After 36 hours, he remains intubated and develops increasing white blood cell count, tachycardia, and fevers. Which of the following statements is most accurate regarding the patient's possible diagnosis of MODS?

A. This patient likely has MODS based the fever and elevated white cell count

B. This patient likely has MODS based on bowel system injury

C. This patient does not likely have MODS without more evidence of organ system injury

D. This patient does not likely have MODS because of his young age

33.4 The best treatment for MODS is:
 A. Preventative
 B. Large volume resuscitation
 C. Dialysis
 D. Lung protective ventilation
 E. Enteral nutrition

ANSWERS TO QUESTIONS

33.1 **D.** This patient is hypoxic and has a diagnosis of ARDS. The essentials of treating ARDS revolve around decreasing the incidence of both volutrauma and barotrauma. The goal is to decrease the tidal volume, increase the PEEP, and maintain adequate oxygenation. Permissive hypercapnia is allowed as long as the pH does not fall below 7.2. The low oxygen saturations in this patient should be treated by decreasing his tidal volume and increasing the PEEP using the ARDS net protocol strategy for lung protective ventilation. Atypical pneumonias are mostly encountered in immunocompromised hosts; therefore, not a likely diagnosis in this otherwise healthy man.

33.2 **E.** While the other mechanisms may be the instituting and contributing factors, the systemic inflammatory response is secondary to the release of cytokines from monocytes that have been activated. Under normal circumstances, the cytokine release decreases as the patient's inciting pathology improves. Occasionally, the inflammatory cascade does not subside and becomes a positive feedback loop. This is the beginning of MODS.

33.3 **C.** Increasing WBC, fever, and tachycardia in this patient can represent a number of possible complications. Given the circumstances of his injury, missed intra-abdominal injury and intra-abdominal infections are distinct possibilities. Similarly, this patient who is a trauma victim and who recently underwent emergency laparotomy for intraabdominal injuries is at risk for the development of pneumonia. The timing of these symptoms do not fit the typical picture of MODS, which generally occurs days to weeks following the initial insult. Additionally, there is currently no evidence of acute kidney injury or hepatic injury or pulmonary injury.

33.4 **A.** The best treatment for MODS is supportive and prevention. Resuscitation, dialysis, enteral nutrition, and lung protective ventilation are all treatment or supportive modalities used when treating a patient with MODS. However, identifying which patients are at risk for developing MODS and instituting early and appropriate care before MODS starts is the best treatment. Once MODS occurs, supportive care through the above modalities is often necessary.

REFERENCES

Barie PS, Hydo LJ, Pieracci FM, Shou J, Eachempati SR. Multiple organ dysfunction syndrome in critical surgical illness. Surg *Infect (Larchmt)*. 2009 Oct;10(5):369-377.

Dewar D, Moore FA, Moore EE, Balogh Z. Postinjury multiple organ failure. *Injury*. 2009 Sep;40(9): 912-928.

Mizock BA. The multiple organ dysfunction syndrome. *Dis Mon*. 2009 Aug;55(8):476-526.

CASE 34

A 69-year-old man was admitted to the hospital 10 days ago for a colonic volvulus complicated by colonic perforation and fecal peritonitis. He underwent surgery, and was placed on IV antibiotics and mechanical ventilation. Yesterday, he was extubated from mechanical ventilation, and had been doing well up to this morning. This morning, the patient has persistent pulse rates ranging from 100 to 110 beats/minute, and he is noted to be somnolent and does not interact with his family. The patient's visiting family members are concerned because they feel that he is "not the same person as usual." A CT scan of the brain is performed and demonstrates no abnormalities.

- What are the potential causes of this patient's condition?
- What are the manifestations of endocrine disorders associated with critical illnesses?

ANSWERS TO CASE 34:
Endocrinopathies in the ICU Patient

Summary: A 69-year-old man is recovering from sepsis due to peritonitis from a GI process; the patient is noted now to have altered mental status and tachycardia. A normal CT scan of the brain suggests that anatomic causes are unlikely to be responsible for his current condition.

- **Potential causes of patient's current picture:** The cardiovascular and neurological abnormalities observed in critically ill patients can have a variety of possible causes, including hypoxia from pulmonary pathology, analgesics and sedation medication-related changes, and critical illness-induced endocrinopathies.
- **Manifestations of endocrine disorders associated with critical illnesses:** Endocrine-related changes following critical illnesses may include *behavioral changes* (psychomotor, cognitive, and sleep disorders), *cardiovascular changes* (vasodilatory shock, multiple organ dysfunction syndrome), *metabolic changes* (defects in glucose metabolism, protein-wasting), and *immunologic changes* (increased susceptibility to infections caused by increased immune suppression related to the shift of TH_1/TH_2 balances toward an excess of TH_2 cells).

ANALYSIS

Objectives

1. To learn the cardiovascular, metabolic, behavioral, and immune disorders that may be produced by endocrine changes associated with critical illnesses.
2. To learn to recognize the manifestations of endocrinopathies in the ICU.
3. To learn the medications that may contribute to endocrinopathies.

Considerations

This patient has been critically ill in the ICU and has had a prolonged ICU course following intra-abdominal infection and sepsis. Even though he has taken steps toward improvement, his persistent tachycardia and mental status change now requires that we further investigate for the causes. At this point, complete blood count, chemistries, arterial blood gas, chest x-ray, electrocardiogram, and cardiac enzymes may be useful in identifying cardiopulmonary causes. Potential new sources of infections may be evaluated with a thorough physical examination, appropriate cultures, and imaging studies. In addition, anatomic causes should be evaluated with a brain CT.

The possibility of endocrinopathies should also be entertained when a patient with critical illness develops cardiovascular, metabolic, and neuropsychiatric derangements, as critical illness can affect the homeostatic processes in several organ systems. A severe septic insult can initially overwhelm the body's innate stress responses primarily regulated by the sympathetic nervous system and hypothalamus-pituitary-adrenal (HPA) axis, leading to early hemodynamic instability that is often associated with mental status changes. Subsequent to these initial responses, critically ill individuals may enter into a state of hypercatabolism, which could be produced by thyroid dysfunction and manifest clinically as tachycardia, atrial fibrillation, or agitation. In older individuals, hyperthyroidism may also manifest as lethargy. Elevated metabolic activity secondary to hyperthyroidism can be evaluated by thyroid function studies. Delirium and cognitive impairment occur quite frequently among individuals following recovery from ARDS, where significant cognitive dysfunction, anxiety, and depression are often reported. The exact causes of these neuropsychiatric changes have not been determined; however, it has been theorized that intense inflammatory mediator and cytokine responses may alter neurohormonal homeostasis and lead to neuropsychiatric dysfunctions.

APPROACH TO: Endocrinopathies in the ICU Patient

CLINICAL APPROACH

Sepsis in the Critically Ill Patient

A systematic guideline as delineated by the Surviving Sepsis campaign provides a multidisciplinary approach to optimize treatment of septic patients. In the initial management, fluid resuscitation begins with isotonic crystalloid for the goals of mean arterial pressure (MAP) >65 mm Hg, central venous pressure 8 to 12, and urine output >0.5 mL/kg/h. Vasoactive agents such as norepinephrine or dopamine are started when patients are unable to maintain MAP >65 mm Hg despite adequate fluid administration. Transfusion of packed red blood cells may also be initiated for a general hemoglobin goal of 7 to 9 g/dL; however, for patients with lactic acidosis, hemorrhage, or coronary ischemia, the hemoglobin goal should be 10 g/dL. Source control with broad-spectrum antibiotics should be started immediately, with subsequent narrowing of coverage as soon as culture results are available. In managing critical illness, physicians should remain vigilant in considering endocrine derangements such as adrenal insufficiency, hyper- or hypoglycemia, vasopressin deficiency, and thyroid dysfunction.

Endocrine Response to Critical Illness

Two physiologic pathways are activated during periods of acute stress: the sympathetic nervous system and the endocrine system. The sympathetic nervous system is activated via secretion of catecholamines from the adrenal medulla, leading to changes in the cardiovascular, metabolic, immunologic, and endocrine systems. **In the acute phase of illness, the endocrine system is responsible for an adaptive response to maintain organ perfusion, decrease anabolism, and up-regulate the immune response. In the chronic phase of illness, the endocrine system may play a role in the development of persistent hypercatabolism and contribute to organ dysfunction.**

Sympathetic Nervous System and Arginine Vasopressin

The "fight or flight" response from the sympathomimetic system is produced by norepinephrine, epinephrine, and dopamine release from the adrenal medulla. These hormones produce complex adaptive responses throughout the body, leading to increased alertness, skin vasoconstriction, vasodilation of skeletal and coronary arteries, bronchodilatation, tachycardia, tachypnea, pupillary dilatation, and glycogenolysis. Catecholamines are also released from mesenteric organs during stress, which contribute to a significant percentage of total levels in the body. Catecholamine release from a typical SIRS reaction typically decreases within 3 to 5 days, which may be inadequate in periods of severe stress such as in septic shock. **Three major pathways are theorized to contribute to development of vasodilatory shock: (1) overproduction of nitric oxide (NO), (2) hyperpolarization of vascular smooth muscle membranes, and (3) relative deficiency of vasopressin.**

Some patients with sepsis have insufficient host catecholamine responses and therefore, may benefit from exogenous administration of vasoactive medication to maintain end-organ perfusion. Dopamine or norepinephrine is often given as a first-line agent when septic shock patients are refractory to appropriate fluid management. Arginine vasopressin is a neurohypophyseal hormone that acts on V_1 vascular smooth muscle cell receptors and V_2 renal tubular cell receptors to cause hemostasis, arterial vasoconstriction, and antidiuresis. With sepsis, some patients may develop relative vasopressin deficiency with down-regulation of V_1 receptors, and may benefit from low-dose exogenous vasopressin. Thus, patients with septic shock that is refractory to fluid management and high-dose conventional vasopressors may be candidates for vasopressin.

Hypothalamic-Pituitary-Adrenal Axis

Acute stress also activates the hypothalamic-pituitary-adrenal (HPA) axis, which is essential for survival. Initiation of this pathway begins with the increased secretion of corticotrophin-releasing hormone from the paraventricular nucleus of the hypothalamus, which in turn stimulates the anterior pituitary to produce ACTH. ACTH then signals for the adrenal cortex to produce cortisol. Cortisol has several important physiologic actions on metabolism, including stimulatory effects on the cardiovascular and immune system. During stress, cortisol increases blood glucose concentration by activating hepatic gluconeogenesis and inhibiting glucose uptake by peripheral tissues. Cortisol also activates lipolysis in adipose tissue to increase free fatty acid release. Cortisol increases blood pressure by sensitizing vascular smooth muscle to catecholamines. Immunologically, cortisol produces anti-inflammatory effects by reducing the number and function of T and B lymphocytes, monocytes, neutrophils, and eosinophils at the site of inflammation.

Approximately 10% to 20% of critically ill patients may exhibit some adrenal insufficiency, with the incidence reported as high as 60% among patients with septic shock. Glucocorticoid resistance is a phenomenon described in septic patients. Observations suggest that mediators released in patients with critical illness, and sepsis in particular, may either stimulate or impair the synthesis and activation of cortisol via actions on the HPA axis and the glucocorticoid receptor signaling system.

Three laboratory assays are applied for the detection of adrenal insufficiency. The first is serum **cortisol** level, which reflects total hormone concentration. The disadvantage of analyzing serum cortisol level is that free cortisol, rather than the protein-bound fraction is actually responsible for the physiologic activities of the hormone. In most critically ill patients, corticosteroid-binding globulin levels are decreased. Furthermore, with acute stimulation of the adrenal gland, free cortisol increase is substantially more pronounced than the increase of total cortisol concentrations. Consequently, the total serum cortisol level may not accurately reflect free cortisol levels and adrenal functions in critically ill patients. Free cortisol level measurements would be preferable; however, this assay is not widely available. **The cosyntropin stimulation test is a measurement of change (increase) in serum cortisol following the administration of 250 μg dose of synthetic ACTH. An increase <9 μg/dL within 60 minutes is indicative of an inability for the adrenal glands to appropriately respond to ACTH stimulation**. However, this test has its limitations, as it does not assess the integrity of the HPA axis, the response of the HPA axis to other stresses such as hypotension or hypoglycemia, or the adequacy of stress cortisol levels.

In a multicenter, randomized controlled trial, Annane and colleagues reported improved survival in catecholamine-dependent patients with septic shock that was unresponsive to cosyntropin who were given a 7-day course of steroids. In another randomized control trial reported in 2008 (The Corticus Trial), no difference in mortality was found with steroid administration in septic patients with or without appropriate responses to cosyntropin stimulation. This study did find a shorter duration for shock reversal in the steroid-treated patients when compared to patients receiving placebos. These apparently conflicting results may be explained by the sicker patients in the Annane study. In 2008, based on a meta-analysis of 6 randomized control trials, the American College of Critical Care Medicine issued a consensus statement that **hydrocortisone should be considered in the management of patients with septic shock, particularly those patients who have responded poorly to fluid resuscitation and vasopressor agents**. The decision to treat septic patients with corticosteroids should be based on clinical criteria and not on results of cosyntropin stimulation test or other adrenal function testing.

Insulin

Critical illness and sepsis frequently cause hyperglycemia in patients with or without a history of diabetes mellitus. The causes of critical illness–induced hyperglycemia include catecholamine-mediated inhibition of insulin release, glucocorticoid and proinflammatory cytokine induced glucose synthesis and release. In addition, pancreatic β-cell dysfunction, hepatic glucose production dysfunction, and peripheral insulin resistance are other factors that contribute to the hyperglycemia. In critically ill patients, hyperglycemia contributes to increased morbidity and mortality through a variety of mechanisms, including augmentation of oxidative burden, activation of stress-signaling pathways, and impairment of neutrophil function. Furthermore, hyperglycemia is associated with the increase in risk for myocardial infarction, impairment of wound healing, and increased mortality in patients following surgery, trauma, or neurotrauma.

Intensive insulin therapy was found to have reduced mortality benefits in a randomized control trial involving mechanically ventilated cardiac surgical patients. These benefits were observed in patients with and without known diabetes, and the benefits appeared to be most significant among patients with sepsis-induced multiple-organ failure, and an ICU stay of >5 days. **Target glucose values of 80 to 110 mg/dL were originally suggested as being most beneficial for ICU patients**

based on the above-mentioned study; however, more recent evidence suggest that target value of 140 to 180 are more appropriate and produce fewer hypoglycemia-related complications when compared to target glucose values of 80 to 110 mg/dL.

Hypothalamic-Pituitary-Thyroid Axis

Thyroid hormones produced by the thyroid gland are regulated by thyrotropin-releasing hormone (TRH) and thyroid-stimulating hormone (TSH) released by the hypothalamus and anterior pituitary, respectively. Thyroid hormones act to increase the basal metabolic rate, affect protein synthesis, and increase the sensitivity of tissues to catecholamines. Thyroxine (T_4) is the principal hormone produced by the thyroid and can be subsequently deiodinated to the active form, triiodothyronine (T_3) in extrathyroidal tissues. Approximately 99% of all T_3 and T_4 are bound to thyroxine-binding globulins and other plasma proteins; its physiologically active form is unbound, the level of which can be measured via laboratory testing.

Euthyroid sick syndrome, also known as low T_3 to T_4 syndrome or nonthyroidal illness syndrome, is commonly identified in critically ill patients. This is characterized by an acute decrease in T_3 followed by a decrease in T_4 within 24 to 48 hours. This caused by inhibition in T_4 to T_3 conversion, leading to an increase in reverse-T_3 (rT_3). TSH often increases briefly at onset, but usually remains within the low-normal range without a circadian rhythm. Although this may reflect an adaptive mechanism aimed at reducing hypercatabolism, this disease process is associated with an increased mortality despite a lack of overt hyper- or hypothyroid symptoms. A small randomized control trial found no mortality benefit in exogenous administration of T_4 versus placebo in critically ill patients with this disorder. Another nonrandomized cohort study showed no clinical outcome difference in patients undergoing continuous thyrotropin-releasing hormone infusion. Current recommendations call for no intervention to correct the thyroid hormone levels in euthyroid sick syndrome.

Somatotropic Axis

Growth hormone (GH) is secreted by the anterior pituitary in a pulsatile fashion and has anabolic effects in the body, increasing lipolysis, protein synthesis, and reducing glucose uptake in hepatocytes. Its activity is mediated by insulin-like growth factor 1 (IGF-1), which is bound by IGF-binding proteins (IGFBP), thereby reducing its bioavailability but prolonging its half-life. The acute phase of critical illness is characterized by a reduced pulsatile release of GH, high basal GH levels, and low levels of IGF-1 and IGFBP. Cytokine release during stress causes a widespread GH resistance with the down-regulation of GH receptors, causing reduced anabolic activity, and providing metabolic energy while wasting muscle protein. This has deleterious effects in critically ill patients, including delaying wound healing, depressed immune function, and respiratory muscle dysfunction. Two large clinical trials investigating whether exogenous GH would reverse hypercatabolism found no benefit, and in fact, an increased risk of infection and death. Currently, there is no evidence to show that pharmacologic agents acting on the somatotropic axis has any benefit on clinical outcome in critically patients.

Hypothalamic-Pituitary-Gonadal Axis

Gonadal hormones, which interact with androgen and estrogen receptors, are mediated by luteinizing hormone (LH) and follicle-stimulating hormone (FSH) released by the anterior pituitary; LH and FSH in turn are regulated by gonadotropin-releasing hormone secreted by the hypothalamus. In males, a low level of testosterone is associated with acute and chronic critical illness and is directly associated with mortality. Female patients may experience the "hypothalamic amenorrhea of stress." Although estrogen supplementation has been shown to be beneficial in critically ill patients, current recommendations do not endorse routine use of sex hormone replacement. Furthermore, estrogen use can increase the risk of venous thromboembolism.

Sleep Disturbances in the ICU

Sleep disturbances in the ICU are common, and these disturbances may include decreased nocturnal sleep, reduced or absence of deep sleep, and disrupted circadian patterns. In addition, ICU patients commonly report anxiety, fear, and nightmares associated with sleep during and after their ICU stays. The normal sleep–wake cycle is controlled by complex interactions between neurotransmitters such as catecholamines, glutamate, histamine, melatonin, and acetylcholine. Melatonin production by the pineal gland follows a diurnal variation pattern and is responsible in promoting nocturnal sleep. Septic patients have been found to have a continuous, non-fluctuating secretion of melatonin. Altered melatonin production is believed to be beneficial during sepsis, as it possesses antioxidant properties. ICU patients may also have sleep disruption due to disturbances in the HPA axis activity, which modulates cortisol release following stress. Cortisol is known to inhibit sleep. Because of these endogenous changes as well as the external stimuli, 60% of all ICU patients report sleep disturbances.

Drug-Induced Endocrine Disorders

Drug-Induced Pituitary-Adrenal Axis Dysfunction **Etomidate** is often used for rapid-sequence induction during intubation. Continuous infusion of etomidate had been utilized during the 1980s, but this practice was discontinued when it was found to be associated with increased mortality due to adrenal dysfunction. Single dose etomidate has been reported to contribute to adrenal dysfunction; however, its uncommon occurrence suggests that the risk is minimal. The patients in which single-dose etomidate may produce clinically significant adrenal insufficiency are the septic patients, in whom any level of adrenal dysfunction could contribute to worse clinical outcomes; therefore, the current recommendations suggest that ketamine may be a more appropriate agent for rapid-sequence induction in the septic patient population. The etomidate effect on adrenal dysfunction is believed to be due to a dose-dependent blockade of the enzyme involved in the final conversion of cholesterol to cortisol.

Chronic glucocorticoid therapy is common in ICU patients. Patients with a history of chronic glucocorticoid therapy are at risk for the development of adrenal insufficiency during stress states; however, the dose and duration of prior steroid use do not predict the likelihood of insufficiency. It is recommended that patients in shock and with history of chronic steroid use receive steroid repletion, and patients without shock should be closely monitored for signs of insufficiency rather than receiving empiric replacement.

Drugs causing up-regulation of cytochrome P-450 (CYP-450) activity may increase cortisol metabolism (breakdown) and contribute to adrenal insufficiency. Examples of this class of agents are rifampin, phenobarbital, and phenytoin. The medication effects can be observed within 7 days of therapy initiation and require close monitoring of clinical effects.

Antifungal agents causing CYP-450 inhibition may produce adrenal insufficiency by suppressing CYP-450-dependent steroidogenesis. Ketoconazole is the most well-documented antifungal agent associated with adrenal insufficiency. Fluconazole and itraconazole are agents that produce adrenal insufficiency much less frequently in comparison to ketoconazole. Due to the potential of causing clinically significant adrenal insufficiency, patients receiving antifugal therapy should be closely monitored.

Drug-Induced Thyroid Dysfunction **Dopamine infusion** is associated with the occurrence of **nonthyroidal illness syndrome**. This effect is related to the reduction of TSH concentration and reduction in thyroxine production. Dopamine effects on thyroid functions can be observed within 24 hours after the initiation of dopamine infusion, and these effects are completely reversed within 24 hours following termination of dopamine infusion.

Lithium is concentrated in the thyroid and may cause a **decrease in thyroxine release.** Hypothyroidism and goiter formation may occur in individuals with prolonged lithium intake; hypothyroidism is reported in approximately 20% of individuals taking lithium for 10 years or longer.

Amiodarone is frequently prescribed for the management of atrial or ventricular arrhythmias. By weight, **37% of amiodarone is made up of iodine,** and this medication is structurally similar to thyroxine. Long-term and short-term administration of amiodarone have the potential of producing **thyrotoxicosis**. Amiodarone-induced thyrotoxicosis 1 (AIT-I) describes the amiodarone-induced thyrotoxicosis that occurs in individuals with preexisting thyroid diseases. This problem is treated with antithyroid medications such as methimazole or propylthiouracil. ATI-II is an amiodarone-induced thyroiditis causing destruction of the gland and release of thyroid hormone; this condition is best treated with glucocorticoids. Due to the long half-life of amiodarone (50-100 days), ATI diseases may occur long after discontinuation of the medication.

Interestingly, **amiodarone can also cause hypothyroidism**; however, the mechanisms that cause amiodarone-induced hypothyroidism are undetermined at this time. Women and those with a history of Hashimoto thyroiditis are at increased risk for amiodarone-induced hypothyroidism. Most cases of hypothyroidism are mild and can be managed with thyroxine replacement or the discontinuation of amiodarone.

CLINICAL CASE CORRELATION

- **See also Case 15 (Cardiac Arrthythmias), Case 19 (Sepsis), and Case 33 (Multiorgan Dysfunction).**

COMPREHENSION QUESTIONS

34.1 A 44-year-old man is hospitalized for septic shock due to pneumonia, and he has received crystalloid resuscitation to achieve a CVP of 18 mm Hg. Thereafter, a norepinephrine drip was initiated. Despite these measures, his mean arterial pressures remained below 65 mm Hg. Vasopressin drip at 0.03 U/min was initiated without improvement. He is believed to be on the appropriate antimicrobial regimen for his infection. Which of the following is the most appropriate management in this patient?

A. Proceed with a cosyntropin stimulation test and give hydrocortisone if the patient is demonstrated to have insufficient adrenal response.

B. Give 100 μg of thyroxine.

C. Measure plasma vasopressin level.

D. Administer cortisol 100 μg intravenously.

E. Transfuse 2 U of pack red blood cells.

34.2 A 55-year-old woman with a history of goiter develops fever, tachycardia, and anxiety 12 hours following the initiation of amiodarone drip for ventricular arrhythmias. Her serum TSH is noted to be <0.01. Which of the following statement best describe her current condition?

A. This patient is experiencing amiodarone-induced hypothyroidism.

B. This condition is best treated by corticosteroid administration.

C. This patient is experiencing amiodarone-induced thyroiditis.

D. This patient's condition is best treated with propylthiouracil.

E. This condition is best treated with iodine administration.

34.3 Which of the following statements best describe the current recommended approach to glycemic control in the ICU?

A. Strict glucose control targeting glucose levels of 80 to 110 is strongly recommended for postoperative patients.

B. Glucose control targeting glucose levels of 140 to 180 is associated with lower morbidity and mortality than glucose target levels of 80 to 110.

C. Glycemic control in the ICU has not been shown to provide clinical benefits.

D. Hyperglycemia is generally not a problem unless individuals are receiving total parenteral nutrition.

E. Serum glucose levels >180 is associated with improved neurological outcomes following head injury.

ANSWERS TO QUESTIONS

34.1 **D.** This patient has persistent septic shock despite sufficient fluid resuscitation to restore intravascular volume. He remains refractory to norepinephrine and low-dose vasopressin infusions. Based on the meta-analysis findings of 6 randomized control trial and the American College of Critical Care Medicine consensus recommendations, hydrocortisone should be considered in this individual. Thyroxine replacement and blood transfusions do not play a role in the treatment of vasopressor-refractory septic shock. Measurement of serum vasopressin levels does not play a significant role in clinical decision-making in this setting.

34.2 **D.** This patient has clinical and biochemical evidence of hyperthyroidism. The condition may or may not be the result of amiodarone-induced hyperthyroidism. In either case, the appropriate treatment is antithyroid medications such as propylthiouracil. Amiodarone can also produce hyperthyroidism by causing an autoimmune thyroiditis; however, this process generally takes more than 12 hours to appear.

34.3 **B.** Current evidence suggest that glycemic control targeting glucose levels of 140 to 180 mg/dL rather than 80 to 110 mg/dL is associated with fewer occurrences of hypoglycemia-associated complications.

CLINICAL PEARLS

- Dopamine and norepinephrine are first-line agents to maintain end-organ perfusion in septic shock after patients have been adequately volume resuscitated.
- Arginine vasopressin may be indicated in patients who are refractory to high-dose vasopressors in critically ill patients who are suspected to have relative vasopressin deficiency.
- Hydrocortisone should be considered in septic shock when hypotension is refractory to fluid and vasopressor agents, and the patient has clinical evidence of adrenal insufficiency.
- Treatment of septic patients with corticosteroids should be a clinical decision and should not be determined on the basis of adrenal function testing results.
- Insulin therapy with target glucose levels of 140 to 180 mg/dL is beneficial in critically ill patients.
- Nonthyroidal illness syndrome may occur in critically ill patients; however, no intervention is currently recommended to restore normal thyroid levels.
- Gonadal steroids have a linear relationship with mortality in critically ill patients; however, current literature does not support exogenous replacement.

REFERENCES

Annane D. Effect of treatment with low doses of hydrocortisone and fludrocortisones on mortality in patients with septic shock. *JAMA*. 2002;288:862.

Bello G, Paliani MG, Pontecorvi A, Antonelli M. Treating nonthyroidal illness syndrome in the critically ill patients: still a matter of controversy. *Curr Drug Targets*. 2009;10:778-787.

Bougle A, Annane D. Endocrinopathy. In: Gabrielli A, Layon AJ, Yu M, eds. *Civetta, Taylor, and Kirby's Critical Care*. 4th ed. Philadelphia, PA: Lippincott Williams & Wilkins; 2009:2411-2427.

Marik PE, Pastore SM, Annane D, et al. Recommendations for the diagnosis and management of corticosteroid insufficiency in critically ill adult patients: consensus statements from an international task force by the American College of Critical Care Medicine. *Crit Care Med*. 2008;36:1937-1949.

Sprung CL, Annane D, Keh D, et al. Hydrocortisone therapy for patients with septic shock. *N Engl J Med*. 2008;358:111-124.

Thomas Z, Bandali F, McCowen K, Malhotra A. Drug-induced endocrine disorders in the intensive care unit. *Crit Care Med*. 2010;38(6):S219-S230.

- Dopamine and norepinephrine are first-line agents to maintain [illegible] organ perfusion in septic shock after patients have been adequately volume resuscitated.
- Arginine vasopressin may be useful in patients who are refractory to high dose vasopressors, particularly in patients who are suspected to have a relative vasopressin deficiency.
- Hydrocortisone should be considered in septic shock when hypotension is refractory to fluid and vasopressor therapy [illegible]
- [illegible]
- [illegible]
- [illegible]

[illegible]

Marik PE, Pastores SM, Annane D, et al. Recommendations for the diagnosis and management of corticosteroid insufficiency in critically ill adult patients: consensus statements from an international task force by the American College of Critical Care Medicine. Crit Care Med. 2008;36(6):1937-1949.

[illegible]

CASE 35

An 18-year-old G1P0 woman at 34 weeks' gestation comes into the obstetrical triage unit complaining of a severe headache. She states that bright lights are bothersome to her. Her prenatal history is unremarkable. Her blood pressures in the first trimester were in the 100/60 mm Hg range. On examination, her blood pressure (BP) is 180/105 mm Hg, heart rate (HR) 98 beats/minute, temperature 98.4°F, and respiratory rate (RR) 12/minute. Her heart and lung examinations are normal. The abdomen is nontender, and the fundal height is 27 cm. The fetal heart tones are in the 135 beats/minute range with occasional variable decelerations on external fetal monitoring. There are no uterine contractions. The vaginal examination reveals that the cervix is closed, long, and posterior. During your examination, you notice that she has some facial twitching and now is undergoing a tonic-clonic seizure involving both upper and lower extremities.

- ▶ What is the most likely diagnosis?
- ▶ What are your next steps?
- ▶ What are the important considerations in managing her condition?

ANSWERS TO CASE 35: Eclampsia

Summary: An 18-year-old G1P0 female at 34 weeks' gestation complains of a severe headache and photophobia. Her BP is 180/105 mm Hg, and her fundal height is 27 cm. The fetal heart tones are in the 135 beats/minute range with occasional variable decelerations without contractions. The cervix is unfavorable. During your examination, you notice that she has some facial twitching, and now she is undergoing a tonic-clonic seizure involving both upper and lower extremities.

- **Most likely diagnosis:** Eclampsia. Other diagnoses to consider include epilepsy, drug intoxication, drug withdrawal, alcohol withdrawal, and CNS abnormalities including cerebral infarction, cerebral hemorrhage, venous thrombosis, head trauma, infections, neoplasms, and metabolic disorders.
- **Your next steps:** (1) Maintenance of airway patency, (2) prevention of aspiration via rolling the mother to her left side and elevating the head of the bed, (3) supplemental oxygen (8-10 L/min) via face mask during convulsive episode, (4) obtain IV access, (5) administer magnesium sulfate intravenously or intramuscularly, (6) constant monitoring of respiratory rate, pulse, and blood pressure, and (7) call obstetrician for delivery.
- **Important considerations in managing her condition:**
  The most important goal when managing a patient with eclampsia is to stabilize the mother.
  Fetal bradycardia and/or decelerations in heart rate can occur during the seizure episode. Both generally resolve with cessation of eclamptic event.

ANALYSIS

Objectives

1. To list the hypertensive disorders of pregnancy.
2. To describe eclampsia and prioritize the management.
3. To describe the treatment of eclampsia.
4. To describe the common complications of preeclampsia.

Considerations

This 18-year-old pregnant patient presented with **hypertension** with a blood pressure of 180/105 mm Hg, headache, and photophobia, all of which are concerning for severe preeclampsia. Because she proceeds with a **generalized tonic-clinic seizure,** she now has progressed to **eclampsia, which appreciably increases the risk to both the mother and the fetus.**

- Her blood pressure will need to be controlled, and an obstetrician should be called, but first she must be stabilized and given **magnesium sulfate to prevent further seizures.**

- Eclamptic seizures may be violent; therefore this patient must be protected. Considering she just had a generalized tonic-clonic seizure, she is likely to become motionless and confused due to the post-ictal state that follows seizures. In some eclamptic patients, a coma of variable durations may ensue. Because eclamptic patients can become combative after a seizure or they may have another seizure, the **railings of her bed should be raised and padding placed on the head board and rails. A padded tongue blade may be carefully inserted into her mouth to prevent biting the tongue, but should not cause a gag reflex or injure the teeth. Physical restraints should not be used.**
- To prevent hypoxia to her and her baby, she needs supplemental oxygen via a face mask. Her vital signs should be frequently assessed, as well as urine output, proteinuria, and peripheral edema.
- To prevent further seizures and associated comorbidities, IV magnesium sulfate should be initiated. **Treatment includes a loading dose of 6 g of magnesium sulfate over 15 minutes, followed by 2 to 3 g/h administered continuously.** Since magnesium sulfate has a narrow therapeutic index of 2 to 3.5 mmol/L, the patient must be monitored for **hyporeflexia and respiratory depression.** Because convulsions often continue during labor and delivery, as well as postpartum, the magnesium should be continued for 24 hours postpartum. In the event of status epilepticus that is resistant to magnesium sulfate, she should be intubated and deeply sedated.
- Along with controlling the seizures, the blood pressure should also be controlled with **hydralazine or labetalol** with a goal systolic blood pressure <160 mm Hg and diastolic blood pressure <100 mm Hg. Additionally, the hemoglobin, platelets, serum creatinine, liver enzymes, and lactate dehydrogenase should be monitored for ensuing HELLP syndrome (hemlysis, elevate liver enzymes, and low platelets).
- The **only curative treatment for eclampsia is delivery of the fetus**. Once the mother is stabilized, vaginal delivery is initially pursued to avoid maternal risks from cesarean delivery.
- The patient's fundal height of 27 cm signifies that the fetus is small for gestational age, which is likely caused by deficiency in uteroplacental blood flow secondary to her hypertension. The fetus is at risk of intrauterine growth retardation and adverse fetal events, so regular surveillance is used for careful monitoring.

APPROACH TO: Hypertensive Disease in Pregnancy

DEFINITIONS

CHRONIC HYPERTENSION: Blood pressure **≥140/90 mm Hg** before pregnancy or diagnosed **before 20 weeks' gestation** not attributable to gestational trophoblastic disease or hypertension first diagnosed after 20 weeks' gestation and persistent after 12 weeks postpartum.

ECLAMPSIA: The development of **grand mal seizures** in pregnancy that are not related to a preexisting condition.

GESTATIONAL HYPERTENSION: New-onset hypertension **≥140/90 mm Hg after the 20th week of gestation without the development of proteinuria**, and associated with normal blood pressure within 12 weeks postpartum.

HELLP SYNDROME: Hemolytic anemia, elevated liver enzymes, and low platelets.

MILD PREECLAMPSIA: The development of new-onset hypertension with **BP ≥140/90 mm Hg** and **proteinuria that is >300 mg/24 h** in the mother **that occurs after the 20th week of gestation.**

SEVERE GESTATIONAL HYPERTENSION: New-onset hypertension **≥160/105 mm Hg** after **the 20th week of gestation without the development of proteinuria,** and associated with normal blood pressure within 12 weeks postpartum.

SEVERE PREECLAMPSIA: The development of new-onset hypertension with **BP ≥160/110 mm Hg systolic, ≥5 g of urinary protein excretion per 24 hours,** plus evidence of **other organ system involvement such as impaired liver function, thrombocytopenia, oliguria (≤500 mL in 24 hours), pulmonary edema, epigastric or right upper quadrant pain, cerebral or visual disturbances, and/or fetal growth restriction.**

SUPERIMPOSED PREECLAMPSIA ON CHRONIC HYPERTENSION: New-onset proteinuria ≥300 mg/24 h in a hypertensive woman but no proteinuria before 20 weeks gestation, or a sudden increase in proteinuria, blood pressure, or platelet count <100,000/μL in a woman with hypertension and proteinura before 20 weeks gestation

CLINICAL APPROACH

Epidemiology

The **deadly triad of pregnancy** consists of **embolism, hypertensive disorders, and hemorrhage.** These 3 complications contribute greatly to maternal morbidity and mortality rates with hypertensive disorders complicating 5% to 10% of all pregnancies. **Hypertensive disorders are the most dangerous and deadly complications of pregnancy.** In the Western world, eclampsia ranges from 1 in 2000 to 1 in 3448 pregnancies and is higher in tertiary referral centers, in multifetal gestation, and in patients with no prenatal care. The onset of eclamptic convulsions in the antepartum period range from 38% to 53%, in the intrapartum period between 18% and 36%, and in the postpartum period from 11% to 44%.

Pathophysiology

The definitive pathophysiology of eclampsia is unknown but several investigations have implicated the **placenta as the main cause.** Likely, **placental hypoperfusion secondary to abnormal modeling of the maternal-fetal interface** is the key. Additionally, other factors such as maternal vasculature increased sensitivity to pressor agents lead to **vasospasm (organ** hypoperfusion) and **capillary leakage** (edema).

Furthermore, activation of the coagulation cascade causes microthrombi that further aggravate perfusion. Though **most patients remain asymptomatic**, a myriad of complications may exist and involve multiple individual organ systems. Hypertension causes increased cardiac afterload, and the endothelium is injured with extravasation of intravascular fluid, leading to cardiac abnormalities, hemoconcentration, nondependent edema, and possible pulmonary edema. Complications of the baby include fetal growth restriction from uteroplacental perfusion deficiency caused by defects in trophoblastic invasion and placentation.

Assessment of Blood Pressure

During an obstetric evaluation of a patient, the blood pressure should be measured with an appropriately fitting blood pressure cuff (cuff bladder should encompass two-thirds of the arm). To diagnose hypertension, there must be **2 separate elevated recordings that exceed 140/90 mm Hg.** Hypertension is considered chronic if it is elevated before 20 weeks' gestation (see Table 35–1).

Gestational Hypertension

If a woman develops hypertension with a blood pressure ≥140/90 mm Hg after 20 weeks of gestation on 2 separate occasions **without evidence of preeclampsia (including proteinuria),** she will be diagnosed with gestational hypertension. As indicated, gestational hypertension is diagnosed based on clinical examinations and she should be evaluated for other signs including severe headache, visual changes, epigastric or right upper quadrant pain, nausea, vomiting, or decreased urine output. Once diagnosed, it is treated with **careful surveillance of the mother and fetus.** However if the hypertension is ≥160/110 mm Hg without proteinuria, then the mother has **severe gestational hypertension** and should be treated with **antihypertensive and magnesium sulfate for seizure prophylaxis. Generally 20% of patients with severe gestational hypertension are actually preeclamptic** and will need termination of the pregnancy with delivery.

Preeclampsia

As defined earlier, preeclampsia means a woman develops hypertension and proteinuria after 20 weeks' gestation. Further subcategories include mild and severe preeclampsia depending on the extent of blood pressure elevation. Mild preeclampsia involves a blood pressure that is **≥140/90 mm Hg with proteinuria ≥300 mg in 24 hours while severe preeclampsia causes ≥5 g of proteinuria and signs of organ involvement.** Treatment for both depends on the gestation of the mother. If she is **≥34 weeks then delivery is preferred** while if she is **<34 weeks gestation, then corticosteroids are given to the mother to aid in lung development of the fetus followed with expectant management and delivery.**

Eclampsia

Although preeclampsia can progress to eclampsia, this is not always the case. That is, eclampsia may not develop or it may occur without the setting of preeclampsia. The cause of preeclampsia still remains unknown, though it is thought to be secondary **to vasospasm, endothelial dysfunction, and ischemia.** Preeclampsia has progressed to

Table 35–1 • THE DIAGNOSIS AND TREATMENT OF HYPERTENSIVE DISEASES OF PREGNANCY

Hypertension during Pregnancy	Diagnosis and Treatment
Gestational hypertension	Systolic BP ≥140 or diastolic BP ≥90 mm Hg for the first time during pregnancy No proteinuria BP returns to normal before 12 weeks postpartum Final diagnosis made only postpartum Tx: Outpatient management with weekly antepartum visits
Severe gestational hypertension	Same as above but BP ≥160 or diastolic BP ≥110 mm Hg Tx: Similar to severe preeclampsia. Seizure prophylaxis, antihypertensive medications, delivery if ≥34 weeks' gestation, if <34 weeks then give maternal corticosteroids followed by delivery
Chronic hypertension	BP ≥140/90 mm Hg before pregnancy or diagnosed before 20 weeks' gestation, not attributable to gestational trophoblastic disease *or* Hypertension first diagnosed after 20 weeks' gestation and persistent after 12 weeks postpartum Tx: Anti-hypertensive medications: labetalol or nifedipine
Superimposed preeclampsia on chronic hypertension	New-onset proteinuria ≥300 mg/24 h in hypertensive women but no proteinuria before 20 weeks' gestation A sudden increase in proteinuria or blood pressure or platelet count <100,000/μL in women with hypertension and proteinuria before 20 weeks' gestation Tx: Depends on extent of hypertension and proteinuria
Mild preeclampsia	BP ≥140/90 mm Hg after 20 weeks' gestation Proteinuria ≥300 mg/24 h or ≥1+ dipstick Tx: If ≥34 weeks then delivery is preferred while if <34 weeks then corticosteroids are given to the mother followed with expectant management and delivery.
Severe preeclampsia	BP ≥160/110 mm Hg Proteinuria 2.0 g/24 h or ≥2+ dipstick Serum creatinine >1.2 mg/dL unless known to be previously elevated Persistent headache or other cerebral or visual disturbance, persistent epigastric pain Tx: Seizure prophylaxis, hypertension control with labetalol or hydralazine , delivery if ≥34 weeks' gestation, if <34 weeks then give antepartum corticosteroids followed by delivery
Eclampsia	Seizures that cannot be attributed to other causes in a woman with preeclampsia Tx: Stabilize mother, IV magnesium sulfate, immediate delivery
HELLP	Platelets <100,000/μL Microangiopathic hemolysis—increased LDH Elevated serum transaminase levels—ALT or AST Tx: Delivery if ≥34 weeks' gestation, presence of non-reassuring fetal status, or severe maternal disease. Magnesium sulfate to prevent seizures, and platelet transfusion if significant maternal bleeding or if platelets <20,000

Table 35–2 • COMPLICATIONS OF PREECLAMPSIA/ECLAMPSIA

- Stroke
- Pulmonary edema
- Renal failure
- DIC
- Intrauterine growth retardation

eclampsia once a patient convulses. Speculations maintain that the pathogenesis of eclamptic convulsions include cerebral vasoconstriction and vasospasms, hypertensive encephalopathy, cerebral edema or infarction, cerebral hemorrhage, and metabolic encephalopathy. **Seizures likely result from excessive release of excitatory neurotransmitters, massive depolarization, and bursts of action potentials.** In a normal pregnancy, renal blood flow and glomerular filtration rate increase, but patients with eclampsia have decreased renal perfusion and glomerular filtration resulting from a reduced plasma volume and increased renal afferent arteriolar resistance. This elevates the blood pressure and causes oliguria and proteinuria. Proteinuria is not always seen before a woman develops seizures but will appear at some point in an eclamptic patient. Hepatic changes that take place are periportal hemorrhage in the liver periphery with more severe cases leading to hepatic infarction and death (see Table 35–2 for other complications).

A straightforward diagnosis of eclampsia occurs when a gravida has **generalized edema, hypertension, proteinuria, and convulsions,** but it may not always be this clear since there is a broad spectrum of these signs. The hallmark is the **convulsion which can occur at any time during pregnancy, delivery, or postpartum.** Hypertension is generally severe around 160/110 mm Hg in 20% to 54% of cases but has been shown to be absent in 16%. Symptoms that may occur before or after a convulsion include persistent occipital or frontal headache, blurred vision, photophobia, epigastric and/or right upper quadrant pain, and altered mental status.

Management of Eclampsia

During or immediately after the acute convulsive episode, steps should be taken to ensure the safety of the mother. A **padded tongue blade** should be inserted to prevent trauma to her tongue, her **bedside rails should be padded** and raised, and physical restraints may be used as needed. She should also be placed in the lateral decubitus position with suction available to prevent aspiration. **Her airway, breathing, and circulation** should be carefully monitored and an intravenous line started. Apply a facemask with 8 to 10 L/min oxygen and monitor oxygenation and metabolic status via pulse oximetry and arterial blood gases. An obstetrician should be notified immediately. After stabilizing the mother, the next step is to manage the convulsions. **It is important not to try and stop the first convulsion, but to stabilize the patient** and then administer **magnesium sulfate** with a loading dose of 6 g over 15 to 20 minutes followed by a continuous maintenance dose of 2 g/h to prevent recurrences. Out of the eclamptic women receiving magnesium sulfate, 10% will have another seizure and should be given another 2 g bolus intravenously over 3 to 5 minutes.

If the patient continues to convulse, she may need to be intubated and sedated. The next step is to control the blood pressure while preserving cerebral, cardiac, and placental perfusion. The goal is to maintain **the blood pressure between 140 to 160 mm Hg systolic, and 90 to 105 mm Hg diastolic.** This is generally achieved with **hydralazine, labetalol, or nifedipine.** Diuretics are only used in the case of pulmonary edema. **During a seizure the fetus may experience bradycardia, transient late decelerations, decreased beat-to-beat variability, and compensatory tachycardia, but usually returns to normal after the convulsion. However if fetal bradycardia or repetitive late decelerations persist, placental abruption may have occurred** which is a surgical emergency needing a stat cesarean. Once the mother is stabilized and has regained consciousness, is oriented to name, place, and time, and her convulsions are controlled, delivery is the definitive treatment.

Eclampsia is not an indication for cesarean unless the patient is <30 weeks' gestation or her Bishop score is below 5, indicating that the cervix is unfavorable for induction of labor. **After delivery, the patient must remain on magnesium sulfate for 24 hours and requires close monitoring of vitals, fluid intake and output, and symptoms of end organ damage (headache, blurry vision, epigastric pain).** Because of the endothelial damage and repair and vasospasm that occur in eclamptic women, they are very sensitive to vigorous fluid therapy and to blood loss at delivery.

Brain pathology was described during the era when mortality was high, prior to the widespread use of magnesium sulfate and anti-hypertensive agents. These studies showed that though gross intracerebral hemorrhage was seen in up to 60% of eclamptic patients, and was fatal in about half of these cases. Other neurologic symptoms besides seizures that are seen in severe preeclampsia include headache and scotoma, blindness, and generalized cerebral edema that can cause confusion or coma.

HELLP Syndrome

Hematological abnormalities may develop in some women, including thrombocytopenia and hemolysis. The thrombocytopenia may lead to life-threatening coagulopathy. When accompanied with elevated liver enzymes indicative of hepatic necrosis, the combination of events is referred to as HELLP (Hemolysis, Elevated Liver enzymes, Low Platelets) syndrome. Other changes that may take place in HELLP syndrome include decreased plasma clotting factors, increased Factor VIII consumption, increased fibrin degradation products that in severe cases can lead to DIC. Hepatic hematomas can develop from hepatic infarctions and can bleed profusely they rupture; when unruptured, they can be observed and treated conservatively.

CLINICAL CASE CORRELATION

- **See also Case 30 (Altered Mental Status), 31 (Status Epilepticus), Case 32 (Stroke), and Case 36 (Critical Care and Obstetrical Issues).**

COMPREHENSION QUESTIONS

35.1 A 27-year-old G3P1102 at 29 weeks' gestation comes into the obstetric triage room with her husband who states that 15 minutes ago she had a seizure involving her entire body. She is lethargic and unable to answer questions. Her husband says her second pregnancy was complicated by high blood pressure and their son was delivered preterm. This pregnancy has not had any complications. Her blood pressures in the first trimester was in the 100/60 mm Hg range. On examination, her BP is 180/105 mm Hg, HR 97 beats/minute, temperature 98.4°F, and RR 12 breaths/minute. What is the most important first step in management?

A. Administer loading dose of magnesium sulfate.

B. Help her into a hospital bed and assess her airway, place a face mask with oxygen, and obtain IV access.

C. Deliver the baby by immediate C-section.

D. Give the mother a dose of corticosteroids and wait to deliver the baby for 48 hours.

35.2 A 26-year-old G2P1001 at 38 weeks' gestation presents with headache and contractions every 5 minutes. She is admitted to labor and delivery. She has not had any complications with her pregnancy. On examination, her BP is 180/110 mm Hg, HR 97 beats/minute, temperature 98.4°F, RR 12 breaths/minute, and cervix is 3 cm dilated. Her urinalysis shows 2+ proteinuria. She is started on magnesium sulfate and hydralazine. Two hours later she is afebrile, her BP is 140/90 mm Hg, HR 100 beats/minute, RR is 8 breaths/minute, and she has decreased deep tendon reflexes. What is your next step in management?

A. CT scan of head

B. Stop hydralazine

C. Ca gluconate

D. Stop magnesium sulfate

35.3 A 30-year-old G3P1102 at 29 weeks' gestation comes in for her prenatal appointment. She has not had any complications with her pregnancy. On examination, her BP is 150/95 mm Hg, HR 97 beats/minute, temperature 98.4°F, and RR 12 breaths/minute. Her urinalysis reveals no proteinuria and she denies shortness of breath, headache, changes in vision, or right upper quadrant pain. What is her most likely diagnosis?

A. Moderate preeclampsia

B. Superimposed preeclampsia on chronic hypertension

C. Severe gestational hypertension

D. Gestational hypertension

35.4 What is the next step in management of the patient in Question 35.3?

A. Weekly antepartum visits monitoring blood pressure and urinalysis
B. Start labetalol
C. Start hydralazine
D. IV magnesium sulfate

ANSWERS TO QUESTIONS

35.1 **B.** This patient presents with a tonic-clonic seizure and therefore has eclampsia until proven otherwise. Considering she has a history of hypertension in a previous pregnancy, high blood pressure on presentation, severe headache, and history of generalized tonic-clonic seizure, she most likely has eclampsia and should first be stabilized. She will need magnesium sulfate and delivery of her baby but first she must be stabilized.

35.2 **D.** This patient has severe preeclampsia since her systolic blood pressure is >160 mm Hg and she has 2+ proteinuria. She is appropriately treated with magnesium sulfate, which has a narrow therapeutic index. Toxic levels of magnesium sulfate can cause decreased deep tendon reflexes and respiratory depression to the point of respiratory compromise and death. Therefore, the patient must be vigilantly monitored when on magnesium. In the event of magnesium toxicity, the magnesium should be stopped and then the patient should receive calcium gluconate. CT scan of the head and hydralazine have no effect on magnesium toxicity.

35.3 **D.** This patient has an elevated blood pressure but no proteinuria. Since her blood pressure is <160/110 mm Hg, she has gestational hypertension and not severe gestational hypertension. Moderate preeclampsia not only has an elevated blood pressure, but also involves proteinuria. Superimposed preeclampsia on chronic hypertension occurs in patient with known hypertension before 20 weeks' gestation, with proteinuria occurring after 20 weeks' gestation.

35.4 **A.** The treatment of gestational hypertension involves weekly antepartum monitoring of the mother and the fetus. Hydralazine and labetalol are used for severe hypertension but are not used for hypertension <160/110 mm Hg. Women with gestational hypertension are accustomed to this elevated blood pressure, and decreasing their blood pressure to normal may cause hypoperfusion of vital organs such as the placenta and the brain. Magnesium sulfate is administered for seizure prophylaxis and is usually not given until the blood pressure is >160/110 mm Hg or the patient is experiencing signs of organ dysfunction including headache, changes in vision, oliguria, or right upper quadrant pain.

CLINICAL PEARLS

- Epilepsy is the recurrence of seizures that are unprovoked by any immediate identifiable cause. This diagnosis cannot be made based on a single seizure, even if anticonvulsant treatment is administered.
- Women with eclampsia should be treated with magnesium sulfate rather than other anticonvulsants because it more effectively reduces the rate of recurrent seizures and reduces the rate of maternal death.
- Intravascular magnesium sulfate has a faster therapeutic effect and is less painful compared to intramuscular administration.
- Calcium gluconate 1 g IV should be given to reverse toxicity symptoms of magnesium sulfate such as hyporeflexia and respiratory depression.
- Though delivery is the only curative treatment, the mother should be stabilized after a seizure before proceeding with delivery.
- Cesarean delivery is reasonable in women who are <32 weeks of gestation and have an unfavorable cervix.

REFERENCES

American College of Obstetricians and Gynecologists. Diagnosis and management of preeclampsia and eclampsia, *ACOG Practice Bulletin*. 2002;33.

Benbadis SR. Differential diagnosis of epilepsy: a critical review. *Epilepsy Behav*. 2009;15:15-21.

Cunningham FG, Leveno KJ, Bloom SL, Hauth JC, Rouse DJ, Spong CY. Chapter 34. Pregnancy hypertension. *Williams Obstetrics*. 23e. New York: McGraw-Hill Publishers, 2012. http://www.accessmedicine.com.foyer.swmed.edu/content.aspx?aID=6032899, accessed Oct 14, 2013.

Haddad B, Sibai BM. Expectant management in pregnancies with severe pre-eclampsia. *Semin Perinatol*. 2009;33:143-151.

Sibai BM. Diagnosis, prevention, and management of eclampsia. *Obstet Gynecol*. 2005;105:402-410.

Sibai BM. Managing an eclamptic patient. *OBG Management*. 2005;17(5):37-50.

Yoder SR, Thornburg LL, Bisognango JD. Hypertension in pregnancy and women of childbearing age. *Am J Med*. 2009;122:890.

CASE 36

A 25-year-old woman is noted to be at 26 weeks' gestation. She developed acute pyelonephritis and was hospitalized on intravenous antibiotic treatment the previous day. The patient was doing well until this morning, when she complained of acute and progressive shortness of breath. She has no past medical history of pulmonary problems. On examination, her heart rate (HR) is 130 beats/minute, respiratory rate (RR) is 40 breaths/minute and labored, blood pressure (BP) is 130/85 mm Hg, and temperature 102.6°F. The lung fields reveal diffuse crackles. The patient had an ABG of 7.35, Po_2 62 mm Hg, Pco_2 40 mm Hg, and HCO_3 of 19 mEq/L on 100% oxygen by non-rebreather mask. Shortly after this, the patient is taken to the ICU and intubated and placed on the ventilator.

- ▶ What is the most likely diagnosis?
- ▶ What are the obstetrical issues in this case?
- ▶ Are there any adjustments to the medical management due to pregnancy?

ANSWERS TO CASE 36:
Critical Care and Obstetrical Issues

Summary: A 25-year-old woman at 26 weeks' gestation is being treated for pyelonephritis and has developed respiratory failure and rales on pulmonary examination. The patient had an ABG of 7.35, Po_2 of 62 mm Hg, Pco_2 40 mm Hg, and HCO_3 of 19 mEq/L on 100% oxygen by non-rebreather mask. Shortly after this, the patient is taken to the ICU and intubated and placed on the ventilator.

- **Most likely diagnosis:** ARDS.
- **Obstetrical issues:** The pregnant patient has different normative values of the arterial blood gas. For instance, the normal pH in pregnancy is 7.45 and normal Pco_2 is 30 mm Hg. Thus this patient has significant acidosis and is retaining CO_2. The other factor involves monitoring the fetal status and developing a delivery plan if needed.
- **Adjustments in management due to pregnancy:** In general, treating the medical condition is beneficial for maternal as well as fetal status. Ventilator management is not contraindicated in pregnant women. Some medications should be avoided in pregnancy, such as the quinolone antibiotics and ACE inhibitors.

ANALYSIS

Objectives

1. To describe the effect of pregnancy on critically ill patients.
2. To describe the considerations of management of the critically ill patient who is pregnant.
3. Describe the methods of monitoring fetal status and considerations for fetal intervention in the critically ill patient.

Consideration

This patient is pregnant at 26 weeks' gestation, which is at the lower limits of perinatal viability. The patient was admitted for acute pyelonephritis 1 day previously and has developed acute respiratory failure leading to being intubated and placed on the ventilator. The patient has significant tachypnea and labored breathing, and the ABG is concerning. Pregnancy is associated with physiological alterations in respiratory system, leading to a primary respiratory alkalosis and partially compensated metabolic acidosis. The normal pregnant woman's arterial pH is 7.45. Thus, this patient's arterial pH of 7.35 reflects a substantial acidosis. Likewise, the normal Pco_2 in pregnancy is 30 mm Hg due to the increased minute ventilation. This patient's Pco_2 of 40 mm Hg is consistent with marked CO_2 retention, and impaired ventilation. The patient was appropriately intubated and placed on the ventilator. After stabilization of the maternal status, attention can be paid to fetal status. This is a very important principle: to prioritize maternal well-being prior to addressing fetal issues. A bedside ultrasound to assess for gestational age and fetal weight is important to establish whether the fetus is viable. In general, 24 to 26 weeks is considered to be the lower limits of viability, that is, survival of the baby if delivered. If the fetus is considered potentially viable, then discussion with the patient and family is important to establish whether cesarean intervention for fetal interest would be considered for persistent fetal bradycardia. Additionally, a delivery plan should be established; for instance, should the patient go into preterm labor, whether the delivery would be vaginal or cesarean.

APPROACH TO: The Critically Ill Patient Who Is Pregnant

DEFINITIONS

DELIVERY PLAN: A comprehensive process for vaginal as well as cesarean delivery in the event of labor or need for emergency delivery such as fetal bradycardia.

FETAL MONITORING: Assessment of fetal status with fetal heart rate monitoring, ultrasound for fetal weight, and ultrasound assessment for fetal activity such as breathing, movement, and amniotic fluid volume.

PERIVIABLE: Gestational age at the borderline of viability, usually specified as between 22 to 26 weeks' gestation.

PERIMORTUM CESAREAN: Performing a emergency cesarean on a patient who is either undergoing CPR, or who has or is recently demised.

CLINICAL APPROACH

Physiological Changes in Pregnancy

During pregnancy, the heart is displaced upward and to the left from changes in the shape of the rib cage and from superior displacement of the diaphragm. It also rotates on its long axis. This lateral change in heart position can be misinterpreted on chest x-ray as cardiomegaly. Other changes in the structure of the heart resemble those found as a result of physical training. Physiologic myocardial hypertrophy is a result of expanded blood volume, peaking at 30 to 34 weeks' gestation, and reversing itself after delivery.

Cardiac output (CO) is the product of stroke volume (SV) and heart rate (HR). During pregnancy CO is increased tremendously. By 5 weeks' gestation it rises to 10% over prepregnancy levels and by 34 weeks peaks at some 50% above those levels seen prior to pregnancy. Heart rate begins to rise in the first trimester and continues to rise until it peaks at 15 to 20 beats above normal at 34 weeks. Cardiac output varies greatly with maternal position. It is highest in the knee-chest and lateral recumbent positions and lowest in the supine position (some 30% lower). Late in pregnancy, because of the development of a dilated paravertebral collateral circulation, venous return from the lower extremities is maintained in the supine position even when the vena cava is completely occluded by the pregnant uterus.

In spite of this, 5% to 10% of pregnant women show signs of "supine hypotension," and experience dizziness, nausea, and even syncope when supine. This may represent a failure of those women to develop an adequate paravertebral collateral system.

Systemic vascular resistance (SVR) diminishes in early pregnancy, reaching its nadir at mid-pregnancy. It gradually rises until term but even then remains approximately 20% lower than prior to pregnancy. This phenomenon is thought to be a direct effect of progesterone on the smooth muscle in the capillary beds, and increased levels of circulating nitric oxide and cyclic adenosine monophosphate also play a role. Since the pregnant woman's blood pressure is a product of her cardiac output and SVR, we see a similar change in blood pressure throughout pregnancy.

Venous blood pressure rises in the lower extremities gradually during pregnancy. Femoral venous pressure rises from 10 cm H_2O to 25 cm H_2O at term. Consequently edema, hemorrhoids, varicose veins, and an increased risk of deep vein thrombosis are common.

It is often difficult to distinguish between the signs and symptoms caused by physiologic adaptations to pregnancy and those of true cardiac disease. S_1 becomes louder by the end of the first trimester, and 90% of pregnant women will develop an S_3. Systolic ejection murmurs along the left sternal border develop in more than 90% of pregnant women, and is thought to be caused by increased blood flow across the pulmonic and aortic valves.

Respiratory System Because of increased hyperemia and estrogen levels, the nasopharyngeal mucosa becomes edematous and irritated. Nasal stuffiness, epistaxis, and nasal polyps occur frequently during pregnancy, and resolve spontaneously postpartum.

Due primarily to change in the size and shape of the chest cavity, the following alterations in lung capacities are seen:

1. Respiratory rate—unchanged
2. Vital capacity—unchanged
3. Inspiratory capacity—increased 5% to 10%
4. Tidal volume—increased 30% to 50%
5. Inspiratory reserve volume—unchanged
6. Functional residual capacity—decreased 20%

During pregnancy, increased levels of progesterone cause a state of relative hyperventilation, resulting in a chronic respiratory alkalosis. This relatively low Pco_2 in the pregnant mother is beneficial in clearing CO_2 from the fetal circulation.

Maternal blood volume comprises the plasma volume and the red blood cell mass. This total blood volume begins increasing as early as 6 weeks' gestation and plateaus at 30 to 34 weeks of pregnancy, increasing by some 40% to 50% in most gravidas. Plasma volume begins to increase at 10 weeks' gestation and plateaus at 30 weeks' gestation, while the red blood cell mass begins increasing at 10 weeks and continues its rise until term. The reasons for these expansions remain unknown. The use of iron supplementation has been shown to enhance the increase in RBC mass from 18% to 30% by term. Since at mid-pregnancy the plasma volume increases more than that of red blood cell mass, there appears a transient physiologic anemia of pregnancy. A gradual decline in platelets has been observed throughout pregnancy, but 98% of pregnant women will have platelet counts of >116,000/mm^3. Values below this should be evaluated for causes of thrombocytopenia.

Renal Changes Renal plasma flow begins to rise early in pregnancy becoming 75% higher than prior to pregnancy by 16 weeks' gestation. Glomerular filtration rate rises as early as 5 to 7 weeks and reaches a level 50% greater than in the nonpregnant female. The altered mechanism of handling glucose in the proximal tubules during pregnancy remains to be completely understood. Glucose excretion into the urine occurs in most pregnant women. While the nonpregnant female excretes <100 mg/d, in pregnancy this can reach 1 to 10 g of glucose per day.

Respiratory Diseases in Pregnancy

Asthma exacerbations are typically slightly decreased in pregnant women with mild disease, while those with **severe disease may have worse deterioration.** Because of the uterine pressure on the diaphragm, there is decreased pulmonary reserve. **Treatment of the asthmatic pregnant patient is identical to that of the nonpregnant patient,** beginning with β-agonist respiratory therapy and steroids, and progressing to magnesium sulfate. Methylxanthines are also considered safe for use in pregnancy. Epinephrine is relatively contraindicated in pregnancy due to its possible vasoconstrictive effects on the uterine arteries.

Influenza mortality is increased in the pregnant woman due to respiratory changes as well as the relatively immunocompromised state. Thus, obstetrical patients are one of the key groups that should receive annual influenza immunization. The live attenuated nasal vaccine is contraindicated in pregnancy. Those women who have suspected or confirmed influenza should promptly receive anti-influenza therapy. Oseltamavir (tamiflu) or zanamivir (Relenza) are safe in pregnancy. These agents are best begun within 2 days of the beginning of infection, and are taken for 5 days. The pregnant patient may have fulminant and severe disease, and prompt admission and respiratory support should be enacted if the patient deteriorates. In a large series of patients with H1N1 influenza in pregnant and postpartum women in California, 10% of those with infections were hospitalized, which is 4 times higher than the general population. Eighteen were admitted to the ICU (20% of those hospitalized), and 8 patients died; 75% of these deaths were complicated with medical illnesses, and none had received anti-viral medication within 48 hours of disease.

Airway Difficulties

Several anatomic changes occur throughout pregnancy such as weight gain, including increase in breast size, respiratory tract mucosal edema, and capillary engorgement of nasal and oropharyngeal mucosa and laryngeal tissues. Decreased functional residual volume of up to 50% with concomitant increase in oxygen needs can lead to rapid development of hypoxemia in the hypoventilating patient. The progesterone effect of the GI tract can also lead to delayed gastric emptying and decreased lower esophageal sphincter tone, which increases the risk of aspiration. Laryngeal edema makes intubation more difficult, and many anesthesiologists advocate **"downsizing" the ET tube**. Also, because of the risk of bronchospasm or further distortion of the airway anatomy, there may be only one good attempt to place the endotracheal tube. Use of the laryngeal mask airway (LMA), which is a supraglottic airway device that is designed to fit in the hypopharynx, may be useful. Every obstetrical airway should be considered a difficult airway. Difficult anatomy and rapid oxygen desaturation should be anticipated.

Cardiac Disease in Pregnancy

Hypertensive diseases in pregnancy are common, affecting approximately 8% of obstetrical patients. These can be gestational hypertension which is isolated elevated blood pressure, preeclampsia (hypertension with proteinuria), or superimposed preeclampsia on chronic hypertension. Preeclampsia alters the hemodynamic parameters by increasing systemic vascular resistance and decreasing intravascular volume. Thus, **preeclamptic women are more sensitive to volume changes, either blood loss which can lead to hypotension,** or fluid overload leading to pulmonary edema.

Peripartum cardiomyopathy is a 4-chamber dilated cardiomyopathy of unknown etiology affecting women in pregnancy or postpartum. Affected patients present with congestive heart failure, and noted on chest radiograph to have a markedly enlarged cardiac silhouette. The **cardiac output is below 45%** and other causes of ventricular dysfunction are ruled out. Many cases are discovered late after onset of severe symptoms, and thus, a high index of suspicion is needed. Treatment in pregnancy is aimed at stabilization of maternal status. The mainstays of treatment are **digoxin, loop diuretics, afterload reduction with hydralazine and nitrates, and β-blocker use.** ACE inhibitors and ACBs are contraindicated in pregnancy due to fetal renal effects. Unless a patient is decompensating, expectant management of the preterm patient (less than 37 weeks) is advisable. For those women who are decompensating, careful hemodynamic monitoring and support and coordination of care with anesthesiologist, cardiologist, and high-risk obstetrician in an ICU labor and delivery setting are required. The prognosis depends on recovery of left ventricular function, which occurs in about 50% of patients. Mortality can approach 10% in those patients with worsening heart failure. **As many as 80% of women who become pregnant again may develop congestive heart failure with future pregnancies.**

Liver Disease in Pregnancy

Acute fatty liver of pregnancy is an extremely dangerous condition characterized by microvesicular steatosis of the liver, thought to be due to **mitochondrial dysfunction of fatty acid oxidation,** which leads to fat accumulation in hepatocytes. Liver insufficiency results, and if it is not diagnosed and promptly treated with delivery, then maternal and neonatal morbidity or mortality results. Women with AFLP are more likely to have heterozygous long chain 3-hydroxyacyl-coenzyme A dehydrogenase (LCHAD) deficiency. Patients present with nonspecific symptoms such as malaise, nausea and vomiting, and possibly right upper quadrant pain. **Hypoglycemia** and fulminant liver failure with encephalopathy can also be present. The physical examination may or may not manifest hypertension or jaundice. The laboratory analysis is important and usually shows elevated liver function tests and decreased glucose levels. Disseminated intravascular coagulopathy (DIC) and hyperbilirubinemia may also be present. Delivery is the cornerstone of therapy. Renal function should also be monitored.

Sepsis in Pregnancy

Infection is more common in pregnancy due to the patient's immunosuppressed state. The most common cause of sepsis is **pyelonephritis**, typically due to *Escherichia coli*, particularly caused by to O127 subtype; however, a large number of gram-negative rods are possible etiologies. Endotoxin release causes hypotension due to peripheral vasodilation. The most common cause of sepsis in the postpartum patient is post-cesarean endometritis. Pregnant women have a higher mortality than nonpregnant patients. Early diagnosis, aggressive antibiotic therapy, supportive therapy, and removal of the source of the sepsis are important. The decision of delivery is difficult due to the fact that the gestation may be premature; nevertheless, the pregnancy may alter the cardiovascular hemodynamics such as decreasing the venous return. Fetal status should be monitored carefully. Placental perfusion in fetus depends on maternal mean arterial pressure.

Trauma in Pregnancy

Approximately 6% to 7% of all pregnant patients experience trauma of some type, with the highest risk in the third trimester. Most of these are accidental, although some are intentional. The most common type of trauma is falls, which comprise about half of the cases. The **most common cause of fetal death is maternal shock, and the second most common cause is placental abruption.** Blunt trauma does not seem to increase the risk of death more than that of the nonpregnant patient. Attention to the patient is systematic and similar to that of the nonpregnant individual, initially focused on the ABCs and then addressing overt or hidden hemorrhage. Uterine rupture due to direct abdominal trauma is rare, but it should be suspected in a patient with a history of prior cesarean, uterine tenderness, rapid onset of maternal hypotension or shock, and a nonreassuring fetal heart rate pattern. After maternal status is assured, attention can be directed to fetal well-being. Fetal ultrasound and fetal heart rate monitoring are important. Because of the maternal soft tissue, fetal injury is rare with blunt trauma.

In the case of penetrating trauma, fetal mortality is higher, especially in those with abdominal injury. Fetal injury occurs in up to 70% of third-trimester cases, and fetal loss occurs in approximately half of cases, whereas maternal mortality occurs in <5% of cases. Most experts recommend exploratory laparotomy with penetrating trauma to the abdomen to assess for possible uterine laceration, or fetal injury. Imaging should be performed as needed on the pregnant patient. Plain film radiographs may be performed with appropriate shielding. If available, MRI is preferable rather than CT to decrease radiation exposure. Nevertheless, CT of the chest, for instance, only emits 1 rad of radiation energy; exposure of a pregnancy to <10 rads is not considered to be dangerous to the developing fetus. Diagnostic peritoneal lavage has not been found to be consistently accurate in pregnancy and is typically not used.

Perimortem Cesarean

Perimortem cesarean is performed primarily for 2 reasons: (1) for certain maternal death due to severe head injury or other non-resuscitatable cause, the indication is to save the fetus, or (2) for maternal cardiac arrest due to a potentially resuscitatable cause, for both maternal and fetal benefit. Examples of the second category include cardiac arrest or severe blood loss, and the cesarean section removes the fetus so as to remove a nonvital organ from the maternal circulation. This facilitates the resuscitation, allowing better venous return and easier chest compressions. With either reason, **the cesarean needs to be done within 4 minutes of cardiac arrest to support neurologic function of the fetus.** The key to rapid delivery is the use of large of incisions. A midline vertical incision is made from the xiphoid to the pubis through all layers of the abdominal wall. If the placenta is in an anterior position, the surgeon cuts through it and addresses the bleeding only after the fetus is delivered. Typically, a midline vertical incision through the upper uterine segment is made and the neonate delivered, suctioned, and cord clamped and cut. Thereafter, resuscitation of the pregnant patient can be resumed.

Amniotic Fluid Embolism

Amniotic fluid embolism (AFE) is a rare obstetrical emergency where the suspected etiology is that amniotic fluid and fetal cells and hair entering into the maternal circulation, leading to maternal hypotension and cardiovascular collapse. An anaphylactic reaction presents acutely associated with pulmonary artery spasm and hypertension, elevated right ventricular pressure and hypoxia. Half of affected women will die within 1 hour of presentation. A second phase then ensues if the patient is successfully resuscitated: florid DIC and massive hemorrhage with uterine atony. Therapy is early recognition, and supportive therapy such as oxygenation, CPR, crystalloid, blood products and pressor agents as needed, and aggressive treatment of associated coagulopathy. Emergency cesarean in women with cardiac arrest unresponsive to resuscitation may be required. Unfortunately, AFE is associated with an 80% maternal mortality.

CLINICAL CASE CORRELATION

- **See also Case 8 (Airway Management and Respiratory Failure), Case 19 (Sepsis), and Case 35 (Hypertensive disorders in pregnancy).**

COMPREHENSION QUESTIONS

36.1 A 30-year-old woman is noted to be at 12 weeks' gestation. An arterial blood gas is performed due to symptoms of shortness of breath. In interpreting the ABG, which of the following statements is most accurate regarding its normal value in pregnancy?

A. The arterial pH will likely be lower, and P_{CO_2} unchanged as compared to the nonpregnant patient.

B. The arterial pH is unchanged, and P_{CO_2} will likely be increased as compared to the nonpregnant patient.

C. The pH will be higher and P_{CO_2} will be lower than the nonpregnant patient.

D. The pH and P_{CO_2} are both unchanged as compared to the nonpregnant patient.

36.2 A 28-year-old G1P0 woman at 34 weeks' gestation is noted to have a 2-day history of malaise and nausea and vomiting. On examination, she appears slightly icteric. Her BP is 140/90 mm Hg. Lab results reveal that SGOT is 200 IU/L, and bilirubin is 5 mg/dL. Which of the following would be most consistent with acute fatty liver of pregnancy?

A. Urine protein of 500 mg over 24 hours

B. Peripheral blood smear showing schistocytes

C. Blood glucose of 40 mg/dL

D. Amylase level of 3 times normal value

36.3 A 31-year-old G2P1 woman at 40 weeks' gestation is in active labor. She is on oxytocin augmentation of labor due to slow labor progress. The nurse notes that the patient is not responsive and has no pulse and no blood pressure. CPR is initiated. Which of the following is the most likely diagnosis?

A. Acute fatty liver of pregnancy

B. Amniotic fluid embolism

C. Diabetic ketoacidosis

D. Uterine rupture

ANSWERS TO QUESTIONS

36.1 **C.** The normal arterial blood gas in pregnancy reveals a primary respiratory alkylosis with partial metabolic compensation. Thus, the arterial pH is higher than the nonpregnant state (7.45) and the P_{CO_2} is lower as compared to pregnancy (30 mm Hg vs 40 mm Hg in nonpregnancy). To compensate for this change, the kidneys excrete bicarbonate, and thus the serum bicarbonate is lower than the nonpregnant patient (19 mEq/L vs 24 mEq/L).

36.2 **C.** This patient presents as acute fatty liver of pregnancy with the malaise, and nausea/vomiting, icterus, and mildly elevated blood pressure. Hypoglycemia is often present. With significant disease, the patient can have an elevated serum ammonia level and encephalopathy.

36.3 **B.** Amniotic fluid embolism. This patient presents with the acute onset of hypotension, cardiovascular collapse, and hypoxia. If resuscitated, the patient may enter into a state of hemorrhage and DIC.

CLINICAL PEARLS

- ► The physiological changes of pregnancy must be considered in interpreting the lab results.
- ► As compared to the nonpregnant patient, the intravascular volume and cardiac output increases 50% in pregnant women.
- ► The pregnant woman has a primary respiratory alkalosis and partial compensatory metabolic acidosis.
- ► The priority should be to assess and stabilize maternal status prior to addressing fetal issues.
- ► Fetal status should begin with accurate gestational age determination. A primary decision point is to determine whether the fetus is viable, and whether there would be emergency cesarean intervention for fetal issues.
- ► A delivery plan should be developed should the patient require delivery.
- ► A fetal monitoring status should be developed.
- ► There are few medications that are contraindicated in pregnancy.

REFERENCES

American College of Obstetricians and Gynecologists (ACOG). Asthma in pregnancy. ACOG practice bulletin; no. 90. Washington DC: American College of Obstetricians and Gynecologists (ACOG); Feb 2008.

Louie JK, Acosta M, Jamieson DJ, Honein MA. Severe 2009 H1N1 influenza in pregnant and postpartum women in California. *N Engl J Med.* 2010;326:27-35.

Sliwa K, Hilfiker-Kleiner D, Petrie MC, et al. Current state of knowledge on aetiology, diagnosis, management, and therapy of peripartum cardiomyopathy: a position statement from the Heart Failure Association of the European Society of Cardiology Working Group on peripartum cardiomyopathy. *Eur J Heart Fail.* Aug 2010;12(8):767-778.

Stein PD, Matta F, Yaekoub AY. Incidence of amniotic fluid embolism: relation to cesarean section and to age. *J Womens Health (Larchmt)*. Mar 2009;18(3):327-329.

Tuffnell DJ. United Kingdom amniotic fluid embolism register. *BJOG*. Dec 2005;112(12):1625-1629.

CASE 37

A 46-year-old man was brought to the hospital because family members have noted that he appears lethargic and complains of abdominal pain. The patient has a history of chronic low back pain and has been under the care of a physician for the past several weeks. He has been prescribed acetaminophen/hydrocodone (Vicodin) and has been supplementing this medication with extra-strength acetaminophen (500 mg tablets). His family members reported that they found several empty medication bottles at home. His laboratory studies from the emergency department revealed normal white blood cell count, hemoglobin, hematocrit, and platelet counts. His serum aspartate aminotransferase (AST) and alanine aminotransferase (ALT) are 1300 IU/L and 1700 IU/L, respectively.

- ▶ What is the most likely cause of the patient's current condition?
- ▶ What is the best next step in management?
- ▶ How is this disease process staged?

ANSWERS TO CASE 37: Poisoning

Summary: This patient is a 46-year-old man with lethargy and abdominal pain, found to have elevated liver transaminase enzymes in the setting of significant acetaminophen ingestion. His presentation to the emergency department is consistent with hepatotoxicity secondary to acetaminophen overdose.

- **Likely cause of current condition:** Acetaminophen overdose.
- **Next step in management:** Gastric lavage following massive ingestions may be effective in retrieving undigested pills or pill fragments 30 to 60 minutes after the ingestion. Activated charcoal that absorbs most toxins (due to its large surface area) should only be administered to awake patients or to comatose patients after appropriate airway protection. The dose is 1 g/kg orally or via gastric tube, with the goal of a 10:1 (charcoal:toxin) ratio.
- **Disease stages:** There are 4 distinct stages of acetaminophen-induced hepatotoxicity: (1) preclinical toxic effects (no lab abnormalities); (2) hepatic injury (elevated transaminase enzymes); (3) hepatic failure; and (4) recovery. Each stage has a different prognosis and management strategy. This patient would appear to be stage 2 based on his initial evaluations.

ANALYSIS

Objectives

1. To learn the clinical manifestations, management, and outcome of **acetaminophen**, **salicylate**, **tricyclic antidepressants**, **alcohol**, **oral hypoglycemics**, **cyanide**, and **propofol**.
2. To learn when activate charcoal is indicated in the management of substance ingestion/overdose.
3. To recognize the importance of airway, breathing, and circulation management in patients with substance ingestion/overdose.

Considerations

This 46-year-old patient was given a prescription for acetaminophen/hydrocodone (Vicodin) and was supplementing this medication with extra-strength acetaminophen to treat his back pain. The additional over-the-counter acetaminophen is sufficient to exceed the liver's ability to metabolize acetaminophen safely. Significant hepatic injury is evident by the patient's elevated transaminase enzymes. Due to the potential for decreased GI motility from opiates, such as hydrocodone, the acetaminophen toxicity could be potentiated because the compound would remain in the patient's system over a prolonged period of time.

Priorities

Assess the patient's airway, with careful attention to the patient's airway-protective reflexes. The most common factor contributing to increased morbidity related to drug overdose is airway compromise caused by a flaccid tongue, aspiration of gastric content, or apnea from respiratory depression. Securing the patient's airway with endotracheal intubation is necessary if the patient's level of consciousness is compromised. Cardiac monitoring and assessment of respiratory rate and functions may give clues to other potential co-ingestants. Continued monitoring of the patient's level of alertness and assessment of serum glucose are important, as the patient may have also ingested other substances in addition to those mentioned by the family. After stabilization of the patient's airway, breathing, and circulation, the acetaminophen level and time of ingestion will be used in concert with the liver enzyme levels and coagulation studies to determine the course of treatment and the extent of hepatic injury. Additional tests to evaluate for concomitant ingestion of other substances include salicylate level, alcohol level, serum electrolytes, serum osmolality, urine toxicology screens (to screen for drugs of abuse), lactate, serum ketones, and an ECG.

Additional History

Approach all poisoned patients as if they have potentially life-threatening polysubstance intoxication (ingestion of multiple substances). Additional history is always helpful to determine which other substances the patient could have accessed. Family members, emergency medical personnel (paramedics, fire department), and the patient's primary doctor are often helpful in providing additional insight. The timing of ingestion and dosage of medication is also of extreme importance and will help guide treatments. In this situation, it will be helpful to have a family member retrieve the additional empty pill bottles that were found in the patient's home. It is always helpful to consult your local poison control center for assistance with patient management, once all the suspected or confirmed ingested toxic substances are identified.

Decontamination

The technique for decontamination will largely depend on the timing, amount, and type of substance ingested. Gastrointestinal decontamination may involve gastric lavage, activated charcoal administration, or whole bowel irrigation depending on the circumstance. There is little clinical evidence to support gastric lavage, but it is currently used for massive ingestions of extremely toxic substances. The aim is retrieving undigested pills or pill fragments, usually most effective when begun within 30 to 60 minutes after the ingestion. **Activated charcoal is a highly effective absorbent that functions to absorb most toxins (due to its large surface area), and should be administered to awake patients or to comatose patients with secured airways. The dose is 1 g/kg orally or via gastric tube, with the goal of a 10:1 (charcoal:toxin) ratio.** Repeat doses of charcoal may enhance elimination of substances. Iron, lithium, and heavy metals are poorly absorbed by activated charcoal. Whole bowel irrigation utilizes nonabsorbable surgical bowel cleansing solutions at high flow rates to force intestinal contents out by way of large volume force. This technique is indicated with ingestion of: (1) substances not absorbed by charcoal, (2) drug-filled condoms or packets, (3) sustained-release tablets. Hemodialysis and antidotes may also hasten the elimination of specific substances.

Psychiatric Evaluation

All poisoned patients must be assessed for suicidal ideation, risk factors for depression, prior history of suicide attempts, and prior psychiatric illnesses. This information can be obtained by the patient, if possible, and corroborated by the family. The potential for accidental overdose exists, particularly in the pediatric, elderly, and disabled populations. Therefore, the need for further evaluation by a psychiatrist should be considered after medical stabilization.

APPROACH TO: Poisoning

CLINICAL APPROACH

The American Association of Poison Control Centers estimated that acetaminophen was responsible for over 70,000 visits to health-care facilities and 300 deaths in 2005. Acetaminophen poisoning can be due to ingestion of a single overdose (typically with suicide attempts) or ingestions of excessive repetitive doses or too-frequent dosages, with therapeutic intent.

Pathophysiology of Acetaminophen Toxicity

Acetaminophen is normally metabolized by the liver, primarily via glucuronidation and sulfation into nontoxic metabolites. However, approximately 5% of acetaminophen is metabolized via cytochrome P-450 2E1 to **N-acetyl-*p*-benzoquinone imine (NAPQI), which is extremely toxic to the liver.** When acetaminophen is taken in therapeutic doses, NAPQI is rapidly detoxified by glutathione to form nontoxic metabolites (cysteine and mercapturic conjugates). However, in an acetaminophen overdose, **NAPQI depletes glutathione reserves and this toxic metabolite interacts with hepatic macromolecules to cause liver injury.**

There are 4 distinct stages of acetaminophen-induced hepatotoxicity: (1) preclinical toxic effects (no lab abnormalities); (2) hepatic injury (elevated transaminase enzymes); (3) hepatic failure; and (4) recovery. Each stage has a different prognosis and management strategy. Patients with frank hepatic failure have a mortality rate of 20% to 40%.

Clinical Assessment

The initial assessment of any patient with a potential overdose should focus on evaluating the **airway, breathing, circulation, disability, and decontamination.** Early in acute acetaminophen ingestions, the majority of patients remains asymptomatic, or will complain of nausea, vomiting, and anorexia. However, 24 to 48 hours post-ingestion, patients begin to show signs of liver injury and liver failure.

After stabilization of the airway, breathing, and circulation, the acetaminophen level and time of ingestion will be used in concert with the liver enzyme levels and coagulation studies to determine the extent of injury and course of treatment.

Additional history to pinpoint the time of ingestion is critical in guiding the therapy. Activated charcoal administration should be considered. Perhaps one of the greatest contributions to the management of patients with acetaminophen overdose is the **Rumack-Matthew nomogram** (Figure 37–1). The nomogram, which was first published in 1975, was developed from the acetaminophen levels of untreated

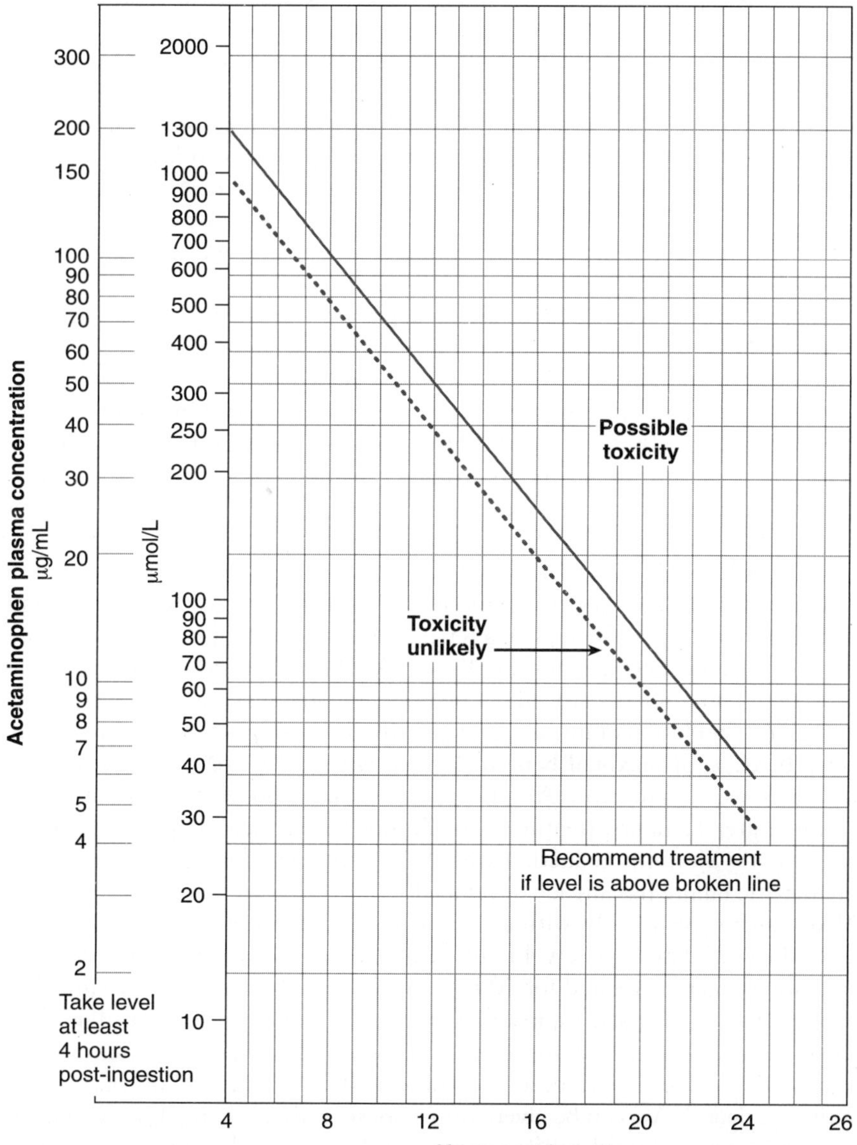

Figure 37–1. Rumack-Matthew acetaminophen nomogram. (Reproduced, with permission, from Tintinalli JE, Stapczynski JS, Ma OJ, et al. *Tintinalli's Emergency Medicine: A Comprehensive Study Guide*. 7th ed. New York, NY: McGraw-Hill Education; 2011. Figure 184–2.)

patients, and describes the mathematic relationship between acetaminophen level, time of ingestion, and the potential for hepatic injury. The upper line of the nomogram defines the toxic level likely to be associated with acute overdose; it is also known as **the "200 line,"** since any level of 200 mcg/mL or greater within 4 hours of ingestion requires antidote treatment. The **lower line ("150 line")** on the nomogram, defines serum levels 25% below those expected to cause hepatotoxicity, and was instituted by the FDA to better improve clinical outcomes with antidote treatment. The nomogram helps the clinician interpret the acetaminophen level. Any acetaminophen level obtained prior to 4 hours post-ingestion is unable to predict the likelihood of hepatotoxicity, but it is able to confirm acetaminophen ingestion.

Acetaminophen levels obtained 4 to 24 hours after ingestion can be plotted on the nomogram to determine the probability of hepatic injury. If the levels plot above the lower line on the nomogram, antidote treatment should be initiated. Any elevated acetaminophen level detected 24 hours after ingestion should be considered toxic and warrants antidote treatment. The majority of poisoned patients present after **polypharmacy** ingestions. When the 4-hour acetaminophen level is nontoxic, an 8-hour level should be drawn in patients who have taken co-ingestants that may delay GI absorption (ie, extended release acetaminophen preparations, opiates, or anticholinergics). Treatment is still guided by the nomogram in these circumstances. **The nomogram is not valid in cases of chronic ingestions.**

N-acetylcysteine (NAC) is the FDA-approved antidote for acetaminophen toxicity, and functions to **aid in glutathione repletion**. Glutathione is synthesized from amino acids glutamate, glycine, and cysteine (cysteine availability is the rate-limiting step in production). *N*-aetylcysteine is readily absorbed and hydrolyzed to cysteine, which provides the substrate for glutathione synthesis. Glutathione functions to convert *N*-acetyl-*p*-benzoquinone (NAPQI) to a nontoxic metabolite that is easily eliminated from the body via renal clearance. NAPQI is capable of causing liver injury by 2 separate mechanisms. First, NAPQI can bind covalently to intracellular proteins and cause hepatocellular necrosis. Second, high rate of NAPQI formation can cause depletion of intrahepatic glutathione stores and cause increased liver toxicity. **NAC is of maximal benefit if given within 8 to 10 hours of ingestion**, since this is usually prior to NAPQI accumulation. Although the benefit of NAC diminishes after 12 hours, treatment should not be withheld despite a delay of 24 hours or more. Mortality reduction with NAC treatment has been shown in cases where hepatic failure has already developed.

NAC can be given orally, with a loading dose of 140 mg/kg, followed by a maintenance dose of 70 mg/kg every 4 hours. Uncomplicated cases with no evidence of hepatic injury may be treated for 20 hours with 5 maintenance doses. However, if there is evidence of hepatic injury, NAC treatment should be continued until liver function tests have improved. Intravenous NAC is indicated if the patient is unable to tolerate the oral formulation, such as those with decreased level of consciousness, vomiting, or ileus. NAC can be given intravenously with a loading dose of 150 mg/kg over 15 minutes, followed by 50 mg/kg over 4 hours, and then 100 mg/kg over 16 hours. Liver enzymes, as well as coagulation studies are monitored until 36 hours post-ingestion. If evidence of liver injury develops, intravenous NAC treatment is continued until liver improvement in function tests occurs.

OTHER COMMON TOXIC INGESTIONS

Management of Salicylate Toxicity

Salicylates are commonly used for their anti-inflammatory and analgesic properties and can be found in Aspirin, Pepto-Bismol, over-the-counter cold medicines, and topical muscle and joint preparations (Aspercreme, Bayer Joint Cream, Icy Hot Cream). The daily therapeutic dose ranges from 40 to 60 mg/kg/d. Mild toxicity can be seen with doses of 150 to 200 mg/kg/d with marked toxicity at 300 to 500 mg/kg/d.

Toxicity from salicylate occurs via 2 main mechanisms: (1) respiratory alkalosis and (2) metabolic acidosis. Salicylates may directly stimulate the central respiratory centers causing hyperventilation, which leads to respiratory alkalosis and a compensatory metabolic acidosis. This metabolic acidosis is further exacerbated by the interruption of glucose and fatty acid metabolism, leading to increased carbon dioxide production. Mild salicylate toxicity may result in respiratory alkalosis with compensatory metabolic acidosis as bicarbonate excreted in the urine. However, with **moderate to severe toxicity, the respiratory alkalosis is accompanied by a high anion gap metabolic acidosis**, as the kidneys deplete sodium bicarbonate and potassium.

Patients typically present with **nausea, vomiting, tinnitus, tachypnea, and lethargy.** Pulmonary edema, coma, and cardiovascular collapse can occur with severe toxicity. Management is aimed at supporting the patient's airway, breathing, and circulation with close attention to ensure adequate ventilation to allow the compensatory mechanisms to maintain a suitable arterial pH. Activated charcoal administration should be considered. Laboratory tests of significance include a salicylate level, electrolytes (to calculate the anion gap), arterial blood gas, and ECG (evidence of hypokalemia). Treatment is aimed at enhancing the elimination of salicylates by the kidneys, which is dependent on hydrogen ion gradients. Therefore, the treatment of choice remains sodium bicarbonate, which functions to treat the metabolic acidosis and enhance renal clearance. Sodium bicarbonate is given as a continuous infusion with a targeted urine pH of 7.5 to 8.0. Potassium supplementation should be added to IV fluids as potassium is rapidly depleted in salicylate toxicity. **Hemodialysis should be considered in acute intoxication with serum salicylate levels of 100 mg/dL in association with severe acidosis.**

Tricyclic Antidepressant Toxicity

Tricyclic antidepressants (TCAs) were traditionally used to treat depression, but they are currently more commonly used to treat **chronic pain syndromes and migraine prophylaxis** in adults, and enuresis, attention deficit disorder, and obsessive-compulsive disorder in children. TCAs have a narrow therapeutic window, and have **anticholinergic** properties that may delay GI absorption. TCAs also have α-adrenergic blockade effects and can cause hypotension and contribute to acidemia along with respiratory depression from CNS effects. However, the most serious complications are its cardiovascular and CNS effects. **Conduction defects** occur as a result of the membrane-depressant qualities due to myocardial fast sodium channel blockade, leading to prolonged PR, QRS, and QT intervals. Hypotension may occur from α-adrenergic blockade. **Anticholinergic** properties may cause tachycardia.

CNS effects mainly manifest as lethargy and coma (due to the anticholinergic properties), in addition to seizures (attributed to central CNS activity).

Supportive care should be immediately initiated to stabilize the airway and support breathing. Intravenous fluids and cardiac monitoring should be instituted for circulatory support. Decontamination with activated charcoal should be considered. Sodium bicarbonate should be administered for patients with QRS prolongation or hypotension. Sodium bicarbonate is believed to reverse the sodium blockade and subsequent myocardial suppressant effects of TCAs. Sodium bicarbonate may also be utilized for serum alkalinization with a goal of achieving serum pH of 7.45 to 7.55, which has been shown to elevate blood pressure and shorten the QRS interval.

Alcohol Toxicity

A variety of alcohols can be found commercially available in liquor, cold medicines, mouthwash, food extracts, colognes, after-shave solutions, antifreeze, and rubbing alcohol. Up to 15% of the US population is considered to be at risk for alcohol dependence. **Alcohol dehydrogenase** is the primary enzyme that metabolizes ethanol, isopropyl alcohol, methanol, and ethylene glycol. The genetic polymorphisms of alcohol dehydrogenase will determine the rate of alcohol metabolism. Patients with alcohol toxicity are typically grossly inebriated, with evidence of slurred speech, ataxia, impaired judgment, and lack of coordination. Severe toxicity may present with progressive CNS depression and coma. **Methanol** toxicities typically cause changes in **vision** in addition to inebriation. Isopropyl alcohol and ethylene glycol typically present gross intoxication similar to that associated with ethanol toxicity.

Ethanol toxicity typically causes CNS depression, which is additive when in combination with benzodiazipines, barbituates, or opiods. **Hypoglycemia** occurs commonly due to impaired gluconeogenesis along with **poor nutrition** in patients with history of chronic alcohol abuse. Occult head injury, hypoxemia, aspiration, and underlying metabolic disturbance must also be considered in all intoxicated patients. **Treatment is mainly supportive with intravenous fluids, glucose, and thiamine.** In cases of alcoholic ketoacidosis (defined by anion gap metabolic acidosis and elevated β-hydroxybutyrate), supplemental glucose and volume replacement are essential. There is no specific antidote for ethanol or isopropyl alcohol intoxication. However, **methanol and ethylene glycol toxicity should be treated with fomepizole or ethanol to saturate the alcohol dehydrogenase enzyme and prevent further production of toxic metabolites.** Methanol may also be eliminated by hemodialysis in cases of severe toxicity.

Hypogylcemic Agent Toxicity

There are several oral agents used to lower serum glucose in the treatment of type 2 diabetes mellitus. Typically, these medications are divided into 2 categories: hypoglycemics and antihyperglycemics. Agents referred to as antihyperglycemics work to reduce glucose levels, but rarely cause hypoglycemia, even when used in excess; these agents include metformin (glucophage), alpha-glucosidase inhibitors, and glitazones. The aforementioned agents work by reducing hepatic glucose production (metformin and glitazones), as well as decreasing intestinal glucose absorption (metformin and α-glucosidase inhibitors). On the other hand, hypoglycemics, namely sulfonylureas, typically cause hypoglycemia in cases of overdose or decreased elimination. Sulfonylurea lowers blood glucose by increasing insulin release from the pancreas and enhancing peripheral sensitivity to insulin.

Sulfonylurea toxicity may cause hypoglycemia, which presents as diaphoresis, delirium, progressive decreased level of consciousness, syncope, or coma. The method of toxicity may be an intentional or unintentional overdose, or decreased elimination secondary to renal insufficiency. The duration of action for many sulfonylureas exceeds 24 hours. Therefore, patients are typically admitted to the hospital and treated with dextrose-containing intravenous fluids in addition to close glucose monitoring. Patients may require intravenous **octreotide** when they are unresponsive to intravenous dextrose. Octreotide is a synthetic somatostatin analog, which suppresses pancreatic insulin release. Adjunctive therapy for patients with sulfonylurea overdose includes alkalinization of the urine to increase renal elimination of sulfonylureas.

Although antihyperglycemics rarely cause hypoglycemia at toxic levels, these agents do exhibit toxicity through other mechanisms. For instance, **metformin is known to cause lactic acidosis with overdose and with renal insufficiency.** Severe cases of acidosis may warrant hemodialysis.

Cyanide Toxicity

Cyanide toxicity is most commonly encountered in victims of **smoke inhalation** from industrial or residential fires. It is caused by the formation of gaseous hydrogen cyanide from burning plastics. Cyanide toxicity can also occur in the ICU as a result of high-dose or prolonged **nitroprusside** infusions. Nitroprusside releases cyanide during metabolism, and is normally converted to a nontoxic metabolite in the liver. However, cyanide may accumulate with prolonged use or high dosages. A rare cause of cyanide toxicity in the United States is the ingestion of cyanide-containing foods, such as cassava, apricot seeds, apple seeds, and spinach.

Cyanide uncouples oxidative phosphorylation, which causes cellular metabolism to switch from aerobic to anaerobic processes, resulting in lactic acidosis. Patients typically present with malaise, headache, confusion, and generalized weakness. Cardiovascular collapse, syncope, and coma may occur with severe toxicity. The safest antidote for cyanide toxicity is **intravenous hydroxocobalamin,** which combines with cyanide to form cyanocobalamin (vitamin B_{12}), which is subsequently excreted by the kidneys. The cyanide antidote kit should be used if hydroxocobalamin is not accessible. The cyanide antidote kit consists of amyl nitrites, sodium nitrites, and sodium thiosulfate. Amyl nitrite pearls and intravenous sodium nitrite are capable of inducing methemoglobinemia in cells, which binds cyanide. However, **nitrites should be avoided in cases of smoke inhalation, where carboxyhemoglobinemia may coexist.** Instead, if hydroxocobalamin is not available, sodium thiosulfate should be administered intravenously, which enhances the conversion of cyanide to thiocyanate that is also excreted by the kidneys.

Propofol Toxicity

Propofol is a lipid-soluble, sedative-hypnotic agent, and is commonly used in surgical and critical care units. It is metabolized by the liver via oxidation by CYP-450

2B6, excreted by the kidneys. Its primary site of action is at the GABA-A receptors. Due to its rapid onset of action and quick metabolism (mean duration of action is 3-5 minutes for a single bolus), propofol is used with increasing frequency in the ICU in patients on mechanical ventilation. It is **contraindicated in patients with egg or soybean allergies** because of the additives in the formulation of the emulsion in which it is administered. Standard dosing of propofol for sedation is 25-75 μg/kg/min (or 1.5-3 mg/kg/h).

Adverse effects with use of propofol range from pain at the site of injection to death. Patients may experience hypotension, arrhythmias (both bradycardia and supraventricular tachyarrhythmias have been described), acute pancreatitis secondary to hypertriglyceridemia, and/or bronchospasm as a result of propofol administration. **Propofol infusion syndrome includes rhabdomyolysis, acute renal failure, lactic acidosis, and hemodynamic instability as a result of prolonged (>48 hours), high-dose infusion (>5 mg/kg/h) of propofol.** There is no specific antidote for propofol toxicity. The treatment is immediate discontinuation of the propofol infusion followed by supportive care. Supportive care may include administration of IV fluids, vasopressor, or antiarrhythmic agents.

CLINICAL CASE CORRELATION

- **See also Case 23 (Acute Kidney Injury), Case 24 (Acid-Base Abnormalities I), and Case 25 (Acid-Base Abnormalities II).**

COMPREHENSION QUESTIONS

37.1 A 25-year-old woman is admitted to the ICU for altered level of consciousness after a polypharmacy ingestion. He was noted to have an acetaminophen level of 80 μg/dL, obtained 12 hours after the ingestion. After stabilization of the patient's airway, breathing, and circulation, the ICU team discussed antidote treatment with liver function tests pending. Which statement is most accurate regarding the next step of management for this patient?

A. Sodium bicarbonate infusion should be initiated with a goal serum pH 7.45 to 7.55.

B. N-acetylcysteine treatment should not be considered until the liver function tests are available.

C. Octreotide can be considered if the patient does not respond to IV dextrose administration.

D. N-acetylcysteine treatment should be started and serial liver function tests should be monitored during treatment.

E. Initiate NG lavage of gastric contents.

37.2 A 54-year-old man is admitted to the burn ICU with confusion and decreased level of consciousness, along with several third-degree burns throughout his body at an industrial fire. The patient was intubated for airway protection after soot in the posterior pharynx and airway edema were noted upon arrival. Cyanide toxicity is suspected. What is the best treatment method for cyanide toxicity in this patient?

A. Sodium bicarbonate infusion should be initiated with a goal serum pH 7.45 to 7.55.

B. Amyl nitrite pearls and intravenous sodium nitrite should be administered.

C. Hydroxocobalamin should be administered intravenously.

D. Methemoglobinemia should be the goal of treatment.

E. Nitroprusside should be administered.

37.3 A 33-year-old man was admitted to the ICU after having been found comatose in his home with a suicide note and an empty bottle of aspirin (30 count). His salicylate level returns at 111 mg/dL and his serum pH is 7.01. What is the best treatment plan for this patient?

A. Octreotide can be considered if the patient does not respond to IV dextrose administration.

B. Sodium bicarbonate infusion should be initiated with a goal serum pH 7.45 to 7.55.

C. Hemodialysis should be initiated to enhance elimination and correct the acidosis.

D. N-acetylcysteine treatment should be started and serial liver function should be monitored during the treatment.

E. Potassium supplementation in intravenous fluid.

37.4 A 40-year-old woman with diabetes mellitus was admitted to the emergency department for acute kidney injury with creatinine 3.2 mg/dL. The patient was prescribed a sulfonylurea agent. She was found to have persistent hypoglycemia (glucose initially noted to be 30 mg/dL). Which of the following therapies is the first-line treatment?

A. Intravenous dextrose infusion with close glucose monitoring.

B. Fomepizole therapy should be initiated immediately.

C. Intravenous octreotide should be administered immediately.

D. Sodium bicarbonate infusion should be initiated with a goal urine pH 7.5 to 8.0.

E. Administer calcium chloride.

ANSWERS TO QUESTIONS

37.1 **D.** The patient's alcohol level is clearly past the line indicating probable hepatic toxicity when plotted on the nomogram for 12 hours after ingestion. Therefore, NAC therapy is warranted. Remember that the nomogram functions to assist the medical team with the decision on whether or not to initiate NAC therapy. Serial liver function tests are followed while the patient is receiving NAC therapy, to help determine the length of therapy. Gastric lavage may be of value when initiated within 30 to 60 minutes following ingestion to help evacuate pill fragments. Sodium bicarbonate and octreotide are not indicated for the treatment of acetaminophen toxicity.

37.2 **C.** Hydroxocobalamin (Cyanokit) is the preferred treatment for cyanide toxicity, especially in the setting of smoke inhalation. Amyl nitrites and sodium nitrite should be avoided with smoke inhalation exposures, as carbon monoxide toxicity is also common with these types of exposures. Since amyl nitrite and sodium nitrite function by inducing methemoglobinemia, this may be detrimental to the patient's oxygen-carrying capacity with concomitant carboxyhemoglobinemia. If hydroxocobalamin is unavailable in these situations, treating with thiosulfate is the next best option for cyanide toxicity from smoke inhalation exposures. Sodium bicarbonate is not indicated in the treatment of cyanide toxicity. Nitroprusside administration in high doses or prolonged fashion, can contribute to cyanide toxicity, and its administration has no role in treatment of inhalation-related cyanide toxicity.

37.3 **C.** Hemodialysis is indicated in salicylate toxicity with a serum level above 100 mg/dL with profound acidosis. Sodium bicarbonate is the mainstay of treatment with salicylate toxicity; however, the goal of treatment is to alkalinize the urine to enhance salicylate elimination. Therefore, the goal of sodium bicarbonate therapy is to maintain a urinary pH of 7.5 to 8.0. Octreotide and N-acetylcysteine are not indicated in salicylate toxicity. Potassium supplementation is helpful during treatment of salicylate toxicity as depletion often occurs; however, replacement of potassium does not actually address the salicylate toxicity.

37.4 **A.** The mainstay of treatment for sulfonylurea-induced hypoglycemia is the administration of dextrose-containing IV fluids and close monitoring for > 24 hours. Octreotide is warranted only after patients display that they are unresponsive to dextrose-containing IV fluids. Fomepizole is used for ethylene glycol poisoning. Sodium bicarbonate can be applied as an adjunctive measure to facilitate the elimination of sulfonylurea in the treatment of sulfonylurea toxicity, if the patient's renal functions are adequate. In this patient with a serum creatinine of 3.2 and acute kidney injury, alkalinization most likely does not work. Calcium chloride does not have any therapeutic benefits in a patient with sulfonyurea poisoning.

CLINICAL PEARLS

- Gastric lavage following massive ingestions may be effective in retrieving undigested pill fragments 30 to 60 minute after ingestion.
- The most common factor contributing to mordity related to drug overdose is airway compromise, aspiration from gastric contents, or respiratory depression.
- Activated charcoal is an effective absorbent but should be administered to awake patients, or to comatose patients with secured airways.
- NAC is the FDA-approved medication for patients with acetaminophen toxicity, and it is of maximal benefit when administered within 8 to 10 hours after ingestion. Benefits may be seen even when administered after 24 hours after ingestion.
- Acute ethanol ingestion may serve a protective role against acetaminophen toxicity by occupying the cytochrome P-450 2E1 system and decreasing the metabolism of acetaminophen to NAPQI.
- Chronic ethanol ingestion up-regulates cytochrome P-450 2E1 system and increases the conversion of acetaminophen to the toxic metabolite NAPQI.
- Patients with salicylate poisoning may have a respiratory alkalosis and metabolic acidosis. Sodium bicarbonate corrects the acidosis and enhances renal excretion of the salicylate. Severe cases may require dialysis.
- Sulfonyurea overdoses may lead to profound hypoglycemia. If dextrose treatment is ineffective, IV octreotide may be helpful.
- Propofol infusion syndrome includes rhabdomyolysis, acute renal failure, lactic acidosis, and hemodynamic instability. This syndrome may be the result of prolonged (>48 hours) high-dose infusion (>5 mg/kg/h) of propofol.

REFERENCES

Heard K. Acetylcysteine for acetaminophen poisoning. *N Eng J Med.* 2008;359:258-292.

Olson K. *Poisoning and Drug Overdose.* 5th ed. San Francisco, CA: McGraw Hill; 2004.

Stolbach A, Goldfrank LR. Toxicology. In: Gabrielli A, Layon AJ, Yu M, eds. *Civetta, Taylor, and Kirby's Critical Care.* Philadelphia PA: Linppincott Williams & Wilkins; 2009:987-1014.

CASE 38

A 66-year-old man fell down a flight of stairs. He sustained several rib fractures and a small right frontal-parietal cerebral contusion. While in the emergency center, he developed progressive dyspnea, which led to intubation and mechanical ventilation. Shortly after arrival to the ICU, his nurse notifies you that the patient appears anxious and agitated despite having received 8 mg of morphine sulfate intravenously over the past 1 hour. His heart rate is 110 beats/minute, BP is 146/90 mm Hg, respiratory rate is 28 breaths/minute, Glasgow coma score (GCS) is 10T (E4, M5, V1), and O_2 saturation is 100%. He appears uncomfortable and is attempting to remove his monitoring leads and urinary catheter.

- ▶ What are the appropriate next steps in assessment?
- ▶ What are appropriate interventions at this time?

ANSWERS TO CASE 38: Pain Control and Sedation

Summary: A 66-year-old man fell down the stairs and suffered rib fractures and a small right frontal-parietal cerebral contusion. He is intubated secondary to progressive dyspnea. He now appears agitated, uncomfortable, and in danger of self-harm.

- **Appropriate next steps in the assessment:** Identify potential reasons for pain and agitation in this patient using validated scales and establish treatment goals.
- **Appropriate interventions at this time:** Administer combination of sedative and analgesic medications. An appropriate combination for this patient is propofol for sedation, titrated to Richmond Agitation Sedation Scale (RASS) of 2, and fentanyl for pain control.

ANALYSIS

Objectives

1. To learn the principles and strategies for pain and anxiety monitoring in the ICU.
2. To learn the various medication treatment strategies available for pain and sedation management in the ICU.
3. To learn management considerations for mechanically ventilated patients.
4. To learn management considerations for patients who are at risk for developing alcohol, benzodiazepines, and opioids withdrawal.

Considerations

This 66-year-old patient is clearly agitated and has progressed to become a danger to himself, as evidenced by his attempt to remove his catheters and lines. To avoid further self-inflicted harm, his agitation and pain must be immediately addressed. Prior to the next step in management however, we must consider the patient's comorbidities, current injuries, and goals of care. The patient has experienced head trauma and subsequently a rapid onset/offset agent that will permit reassessment of his neurological status would be optimal. The ICU team must evaluate how long they anticipate the patient to require mechanical ventilation based on the severity of his respiratory failure. This initial assessment must occur quickly and will guide the ICU care providers toward particular agents and techniques of sedation and pain management.

APPROACH TO: Pain and Agitation

CLINICAL APPROACH

The ICU care practitioner is responsible for maintaining the patient's comfort while in the ICU. Mechanically ventilated patients in the ICU can exhibit even further stress superimposed on their acute medical problems; examples of these additional stresses include anxiety related to unfamiliar surroundings, and distress with potential and experienced pain. Agitation, anxiety, and pain can bring about many adverse side effects including increased endogenous catecholamine activity, myocardial ischemia, hypercoagulable and hypermetabolic states, sleep deprivation, and delirium possibly resulting in self-injury via removal of life-sustaining devices. Although such adverse effects should be actively avoided, the care providers must be mindful of the potential detrimental effects associated with pharmacological treatment of pain and agitation. A fine balance must be established to maximize the benefits while minimizing the risks of drug accumulation in tissue stores, which may produce prolonged clinical effects and prolongation of ICU stay.

When considering sedation and pain management, the anticipated duration of treatment and mechanical ventilation should be considered. Addressing the target of intervention will help determine the most practical medication strategies. Very often, **a combination of opioids and benzodiazepines** are used for analgesia and sedation. Alternatively, other agents may be selected depending on the patient's clinical status (Table 38–1). The benzodiazepines (midazolam, lorazepam, and diazepam) have been the cornerstone of anxiolytic, amnestic, and sedative therapy for the ICU patient, while opioids have a long history of efficacy and safety for adequate analgesia in the ICU patient.

Pain is common, and the majority of algorithms incorporate testing for pain, with patient self-report being the most accurate means of assessment if the patient is able to communicate. Self-reporting for pain is facilitated using a numerical rating scale (NRS) or visual aid (Figure 38–1). A number of other tools for pain observation such as the behavioral pain scale (BPS) (Table 38–2) and critical pain observation tool (CPOT) have been validated. These tools utilize facial expression, body movement, muscle tension, and ventilator synchrony to help assess one's pain. Notably, the validity of these scales declines with the increased depth of sedation.

Sedation scales, the most common being **Ramsay Sedation Scale (RSS), Richmond Agitation Sedation Scale (RASS)** (Table 38–3), **and Sedation Agitation Scale (SAS)** (Table 38–4), are used to direct the management of agitation and establish a target level of sedation for medication titration as well as detecting when oversedation is present. The Ramsay score of 2 or 3 is optimal. In the absence of organic or natural causes of obtundation (ie, central nervous system pathology), a Ramsay score of 5 or 6 represents oversedation.

Once a patient is started on a sedative and analgesic medication, the goal should be to minimize the risk of continued infusion of these agents. A focused downward titration of sedative drugs over time can be accomplished with **daily interruption**

Table 38–1 • PAIN MEDICATIONS

Class of Medication	Mechanism of Action	Uses	Adverse Effects	Examples
Opioids	Mu-1 receptors for analgesia in CNS and peripheral tissue Mu-2 receptors mediate respiratory depression, nausea, vomiting, constipation	Mainstay drug for analgesia therapy in ICU	Depress respiratory drive, decrease GI motility—ileus, little cardiovascular effects in euvolemic patients, but can result in significant hypotension in hypovolemic patients, dependence and withdrawal effects with prolonged infusion	• Morphine • Fentanyl • Remifentanil • Methadone • Hydromorphone
Benzodiazepines	Potentiate effects of γ-aminobutyric acid (GABA) via benzodiazepine receptor—suppresses CNS activity	Mainstay for sedation in ICU—do not have analgesic properties	Respiratory depression	• Lorazepam (Ativan) • Midazolam (Versed)
Propofol	Potentiate effects of GABA receptor (different receptor than benzodiazepines), very lipophilic—crosses blood–brain barrier rapidly	Rapid onset and offset action for sedation, used for short-term sedation, to treat status epilepticus and as a common anesthesia induction agent	Highly lipophilic compound—can cause hypertriglyceridemia Pain at injection site Propofol infusion syndrome: rare, seen with high infusion rates >48 hours, characterized by arrhythmias, heart failure, metabolic acidosis, hyperkalemia, rhabdomyolysis	
α_2-Receptor agonists	Binds to α_2-receptors releasing norepinephrine and decreasing sympathetic activity—net effect: sedation, analgesia and amnesia, sedative properties facilitated through locus coreuleus site in CNS and analgesic effects accentuate opioid receptors	Commonly used following cardiac and neurosurgical procedures, not associated with respiratory depression	Biphasic cardiovascular effect: initial bolus may cause vasoconstriction, causing bradycardia and hypertension; continuous infusion associated with hypotension secondary to vasodilation	• Dexmedetomidine • Clonidine

Neuromuscular blocking agents (NMBA)	Block neuromuscular transmission at neuromuscular junction causing paralysis of affected skeletal muscles, clinically relevant drugs act postsynaptically at acetylcholine receptors of motor nerve end-plate	Indicated for patients on modes of mechanical ventilation that produce agitation interfering with ventilation/oxygentation, closed head injury with increased ICP, tetanus, and decreased venous O_2 in hypermetabolic, agitated states	Most feared complication is accidental extubation Considered a causative factor for critical illness myopathy—causing prolonged weakness after use, especially in those patients using steroids	• Rocuronium • Vecuronium • Atracurium • Cisatracurium
Butyrophenones	Inhibit dopamine-mediated neurotransmissions in the CNS	Indications include treatment of agitation, delirium, and hallucinations in ICU patients	Detachment from the environment leading to flat affects. May produce extrapyramidal symptoms, anticholinergic effects, neuroleptic malignant syndrome; prolonged QT interval.	• Haloperidol • Droperidol

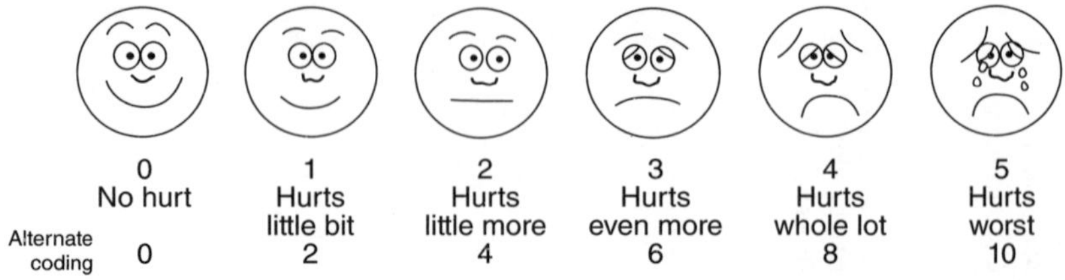

Figure 38–1. Analog Pain Scale. (From Hockenberry MJ, Wilson D: *Wong's essentials of pediatric nursing,* ed 8, St. Louis, 2009, Mosby. Used with permission. Copyright Mosby.)

of sedative infusions (DIS). Mechanically ventilated patients receiving continuous sedation can benefit from daily interruption in the sedation until the patient is awake, as this strategy is associated with decreases in the duration of mechanical ventilation and ICU length of stay. DIS minimizes drug accumulation and shortens the duration of mechanical ventilation. Both sedative and analgesic agents should be interrupted once daily, unless there is evidence for ongoing patient distress. Once drugs are interrupted, the ICU team must be vigilant for evidence of patient distress—overt physical agitation, hemodynamic lability (HTN or tachycardia), or ventilator asynchrony. A bolus should be given to de-escalate symptoms and restart both sedative and analgesic drugs at half the previous infusion doses with subsequent titration. Performing DIS in every patient may not be appropriate, as there is some concern that DIS could provoke brief episodes of intense withdrawal from drugs or alcohol in those patients at high risk. Further research is needed to clarify the most optimal approach to selecting patients for DIS, though at the discretion of the ICU physician, DIS can be beneficial to the right patient.

Selection of Pharmacologic Therapy

In agitated and anxious patients, the clinician can first attempt nonpharmacologic interventions such as comfortable positioning, verbal reassurance, and encouraging the presence of family and friends, though such interventions are often inadequate alone and ultimately require medical intervention. On initial assessment of

Table 38–2 • BEHAVIORAL PAIN SCALE

Score	Facial Expression	Verbalization	Body Position
0	Neutral/positive facial expression, calm	Normal conversation, laugh	Inactive, laying relaxed with all extremities or sitting, walking
1	Negative facial expression, concerned	Completely quiet or sobbing and/or complaining but not because of pain	Restless movements, shifting fashion, and/or touching wound or wound area
2	Negative facial expression, grimace, distorted face	Crying, screaming, and/or complains about pain	Lying rigid and/or drawn up with arms and legs to the body

Table 38–3 • RICHMOND AGITATION SEDATION SCALE

Score	Term	Description
+4	Combative	Overtly combative or violent and an immediate danger to staff
+3	Very agitated	Pulls on or removes tubes/catheters or has aggressive behavior to staff
+2	Agitated	Frequent nonpurposeful movement or patient ventilator dyssynchrony
+1	Restless	Anxious or apprehensive but movements not aggressive or vigorous
0	Alert and calm	
−1	Drowsy	Not fully alert but has sustained (>10 seconds) awakenings, with eye contact, to voice
−2	Light sedation	Briefly (<10 seconds) awakens with eye contact to voice
−3	Moderate sedation	Any movements (but no eye contact) to voice
−4	Deep sedation	No response to voice, but any movement to physical stimuli
−5	Unarousable	No response to voice or physical stimulation

the patient's agitation in the clinical example in this chapter, we can place him at a RASS +3, since he is removing his catheters and is clearly agitated. Because the patient is awake, we can ask him directly about pain, instructing him to quantify his pain numerically if he is able to do so.

Prior to initiating a sedation and pain regimen in an ICU patient, the patient's injuries, comorbidities, and goals of care must always be addressed. The patient discussed earlier has experienced head trauma for which frequent neurologic examinations may be necessary in the immediate observation period. In this situation, propofol may be the best choice given its rapid onset and offset. Midazolam (Versed) can also be used as a sedative in this patient, although its offset is longer than propofol and frequent neurologic examinations would not be as easy to administer. When initiating a sedative agent, a level of sedation should always be identified—that is, using the RASS sedation scale as a guideline. An appropriate level of sedation would allow the patient to be easily awakened and comfortable, consistent with RASS-1 or -2. Sedation and analgesia in the ICU is multidisciplinary, as the bedside nurses

Table 38–4 • THE RAMSAY SEDATION SCORING SYSTEM

Score	Response
1	Anxious and agitated or restless; or both
2	Cooperative, oriented and tranquil
3	Responding to commands only
4	Brisk response to a light glabellar tap
5	Sluggish response to a light glabellar tap
6	No response to a light glabellar tap

will be the crucial component of evaluating the patient's sedation level. As such, it is important to communicate the sedation goals with the entire health-care team.

Opioids are the mainstay of analgesic care in the ICU. These drugs are also very good at palliating coughing and the subjective sense of dyspnea—particularly important for patients who are mechanically ventilated. Among the opioids, fentanyl has a rapid onset of action (1 minute) and rapidly redistributes into peripheral tissues, resulting in a short half-life (0.5-1 hour) after a single dose. As a continuous infusion, fentanyl can be titrated to the patient's comfort as identified by a pain scale as described earlier. If the patient is easily awakened, we can address pain by simply asking the patient to quantify the pain. If the patient is not easily awakened, tools such as facial expression, body movement, and ventilator synchrony can be utilized, again with the bedside nurse being the most important person in this assessment.

After initiation of sedation and analgesia, it is important to continuously reevaluate the clinical status. If the patient appears to be improving from a respiratory standpoint and is prepared to undergo spontaneous breathing trials in preparation for extubation, the patient's sedation should be titrated downward and the patient slowly awoken, as sedation can hinder one's respiratory status. The ICU clinician must be vigilant in this aspect—always reassessing the patient's clinical status and de-escalating medications (or escalating medications if needed) to minimize the risks of medical sedation and analgesia.

Sedation and Analgesic Selection for the Mechanically Ventilated Patients

Patients in need of mechanical ventilation generally require sedation and/or analgesic medication to overcome the stress and discomfort associated with ventilation. As patients who require prolonged ventilatory support progress toward extubation, sedation and analgesic agents are generally decreased. Medication tapering at this time must be done in a way to avoid withdrawal symptoms, avoid over-sedation, and provide adequate comfort so that the patient is able to cooperate with the transitional process.

Agitation Related to Substance Ingestion or Administration

Alcohol abuse contributes to a number of health problems; consequently, it is not uncommon to encounter patients with chronic alcohol ingestion history in the ICU. Chronic excessive alcohol consumption causes depression of the central α- and β-receptors and increase in the inhibitory neurotransmitter GABA. At the same time, chronic alcohol use causes an increase in NMDA receptors, which are responsible for central excitatory activities. When alcohol consumption stops in an individual with a chronic consumption history, the combination of excess excitatory activities and the withdrawal of inhibitory activities can cause symptoms of withdrawal, which include a number of neuropsychiatric and hemodynamic manifestations. Alcohol withdrawal symptoms may include **tremulousness** (onset within hours, peak 10-30 hours, subsides at approximately 40 hours), **seizures** (onset 6-48 hours, peak 13-24 hours), **hallucination** (onset 8-48 hours, may persist 1-6 days), and **delirium tremens** (onset 48-96 hours). Recognition of patients at risk for alcohol withdrawal is important and can be determined based on social history and history of withdrawal episodes. The treatments are supportive care and benzodiazepines administration, and in some cases of delirium tremens, the addition of propofol and neuroleoptics may be considered.

Chronic ingestion and the administration of exogenous opioids lead to diminished endogenous opioid peptides, therefore when exogenous opioids are abruptly discontinued, the patients may develop withdrawal symptoms. Early symptoms of opioid withdrawal may include yawning, rhinorrhea, sneezing, and seating. Later manifestation of withdrawal may include restlessness, irritability, tachycardia, tremor, hyperthermia, vomiting, and muscle spasm. Withdrawal symptoms may begin within 6 to 12 hours after the last dose of short-acting opioid or after 36 to 48 hours of the last dose of long-acting opioids such as methadone. Withdrawal can occur when long-term administration of opioids is discontinued or tapered too rapidly. A course of tapering over days to weeks may be implemented to avoid this problem.

Benzodiazepine withdrawal can occur in the ICU setting when infusions are decreased or interrupted. Patients receiving higher doses of the medications for prolonged periods of time (>7 days) have increased susceptibility for developing withdrawal. Close monitoring and slow tapering schedules may be needed when considering benzodiazepine discontinuation in the ICU patients.

CLINICAL CASE CORRELATION

- **See also Case 8 (Airway Management/Respiratory Failure), Case 9 (Ventilator Management), and Case 30 (Altered Mental Status).**

COMPREHENSION QUESTIONS

38.1 A 45-year-old man with multiple abdominal gunshot wounds is intubated in the ICU and has been receiving continuous infusion of propofol and fentanyl for 3 days. His morning labs reveal a potassium count of 6.3 mEq/L, bicarbonate of 16 mEq/L, and the patient had 3 episodes of unsustained ventricular tachycardia overnight. What is your next step in management?

A. Administer calcium gluconate, insulin, and β-blockers for his hyperkalemia.

B. Opt for cardioversion.

C. Discontinue propofol.

D. Resuscitate with fluids to increase bicarbonate.

E. Opt for hemodialysis.

38.2 A 37-year-old woman is admitted to the ICU for severe pancreatitis complicated by acute respiratory distress syndrome (ARDS) requiring mechanical ventilation. She continues to have difficulty ventilating and agitation on increasing doses of fentanyl and midazolam (Versed) IV infusions. What is the most appropriate next step?

A. Continue to increase midazolam (Versed) as tolerated.

B. Change sedative agent from midazolam (Versed) to propofol.

C. Administer a neuromuscular blocking agent in addition to current regimen.

D. Administer a second analgesic as difficulty in ventilating her and agitation are secondary to poorly controlled pain.

E. Provide a trial of pressure support ventilation.

38.3 A 67-year-old woman with end-stage renal disease and coronary artery disease is admitted to the ICU for respiratory failure secondary to pneumonia. Which analgesic agent is most appropriate for this patient?

A. Ketorolac

B. Fentanyl

C. Morphine

D. Meperidine

ANSWERS TO QUESTIONS

38.1 **C.** Propofol infusion syndrome is a rare but serious and potentially fatal adverse effect, typically seen with infusion rates >83 μg/kg/min for more than 48 hours and carries with it a mortality rate of up to 85%. This syndrome is characterized by dysarrhythmias, heart failure, metabolic acidosis, hyperkalemia, and rhabdomyolysis. High-risk patients include those receiving high doses of the drug, those with history of hypertriglyceridemia, and those concurrently receiving parenteral lipids for nutrition. Treatment consists of immediate cessation of propofol infusion and then correction of hemodynamic and metabolic abnormalities.

38.2 **C.** Some patients may remain delirious, agitated, and have difficulty maintaining ventilation regardless of whether they are on an effective dose of anxiolytic drugs. If the patient is tracheally intubated, mechanically ventilated, and receiving adequate sedation, using a neuromuscular blockade to paralyze the patient is a good option. In patients with ARDS who are difficult to ventilate and often agitated, neuromuscular blockades may be a reasonable alternative to help improve ventilation and gas exchange.

38.3 **B.** Fentanyl is metabolized by the liver which creates inactive metabolites that are excreted by the kidneys. Because the metabolites are inactive, fentanyl a good choice for patients with renal insufficiency. Morphine is conjugated by the liver to metabolites that include morphine-6-glucuronide, a potent metabolite. Both morphine and morphine-6-glucuronide are eliminated by the kidney, thus patients with renal dysfunction may suffer from prolonged drug effects. Like morphine, meperidine is renally excreted. A metabolite of meperidine, normeperidine, is a potent CNS stimulant that can potentiate seizures, especially in patients with renal dysfunction. Ketorolac is an NSAID that reversibly inhibits cyclooxygenase-1 and -2 enzymes and is contraindicated in patients with advanced renal impairment as NSAID use may compromise existing renal function.

REFERENCES

Devlin JW, Roberts RJ. Pharmacology of commonly used analgesics and sedatives in the ICU: benzodiazepines, propofol, and opioids. *Crit Care Clin*. 2009;25:431-449.

Murray MJ, Bloomfield EL. Sedation and neuromuscular blockade. In: Gabrielli A, Layon AJ, Yu M, eds. *Civetta, Taylor, and Kirby's Critical Care*. 4th ed. Philadelphia, PA: Lippincott, Williams & Wilkins; 2009:961-971.

Rajaram SS, Zimmerman JL. Substance abuse and withdrawal: alcohol, cocaine, opioids, and other drugs. In: Gabrielli A, Layon AJ, Yu M, eds. *Civetta, Taylor, and Kirby's Critical Care*. 4th ed. Philadelphia, PA: Lippincott, Williams & Wilkins; 2009:1015-1027.

Zapanis A, Leung S. Tolerance and withdrawal issues with sedation. *Crit Care Nurs Clin N Am*. 2005;17:211-223.

CASE 39

A 56-year-old man was at a mall, where he had a sudden witnessed cardiac arrest. He received immediate cardiopulmonary resuscitation (CPR) from bystanders. When the paramedics arrived, they noted that the patient was in ventricular fibrillation and initiated cardioversion and continued CPR. After several rounds of cardioversion, the patient's rhythm returned to sinus tachycardia with a rate of 120 beats/minute and a blood pressure of 96/40 mm Hg. In the emergency center he was noted to have sinus tachycardia with rate of 115 beats/minute, BP of 98/60 mm Hg, and Glasgow coma score (GCS) of 7T. You have been called to see the patient, since he has been admitted to the ICU.

- ▶ What are your priorities in this patient's management?
- ▶ What are post-resuscitation treatment strategies that have shown to improve outcome?

ANSWERS TO CASE 39:
Post-Resuscitation Management in the ICU

Summary: A 56-year-old man with witnessed ventricular fibrillation-induced cardiac arrest has been successfully resuscitated following CPR, cardioversions, and pharmacological interventions. He is now intubated and admitted to the ICU for further care.

- **Priorities in patient's mamagement:** Minimizing post–cardiac arrest brain injury, addressing his post–cardiac arrest myocardial dysfunction, minimizing his systemic ischemia/reperfusion responses, addressing the problem that caused his cardiac arrest in the first place, and lastly prognostication of outcome.
- **Post-resuscitation strategies that improve outcome:** Coronary reperfusion with either percutaneous intervention and/or thrombolytic therapy has shown to improve survival in cardiac arrest survivors if acute change in coronary plaque morphology is the underlying cause for the cardiac arrest. Other strategies that have shown to improve neurologic outcome in post–cardiac arrest patients include controlled reoxygenation, therapeutic hypothermia, and glucose management.

ANALYSIS

Objectives

1. To learn the post–cardiac arrest syndrome and strategies directed toward its management, including optimization of neurological outcome, optimization of myocardial function, glucose management, and controlled reoxygenation.
2. Describe the use the therapeutic hypothermia to reduce the neurological injury after resuscitation.

Considerations

This 56-year-old man is admitted to the ICU after successful resuscitation from an apparent ventricular fibrillation (VF)-induced cardiac arrest. Neurological and cardiac dysfunction are common complications. Therapeutic hypothermia (TH) is defined as lowering the core temperature to 32°C to 34°C, which can help both post-resuscitation neurological and myocardial dysfunction. Maintaining oxygen saturation in the 96% to 98% range also decreases post-resuscitation sequelae. Finally, hyperglycemia is very common following resuscitation. While prior interventions attempted to more strictly control serum glucose levels, more recent evidence has found that moderate hyperglycemia correlates to better prognosis. Thus, target glucose levels of 144 to 180 mg/dL are sought.

APPROACH TO:
The Post-Resucitation Patient

DEFINITIONS

POST–CARDIAC ARREST SYNDROME: This syndrome includes post–cardiac arrest brain injury, post–cardiac arrest myocardial dysfunction, ischemia/reperfusion injuries, and the underlying disease process that contributed to the event.

THERAPEUTIC HYPOTHERMIA (TH): Therapeutic maneuvers to improve neurological outcomes by reducing core body temperature to 32°C to 34°C following cardiac arrest, with hypothermia maintained for 24 to 48 hours.

POST–CARDIAC ARREST MYOCARDIAL DYSFUNCTION: This is a biventricular dysfunction from multiple reasons that occurs transiently following resuscitation from cardiac arrest.

POST–CARDIAC ARREST ENCEPHALOPATHY: Ischemic brain injury in which the 2 main issues are depressed level of consciousness and seizures.

CLINICAL APPROACH

Introduction

Survival after in-hospital and out-of-hospital cardiac arrest is poor. For the subset of patients with return of spontaneous circulation following resuscitation, the probability of survival is significantly improved. **Approximately one-third of patients admitted to an ICU following cardiac arrest survive to discharge from the hospital.** Post–cardiac arrest syndrome describes a number of complex pathophysiologic processes, which are grouped into 4 major categories: post-resuscitation brain injury, ischemia/reperfusion injuries, myocardial dysfunction, and persistence of the precipitating cause of the cardiac arrest. Neuronal susceptibility to ischemia is not uniform within the brain. These differential responses may be related to the different brain regions' cellular energy requirements and adaptive heat-shock responses. The **hallmark of anoxic encephalopathy is disorder of consciousness and arousal.** In addition to depressed levels of arousal, 10% to 40% of post–cardiac arrest patients develop seizure activities that have to be monitored and treated.

Most of the treatment strategies and rationale are based on recent post-arrest resuscitation literature and include TH and early cardiac intervention. **Several organizations now recommend bundling of post-resuscitation care to include therapeutic hypothermia, early coronary angiography and PCI, hemodynamic support with inotropes or vasopressors, and rapid extubation.**

Therapeutic Hypothermia

TH, lowering the patient's core temperature to 32°C to 34°C, has been shown in several randomized controlled trials to improve neurological recovery in patients following VF-induced cardiac arrest. TH should be instituted as soon as possible with surface cooling using cooling blankets and ice packs. This approach has been **definitively shown to improve neurologic outcomes in patients suffering from**

out-of-hospital VF arrest. Some experts have proposed applying this strategy more broadly to include patients with cardiac arrest from other causes; however, the beneficial effects in these groups have not been demonstrated. TH has been incorporated into the International Consensus Guidelines for Resuscitative Care since 2005. During hypothermia, magnesium, phosphate, potassium, and calcium should be replaced to higher end of normal values. During the rewarming phase, core temperature should increase at a rate of 0.25°C to 0.5°C/h, with continued monitoring and replacement of electrolytes. **Rapid rewarming is associated with increased catabolism and can worsen outcomes.** The potential complications associated with hypothermia include increased infections from leukocyte dysfunction, increased bleeding from platelet and clotting factors dysfunction, and arrhythmias (predominantly atrial fibrillation).

Post-resuscitation myocardial dysfunction is a transient reduction in left and right ventricular function that presents after cardiac arrest for up to 24 to 48 hours. It is now believed that TH also may have beneficial effects in reducing post-resuscitation myocardial dysfunction. Because the majority of out-of-hospital cardiac arrests occur as the result of acute coronary syndrome, patients with successful resuscitation from out-of-hospital cardiac arrest should be considered for intervention. For those candidates, early coronary angiography and percutaneous coronary interventions (PCI) may improve outcome.

Oxygenation

Observations from experimental models suggest that ventilation during and after resuscitation with minimal oxygen fractions to maintain O_2 saturations of 94% to 96% or PAO_2 ~100 mm Hg would lead to reduction in reperfusion injuries. In addition, in a multicenter cohort study, it was observed that adult patients with non–trauma-related cardiac arrests had a mortality odds ratio of 1.8 when hyperoxia (PAO_2 >300 mm Hg) was recorded as the initial blood gas values following arrest. **Based on these principles and clinical evidence, the target oxygenation for this patient during resuscitation and immediately following resuscitation should be 94% to 98% saturation, and not higher.**

Fluids and Vasopressors

The resuscitation of patients with hemodynamic instability from hemorrhagic shock and sepsis are discussed in detail in other sections of this book. The Surviving Sepsis Campaign is a multinational sponsored effort to standardize the approach to the early management of patients with sepsis and septic shock. Fluids and vasopressor support strategies have been well defined based on these efforts. Similarly, recent clinical observations from the casualty management during the ongoing military conflicts in the Middle East have led to developments in the resuscitation of patients with hemorrhagic shock. What remains relatively undefined is management strategies to minimize the harm associated the initial aggressive resuscitation of patients with sepsis, septic shock, and hemorrhagic shock.

The amount of fluids and blood products required to resuscitate patients with hemorrhagic shock or sepsis may produce generalized edema with excess loss of fluid into the extracellular tissue spaces. These fluid shifts produce edema and organ dysfunction, especially in the lungs and gastrointestinal tract. Resuscitation efforts directed at optimizing tissue oxygenation are most valuable during the **initial few hours** following the septic or hemorrhagic insults, whereas extended periods of excess fluid administration in these patients is potentially harmful. Strong efforts should be made to limit fluid administration; those who have had excessive fluids should receive timely diuretic treatment as soon as shock has been corrected. **Early fluid restriction to avoid hypervolemia is associated with improved recovery from acute lung injury and acute respiratory distress syndrome.** Early fluid restriction has been demonstrated to be associated with improved lung injury scores, reduced ventilator days, and reduced ICU lengths of stay. Similarly, judicious fluid management in patients following resuscitation from sepsis or hemorrhage is beneficial as it is associated with improved GI functions and improved tolerance to early (within 24 hours) enteral nutritional support, which has been shown to be associated with immunological and physiological benefits.

Glucose Levels

Hyperglycemia is a common encounter in post–cardiac arrest patients. Recent observations suggest that **strict glycemic control in the ICU patient leads to increase in neurological complications,** and a randomized controlled trial has shown that there was no difference in mortality among out-of-hospital arrest patients managed with glucose values of 72 to 108 mg/dL versus those maintained with glucose levels of 108 to 144 mg/dL. Therefore, suggesting that controlling glucoses to "normal" levels may be harmful. The 2010 American Heart Association Guidelines for Cardiopulmonary Resuscitation and Emergency Cardiovascular Care now recommends **moderate glycemic control targeting glucose values between 144 and 180 mg/dL, to avoid possible hypoglycemia.**

CLINICAL CASE CORRELATION

- **See also Case 3 (Scoring Systems and Patient Prognosis), Case 4 (Hemodynamic Monitoring), and Case 40 (Postoperative Care in ICU).**

COMPREHENSION QUESTIONS

39.1 Which of the following strategies has been shown to improve recovery from the post–cardiac arrest syndrome?

A. Early echocardiography

B. Cooling of core temperature to 28°C to 30°C

C. Maintaining O_2 saturation of 100%

D. Cooling of core temperature of 32°C to 34°C

E. Swan-Ganz catheter–directed goal resuscitation

39.2 Which of the following is the most accurate statement regarding glucose management in the post–cardiac arrest patient?

A. Hypoglycemia is a common cause of in-hospital cardiac arrest.

B. Glycemic control does not play a role in the management of patients following cardiac arrest.

C. Glycemic control to target glucose at 80 to 110 mg/dL is optimal.

D. Glycemic control to serum glucose values of 144 to 180 mg/dL is preferred.

E. Avoidance of glucose-containing intravenous solutions.

39.3 A 64-year-old man, who was being treated in the hospital for acute cholecystitis, is found to be unresponsive. He was found to be in VF and underwent chest compression for several minutes and resuscitated successfully. Which of the following is an important treatment for this patient?

A. Target oxygen saturation for 93%

B. Target glucose level at 110 mg/dL

C. Percutaneous coronary angiography

D. Target core body temperature for 37°C

E. Extended and prolonged fluid resuscitation

ANSWERS

39.1 **D.** Therapeutic hypothermia to core temperatures of 32°C to 42°C for 24 to 48 hours has been shown to improve neurological outcomes in patient following V-fib arrests. Cooling of patients to 28°C to 30°C is associated with increased risk of arrhythmia without additional improvement in neurological outcomes. Maintaining PAO_2 of 100% could result in hyperoxia and has been shown to increase mortality. Even though maintaining euvolemia improves post–cardiac arrest patient outcomes, the use of Swan-Ganz catheter goal-directed therapy has not been proven to have survival benefits in these patients.

39.2 **D.** Hyperglycemia and hypoglycemia are common following resuscitation from cardiac arrest and if unaddressed can contribute to worse neurological outcomes. The AHA guidelines currently recommend moderate glycemic control targeting values of 144 to 180 mg/dL. Randomized trial comparing glycemic control targeting levels of 80 to 110 mg/dL versus target levels of 110 to 140 mg/dL for post–cardiac arrest patients did not demonstrate a survival difference in the ICU setting. Hypoglycemia in the post-resuscitation patient contributes to worsening neurological outcome; therefore, glucose-containing solutions may be indicated if the patient is hypoglycemic.

39.3 **C.** This patient likely has acute coronary syndrome. Early cardiac intervention has been shown to improve prognosis. TH may also help with target core temperature of 32°C to 34°C. Glucose levels should be in the range of 144 to 180 mg/dL. Resuscitation to achieve early hemodynamic goals (first 6 hours) has been shown to improve survival in septic patients; however, prolongation of resuscitation has not been shown to provide survival advantages. Intolerance to feeding, decreased pulmonary compliance, decreased oxygenation, and the development of abdominal compartment syndrome are associated with excess fluid administration and failure to reduce excess fluid administration following initial resuscitation from septic shock.

CLINICAL PEARLS

- The 4 major categories involving post-resuscitation care include post-resuscitation brain injury, ischemia/reperfusion injuries, myocardial dysfunction, and persistence of precipitating cause of the cardiac arrest.
- Core temperature cooling to 32°C to 34°C for 24 to 48 hours has been shown to improve neurologic recovery after successful resuscitation from cardiac arrest caused by VF.
- Core temperature cooling to 32°C to 34°C has been shown in animal models to improve cardiac recovery following cardiac arrest resuscitation.
- Oxygen saturation targets should be in the 96% to 98% range.
- Hyperglycemia is common after resuscitation and glucose levels should not be strictly controlled but allowed to be in the 144 to 180 mg/dL range.
- Goal-directed resuscitation has been shown to be of benefit during the initial 6-hour window.

REFERENCES

Bernard S. Hypothermia after cardiac arrest: expanding the therapeutic scope. *Crit Care Med.* 2009;37 (7 suppl):S227-S233.

Kilgannon JH, Jones AE, Shapiro NI, et al. Association between arterial hyperoxia following resuscitation from cardiac arrest and in-hospital mortality. *JAMA.* 2010;303:2165-2171.

Nolan JP, Soar J. Postresuscitation care: entering a new era. *Curr Opin Crit Care.* 2010;16:216-222.

Sagalyn E, Band RA, Gaieski DF, Abella BS. Therapeutic hypothermia after cardiac arrest in clinical practice: review and compilation of recent experiences. *Crit Care Med.* 2009;37(7 suppl):S223-S226.

The National Heart, Lung, and Blood Institute Acute Respiratory Distress Syndrome (ARDS) Clinical Trial Network. Comparison of two fluid-management strategies in acute lung injury. *N Engl J Med.* 2006;354:2564-2575.

Xiong W, Hoesch RE, Geocadin RG. Post-cardiac arrest encephalopathy. *Semin Neurol.* 2011;31:216-225.

Zia A, Kern KB. Management of postcardiac arrest myocardial dysfunction. *Curr Opin Crit Care.* 2011;17:241-246.

CASE 40

An 81-year-old man with an extensive past medical history including hypertension, type II diabetes mellitus, COPD, and gout was admitted to the hospital with microcytic anemia, and signs and symptoms of large bowel obstruction. The patient has lost approximately 10 lb (4.5 kg) over the past 1 month. A colonoscopy revealed an obstructive carcinoma in the descending colon. The patient subsequently underwent an exploratory laparotomy and left colectomy. He is admitted to the ICU approximately 4 hours postoperatively.

- ▶ How would you optimally manage this patient's fluid status?
- ▶ How would you address the patient's nutritional status at this time?
- ▶ What are the possible complications related to his surgical disease processes, and how would you monitor and identify them?

ANSWERS TO CASE 40: Postoperative Care in the ICU

Summary: An 81-year-old man has an obstructing carcinoma in the descending colon. The mass was removed by an open left colectomy. The patient has extensive multiple medical comorbidities and is admitted to the ICU for close postoperative monitoring and management.

Management of fluid status: This patient needs cautious balance of his fluid status given his age and medical problems. Careful monitoring of urine output via Foley catheter and intravascular status with central venous pressure measurements will help guide management.

Nutritional status: The patient should be allowed to resume oral intake as soon as possible, generally within 48 hours postoperatively if tolerated. If the patient is unable to take in adequate calories orally, he may require supplemental enteral nutrition.

Possible complications: The approach to monitoring and identification:

- **Cardiac:** Myocardial infarction, atrial fibrillation, other cardiac arrhythmias—identified by clinical examination, cardiac monitoring/ECG.
- **Respiratory:** Pulmonary edema, atelectasis, COPD exacerbation, acute respiratory distress syndrome (ARDS)—identified by clinical examination, CXR/chest CT, oxygen saturation, arterial blood gas.
- **Fluids/electrolytes/nutrition:** Third-space fluid shifts, stress-induced hyperglycemia, and poor nutritional status—identified by clinical examination, laboratory workup.
- **Gastrointestinal:** Surgical anastomostic leak, ileus, mechanical bowel obstruction—identified by clinical examination, imaging studies, laboratory workup
- **Genitourinary:** Pre-renal azotemia, acute kidney injuries, and post-renal obstructive processes—identified by clinical examination, laboratory workup, imaging studies.
- **Endocrine:** Insulin-resistance, adrenal insufficiency—identified by clinical examination, laboratory workup.
- **Hematologic/infectious:** Anemia, wound infection, systemic inflammatory response syndrome (SIRS), sepsis—identified by clinical examination, laboratory workup.
- **Musculoskeletal:** Gout flare—identified by clinical examination.

ANALYSIS

Objectives

1. To learn the common complications that may develop in the postoperative patients.
2. To learn the disturbances produced by operative stress.
3. To learn patient assessment, risk stratification, and risk-reduction strategies in the preoperative and perioperative settings.

Considerations

This patient has a descending colon cancer with anemia and large bowel obstruction. Large bowel obstruction from a mechanical cause has a poorer prognosis and higher morbidity since an emergency operation is needed. Additionally, the patient is already nutritionally depleted from the obstructive mass in the intestine as well as from weight loss from malignancy. The added stress of operation will increase his baseline energy expenditure and his nutritional requirements. Attention must be paid to the patient's fluid status as postoperative shifts will place stress on the cardiovascular and pulmonary systems, which are likely already affected by the patient's history of hypertension, anemia, and COPD. The presence of type 2 diabetes may mean that some degree of renal insufficiency is present and that there may be an increased risk for infection. An acute flare of gout is possible from the catabolic state after surgery or as a result of the fluid shifts caused by surgery. To minimize this patient's postoperative complications and facilitate his postoperative recovery, meticulous ICU care will be important to monitor several important organ system functions.

APPROACH TO:
Postoperative Patients in the ICU

DEFINITIONS

CENTRAL VENOUS PRESSURE: The pressure in the superior vena cava, measured with a central venous catheter inserted into the internal jugular or subclavian vein. This estimates the right atrial pressure, reflecting the amount of the blood in the venous system returning to the heart.

ATELECTASIS: Collapse of lung alveoli or fluid consolidation that prevents effective gas exchange where the alveoli are deflated. This can affect varying proportions of the lungs and is commonly seen after injury or surgery, especially if breathing is restricted by pain or fatigue.

PULMONARY EDEMA: Fluid accumulation in the lung parenchyma either due to the inability of the heart to adequately remove fluid from the lung circulation (cardiogenic) or due to lung parenchyma injury (noncardiogenic). It can be caused iatrogenically by over-infusion of intravenous fluid.

ACUTE RESPIRATORY DISTRESS SYNDROME: Inflamed lung parenchyma associated with a systemic inflammatory response causing severe hypoxemia, often requiring mechanical intubation. It may be present by itself or as part of the multiple organ dysfunction syndrome (MODS). ARDS is defined as an acute process with a ratio of arterial partial oxygen tension (PAO_2) to fraction of inspired oxygen (FIO_2) <200, with bilateral infiltrates on chest x-ray, in the absence of elevated cardiac filling pressures.

THIRD SPACE FLUID LOSS: During inflammation, sepsis, or shock, fluid can be sequestered in extravascular spaces as proteins and fluid move to interstitial compartments, depleting intravascular volume. Examples include pulmonary edema, bowel wall edema, and fluid forced into the bowel lumen in cases of obstruction and retroperitoneal fluid sequestration with pancreatitis.

CLINICAL APPROACH

The intensive care providers in the ICU need to be familiar with the complications related to procedures, surgical diseases, and operative stresses. Understanding of these issues is critical for the anticipation and treatment of complications, addressing the needs of the postoperative patients, and optimizing communications between the intensive care providers and the surgical specialists. Postoperative problems can range from being relatively minor to life threatening. It is important for the clinician to be aware of the complications that can occur and to be vigilant about looking out for those that can cause serious morbidity and even mortality. The most important aspect to remember about postoperative complications is that complications in the postoperative patients are nearly always related to the operative procedures (known complications of the procedures and/or underlying disease conditions that necessitated the operations, and/or complications related to the exacerbation of 1 or more of the patient's comorbid conditions). The various systems that can be affected by surgical stresses are listed later.

Complications Categorized by Systems

Cardiac complications include acute coronary syndrome, myocardial infarctions, cardiac arrhythmias, and congestive heart failure. The increased stress on the heart increases the risk for myocardial infarction. Arrhythmias such as atrial fibrillation often occur due to fluid shifts throughout the body after an operation, placing more stress on the atria of the heart. These fluid shifts can also cause or worsen congestive heart failure.

Pulmonary complications can be closely linked to cardiac dysfunction in which the ability to adequately distribute intravascular fluid may be lost, causing a backup of fluid in the lungs, as in the case of pulmonary edema. Other common pulmonary complications include atelectasis, pneumonia, ARDS, and exacerbation of any underlying lung disease, such as COPD or emphysema.

Renal complications mainly present as oliguria, or low urine output. Acute kidney injuries can be classified into pre-renal, renal, and post-renal categories. Pre-renal causes are due to hypoperfusion of the kidney as seen in dehydration, fluid losses from vomiting/diarrhea, or as a result of an operation, poor intake or inadequate repletion, and cardiogenic shock or significant blood loss. Insensible fluid losses are increased during an operation, especially if the abdomen is left open postoperatively.

Bowel obstruction causes third spacing, further reducing intravascular volume. Renal causes of oliguria are from damage to the kidney itself, such as acute tubular necrosis from ischemia or medication toxicity. Post-renal causes are due to obstruction of urine flow, such as Foley catheter blockage, prostatic hypertrophy or compression from tumor, hematoma, or fluid collection. If the FE_{Na} (fractional excretion of sodium) is <1 along with other signs that the body is trying to retain water (high serum osmolality, low urine sodium), this indicates a pre-renal state whereas proteinuria and cells or casts on urinalysis may point toward direct renal damage or ATN. Causes of post-renal (obstructive) oliguria can usually be found via physical examination or imaging.

Fever can be a sign of complications and can be divided into 3 categories based on timing. Immediately postoperative fever (<24 hours) may be a response to surgery or atelectasis, although in some cases a necrotizing wound infection (*Clostridium* or group A *Streptococcus*) can be the cause. Fevers occurring from 24 to 72 hours may be residual atelectasis but should prompt a search for other sources of infection such as pneumonia, urinary tract infections (especially if a Foley catheter is in place), or IV line infection/phlebitis. After 72 hours, fever is likely due to the infectious sources mentioned above or wound infections, deep internal abscesses, anastomotic leaks, prosthetic infections, or deep vein thrombosis. Rarely, entities such as acalculous cholecystitis, most often seen in critically ill patients, can also be a cause of fever. The workup includes physical examination of the patient, the incision site, and any IV lines or catheters as well as blood, sputum, urine, and wound cultures. Imaging may be helpful. For example, a chest x-ray may reveal a pulmonary consolidation in pneumonia or an effusion, a Doppler ultrasound of the legs or chest CT may identify a DVT or pulmonary embolus, or an abdominal CT scan may find a deep abscesses. Appropriate treatment depends on the cause, varying from incentive spirometry and mobilization for atelectasis to removal of catheters and IVs, antibiotics, and operative drainage of deep abscesses if necessary.

Wound complications may occur in any patient although appropriate preoperative antibiotics, meticulous operative technique, and hemostasis are the most effective prevention. There is no additional benefit in the extension of prophylactic antibiotics beyond the immediate postoperative period. High-risk patients for wound complications are individuals with contaminated surgical fields, impaired blood flow to healing tissues from hypotension, diabetes, obesity, or smoking, and those who are immunocompromised. Wound complications include hematomas and seromas, infection in either superficial or deep spaces, and fascial dehiscence or incisional hernias. Wounds or hematomas/seromas that appear infected (tenderness, erythema, purulence) should be opened, drained, and packed loosely. Extensive wound dehiscence at the fascial level may require repair in the operating room. Close communication between the intensive care provider and the surgeons are critical for the management of wound-related complications.

Neurologic complications after operation are often related to the treatment of postoperative pain. While hypoxemia and stroke can cause neurological changes, electrolyte abnormalities and medications are also common causes. Medications for treatment of pain, including opiates, and sedatives in critically ill patients may cause delirium, agitation, and somnolence. Elderly patients tend to have greater susceptibility to these effects. Patients in the ICU may also experience delirium, ICU psychosis or "sundowning," which may be brought on by fragmented sleep patterns, disturbances in the day–night cycles, and loss of familiarity with one's surroundings.

Disturbances Produced by Operative Stress on the Various Systems

Cardiovascular: Due to increased postoperative metabolic demands, cardiac output increases, leading to higher oxygen requirements of cardiac myocytes. Operative stress coupled with hypovolemia, infection or traumatic injury, as well as any anesthetic or vasoactive medications, may prevent the patient's cardiovascular system from fully compensating for the increased demand, leading to myocardial ischemia, infarction, fluid overload, cardiac failure, and arrhythmias. Despite the increased cardiac demands, recent data suggest that postoperative acute coronary syndrome is just as likely to be produced by coronary artery plaque instability and rupture, which is believed to be due to increased catecholamine and inflammatory mediators' responses in the postoperative period.

Pulmonary: Oxygen consumption demands are increased postoperatively due to increased metabolic demands. Ventilation and oxygenation problems in the postoperative period may arise from the combination of increased O_2 demand and compromised vital capacities. For example, upper abdominal and thoracic incisions significantly decrease the patients' vital capacities secondary to pain associated with the respiratory effort; this can then result in subsequent atelectasis and increased risk for pneumonia. Decreased mentation following general anesthesia and/or sedation medications may increase patients' susceptibilities for pulmonary aspirations. Lung parenchymal injuries may develop following systemic inflammatory response, leading to acute lung injury (ALI) and ARDS. Surgical stresses and immobility render the patients susceptible to venous thromboembolic complications. Conditions such as asthma or COPD can be exacerbated postoperatively and require treatment with steroids and/or bronchodilators.

Metabolic: The patient' metabolic responses to surgery are variable and are related to the type and magnitude of the surgical stresses. Conditions such as trauma, sepsis, and burns further contribute to the increase in metabolic demands. Critically ill patients have accelerated breakdown of muscle protein for the reprioritization of acute-phase protein synthesis. **Hyperglycemia in the postoperative patient is common and is caused by both increase in glucose production by the liver and decrease in uptake of glucose by insulin-dependent tissues.** Untreated hyperglycemia contributes to glycosuria, excess fluid losses, and impairment of leukocyte function leading to infections. Glucose monitoring and treatment with insulin are essential in the postoperative patients. Insufficient adrenal functions can be exacerbated by surgical stresses and/or sepsis. This may be manifested by hypotension that is unresponsive to standard fluid administration. In some instances, adrenal dysfunction can manifest as unexplained fever, hypoglycemia, confusion, lethargy, and abdominal pain. By far, the most common reason for adrenal insufficiency is iatrogenic. A patient with long-term steroid medication use history is vulnerable to the development of adrenal insufficiency in the face of surgical stress, sepsis, or trauma.

Gastrointestinal: Patients who are not intubated can be expected to resume oral intake shortly after an operation. While the traditional practice is to maintain a nil per os (NPO) policy until there is return of bowel function documented by passage of flatus or bowel movement, a growing body of literature suggests that there are potential benefits to reinstating some form of oral intake within 48 hours of operations in patients who can tolerate it. In patients who are intubated and/or those who are not expected to take in adequate oral calories for prolonged periods of time, supplemental nutrition via enteral tube should be anticipated and implemented. Operative manipulation of the bowel and medications for pain can contribute to ileus and delayed GI functions. Narcotics can contribute to constipation and fecal impaction. It is possible for adhesions to form and bowel obstructions to occur within days after surgery, although most obstructive complications secondary to adhesions occur later. Critically ill patients are also at risk for stress ulcers, where hypoperfusion, loss of host gastric barrier functions, and gastric acidity can produce mucosal injuries. ICU patients in shock, sepsis, respiratory, hepatic, renal, or hematologic failure are benefited by stress ulcer prophylaxis with H_2-antagonists or sucralfate.

Perioperative Assessment, Risk Stratification, and Risk Reduction

Patient assessment: Many healthy patients are able to undergo operative procedures uneventfully. However, those who are medically compromised require more careful pre- and perioperative evaluations to assess for fitness for surgery and ensure favorable outcomes.

Several methods are commonly used to assess patients' medical status prior to an operation. The **American Society of Anesthesiologists' (ASA) classification** is based on the patient's condition where Class I patients are healthy, Class II have mild systemic disease, Class III have severe systemic disease which limits activity but is not incapacitating, Class IV is incapacitating systemic disease which is a constant threat to life, Class V is a moribund patient not expected to survive 24 hours with or without operation, and Class VI is an organ transplant donor. The designation of "E" is added to any class if the case is an emergency. Goldman calculated a cardiac risk index in which a varying number of points is awarded for clinical factors present, with 11 points for an S_3 gallop/JVD and 10 points for a myocardial infarction within 6 months as the 2 biggest contributors to cardiac risk. The highest risk (Class IV) patients had a 22% incidence of major cardiac complications and a 56% mortality rate. More recently, Lee developed the Revised Cardiac Risk Index in which 6 independent predictors of perioperative cardiac complications were established—ischemic heart disease, congestive heart failure, cerebrovascular disease, diabetes requiring preoperative insulin treatment, serum creatinine >2.0 mg/dL, and whether the patient was undergoing a high-risk operation. A high-risk operation includes intraperitoneal, intrathoracic, or suprainguinal vascular (such as aortic) operation.

Risk stratification: Preoperative evaluation provides the anesthesia and surgical teams' information regarding the patient's current medical status, risk profile, and recommendations for management during the perioperative period. Tests should only be ordered if the results could change the treatment and management plan. Examples include an electrocardiogram, or a cardiac stress ECG to examine the patient's cardiac response to increasing oxygen demand with exercise or dipyridamole-thallium scanning for those patients unable to exercise. Echocardiography gives an analysis of ventricular wall motion, ejection fraction, and ventricular hypertrophy. Pulmonary function tests are useful in patients who may need to undergo lung resection. On admission to the ICU, the APACHE (acute physiology and chronic health evaluation) score may be used to risk-stratify patients, and it is calculated from 12 different physiological measurements. Although it is used for risk stratification and to compare the morbidity of patients, due to its complexity it is cumbersome to use.

Risk reduction: The ultimate goal of pre- and perioperative assessment is to optimize patient outcome. Patients may certainly benefit from having their medical comorbidities optimized preoperatively; examples include controlling hypertension, cardiac arrhythmias, and diabetes before surgery. Improving the patient's preoperative nutritional status is also important. Percutaneous coronary intervention (PCI) and coronary artery bypass grafting (CABG) have not been shown to be effective in reducing perioperative cardiac morbidity except perhaps in patients with left main coronary artery disease. **The use of β-blockers in at-risk patients has been shown to reduce the risk of perioperative cardiac ischemia and death, but the timing of stopping the β-blocker postoperatively remains controversial.** If the patient does not have an emergency condition, a preoperative workup may elucidate a need to modify the original anesthetic or operative plan and defer or change the operative approach. Intraoperative risk reduction strategies include keeping the patient warm, maintaining euglycemia, administration of perioperative antibiotics within an hour of skin incision, and sequential compression devices for prevention of DVT. Postoperatively, patients should be have continued DVT prophylaxis with sequential compression devices (SCDs), heparin, or low molecular weight heparin until they are able to mobilize, as well as oral hygiene, aspiration precautions, incentive spirometry to prevent atelectasis and pneumonia, frequent turning to prevent pressure sores, and ulcer prophylaxis if indicated.

CLINICAL CASE CORRELATION

- **See also Case 3 (Scoring Systems and Patient Prognosis), Case 8 (Airway Management), Case 14 (Acute Coronary Syndrome), Case 23 (Acute Kidney Injury), and Case 33 (Multiorgan Dysfunction).**

COMPREHENSION QUESTIONS

40.1 A 92-year-old woman underwent a laparoscopic cholecystectomy for cholecystitis. She had some mild hypotension to the 80/40 mm Hg range postoperatively and received fluid resuscitation. Her weight is 45 kg. Which of the following findings are most consistent with inadequate resuscitation?

A. Urine/serum creatinine ratio of 45

B. CVP of 13 mm Hg

C. Urine output of 25 mL in the last hour

D. Bilateral pulmonary crackles on auscultation

E. Fractional excretion of sodium of 1.3%

40.2 A 78-year-old patient develops a temperature of 101.4°F 2 days after undergoing an elective right hemicolectomy for a small, nonobstructing cancer that was found on colonoscopy. Which of the following is the *least* likely cause of her fever?

A. Pneumonia

B. Urinary tract infection

C. Atelectasis

D. Wound infection

E. Intra-abdominal abscess

40.3 A 34-year-old obese man underwent an emergency midline laparotomy after sustaining a gunshot wound to the abdomen. A short segment of small bowel was resected due to damage from the bullet. Several days later, the patient has made a good recovery. However, when he stands to walk to the bathroom, he experiences a large gush of serosanguinous fluid from his abdominal wound. Examination of the wound shows a 4-cm fascial dehiscence. The most appropriate management is:

A. Reapproximation of the wound with sterile tape

B. Abdominal binder and placing the patient on bed rest

C. Further opening of the wound to allow adequate drainage and packing with gauze

D. Return to operation room for repair

E. Culture of the wound fluid and antibiotic treatment

40.4 A 55-year-old patient has hypertension that is controlled with hydrochlorothiazide and metoprolol. What is his ASA classification?

A. I

B. II

C. III

D. IV

E. V

40.5 A 68-year-old patient who has a history of insulin-dependent diabetes and stable angina takes chronic steroids for rheumatoid arthritis, and has a history of colonic diverticuli. She underwent an emergency diverting colostomy for perforated diverticulitis with fecal spillage, remains intubated in the ICU, and is on broad-spectrum antibiotics. Two days postoperatively, she becomes acutely febrile to 102.6°F with confusion and lethargy. Her heart rate is 110 beats/minute with a blood pressure of 79/58 mm Hg. She remains hypotensive despite starting on fluid resuscitation and vasopressors. Her laboratory tests show a glucose of 46 mg/dL. What is the most likely cause of her clinical picture?

A. Myocardial infarction
B. Diabetic ketoacidosis
C. Hypovolemia
D. Adrenal insufficiency
E. Sepsis

ANSWERS TO QUESTIONS

40.1 **A.** In a hypovolemic patient, the CVP would be low (<5), she would not have bilateral crackles suggestive of pulmonary edema, and the fractional excretion of sodium would be <1%. Although a urine output of 25 mL may seem low, for a patient weighing only 45 kg, 0.5 mL/kg/h equals an expected urine output of 22.5 mL/h. The kidney would be trying to retain volume so the urine sodium would be low (<20 meq/L), the serum osmolality would be high (>500 mOsm/kg), and the urine/serum creatinine ratio would be >40. Thus, the urine to serum creatinine ratio of 45 in this patient indicates a "prerenal" picture of hypovolemia.

40.2 **E.** The patient has developed a fever within 72 hours of undergoing surgery. This may still be due to atelectasis if the patient is not expanding her lungs well due to being in bed or to pain. However, infectious sources may be the culprit by this time frame. Pneumonia, urinary tract infection, wound infection, and IV line infections may all be possibilities. Intra-abdominal abscesses generally take a few more days to form and are less likely at this relatively early time point.

40.3 **D.** This patient has experienced a fascial disruption with the serosanguinous fluid coming from the peritoneum. Because the dehiscence is larger than just 1 or 2 cm, the patient is at high risk for infection and evisceration as well as a ventral hernia. Prompt operative repair will minimize these risks and allow the patient to recover and resume normal activity sooner.

40.4 **C.** Hypertension is classified as a systemic disease. The patient requires medication to treat his disease, which makes his condition more serious than a Class II. However, his hypertension is controlled on his medications, so he is ASA Class III rather than Class IV.

40.5 **D.** Acute adrenal insufficiency often presents as unexplained fever, persistent hypotension, mental status changes, and hypoglycemia. This presentation can be similar to sepsis but sepsis tends to present with hyperglycemia in its early stages. While the etiology of adrenal insufficiency can be primary in nature, abrupt cessation of steroids is the most common cause. Treatment consists of IV fluids and hydrocortisone 100 mg IV for adrenal crisis, with steroid taper as tolerated as the crisis resolves.

CLINICAL PEARLS

- Most postoperative complications are related to the surgery or the underlying diseases that led to the operation.
- Risk assessment in the preoperative setting help identify patients that are at risk for specific complications and provide opportunities for the implementation of risk-reduction strategies.
- Older age and preexisting conditions contribute to reduced functional reserve and increased susceptibility to injury-induced organ dysfunctions.

REFERENCES

Fleisher LA. Cardiac risk stratification for noncardiac surgery: update from the American College of Cardiology/American Heart Association 2007 Guidelines. *Cleveland Clin J Med*. 2009;76(suppl 4): S9-S15.

Lee TH, Marcantonio ER, Mangione CM, et al. Derivation and prospective validation of a simple index for prediction of cardiac risk of major noncardiac surgery. *Circulation*. 1999;100:1043-1039.

Marquardt DL, Tatum RP, Lynge DC. Postoperative management of the hospitalized patient. In: Souba WW, et al, eds. *ACS Surgery: Principles and Practice*. 6th ed. Philadelphia, PA: Decker Publishing, 2007.

Walsh F, Ali J. Chapter 88. Preoperative assessment of the high-risk surgical patient. In: Hall JB, Schmidt GA, Wood LDH, eds. *Principles of Critical Care*. 3rd ed. http://www.accesssurgery.com/content.aspx?aID=2296894, accessed July 2, 2013.

CASE 41

A 20-year-old man is brought from the operating room to the ICU following a damage-control operation for multiple gunshot wounds. The patient was reportedly unstable throughout the entire operation. The injuries indentified include transection of the left superficial femoral artery (SFA) and multiple small bowel perforations. During the operation, the patient had 3 small bowel segments resected and had placement of a temporary intraluminal shunt in the SFA to control the bleeding and reestablish blood flow to his leg. At the time he arrives to the ICU, his temperature is 34.6°C, pulse rate is 128 beats/minute, and blood pressure is 90/70 mm Hg. He is intubated and mechanically ventilated. The patient is bleeding externally from his wounds and multiple intravenous catheter sites.

- ▶ What is the most likely diagnosis?
- ▶ What are the causes of the patient's current condition?
- ▶ What are the priorities in this patient's management?

ANSWERS TO CASE 41:

Hemorrhage and Coagulopathy

Summary: A 20-year-old man has gunshot wounds through his abdomen and extremity. The bowel injuries have been controlled with resection, and the vascular injury has been controlled with a temporary shunt. He was noted to be unstable throughout the surgery. His presentation to the ICU is consistent with shock and coagulopathy.

- **Most likely diagnosis:** Hemorrhagic shock and coagulopathy.
- **Causes of patient's condition:** Trauma with massive blood loss and transfusion and hypothermia.
- **Priorities in this patient's management:** Warm the patient, resuscitate with packed red blood cells (PRBCs), fresh frozen plasma, and platelets to correct coagulopathy and acidosis.

ANALYSIS

Objectives

1. To learn the principles of massive transfusion.
2. To learn the conditions that contribute to coagulopathy following massive transfusions.
3. To understand the limitations of laboratory studies for the evaluation of patients with this condition.

Considerations

This patient suffered significant penetrating trauma that required a damage-control operation and temporary shunting of the SFA. On admission to the ICU, he is hypotensive, tachycardic, and is bleeding from his wounds and catheter sites. His surgical bleeding site has been controlled (shunting of the SFA), but he continues to bleed from his wounds, indicating that he has a significant coagulopathy. During the operation, he has lost not only red blood cells, but also the coagulation factors that are present in his plasma. Additionally, he is **hypothermic**, which is common among trauma victims.

The hypothermia usually starts in the emergency department during the initial resuscitation and continues while in the operating room. Trauma patients have all of their clothes removed and are infused with normal saline and PRBCs that may not be warm. In the operating room, their chest and/or abdomen may be open, increasing their heat loss. They also may be paralyzed for intubation, which prevents shivering. All of these mechanisms can lead to profound hypothermia. The hypothermia actively slows down the coagulation process, exacerbating coagulopathy and continued nonsurgical bleeding (ie, bleeding that cannot be controlled by suture ligation). It is likely that this patient is also acidotic from incomplete resuscitation, which can also worsen the coagulopathic state. **The combination of acidosis, hypothermia, and coagulopathy is often referred to as the "triad of death."**

APPROACH TO:
Hemorrhage and Coagulopathy

DEFINITIONS

HEMOSTATIC RESUSCITATION: Hemostatic resuscitation is a relatively new concept that evolved largely based on clinical observations from injuries managed during the conflicts in Iraq and Afghanistan. This begins with limitation of fluids in the field, application of tourniquets and hemostatic agents for direct bleeding control. Once victims arrive to the medical care facility, the resuscitation is directed to preserve coagulation functions rather than restoring normal vital signs.

MASSIVE TRANSFUSION: A commonly used definition is the transfusion of ≥10 U of PRBCs in 24 hours. Patients who require massive transfusion have suffered a large amount of blood volume losses; therefore, they require the replacement of PRBCs, fresh frozen plasma, and platelets in a short time period. These components are often given in ratios that mimic whole blood concentrations.

FACTOR VII: Coagulation factor that can be made in recombinant fashion and administered to patients who are coagulopathic.

THROMBOELASTOGRAPHY: Method for real-time measurement of coagulation status. The results report the time to clot formation and the clot strength. They can be used for goal-directed administration of blood products.

PLATELETPHERESIS: Process whereby the platelets are separated from the other blood components and the remaining components are returned to the donor. Thus, a unit of plateletpheresis consists of approximately 6-7 units of random platelet units.

CLINICAL APPROACH

Massive Transfusion Principles

Hemorrhage remains one of the leading causes of preventable deaths in trauma patients. The cause of death goes beyond just exsanguination. Up to one-third of all trauma patients who present to the hospital already have a coagulopathy due to tissue injury, hypoperfusion, and loss of clotting factors and platelets via hemorrhage. Accentuation of this initial coagulopathy may also be mediated by an increase in fibrinolysis via a protein C pathway. Surgical control of the hemorrhage is the primary therapy of ongoing bleeding. Until surgical control of hemorrhage is accomplished, the patient should be resuscitated with volume. Historically, the correction of hypovolemia caused by hemorrhage was infusion of large volumes of crystalloids. Normal saline was the crystalloid of choice, but **infusion of large volumes of normal saline has untoward complications;** dilutional coagulopathy, thrombocytopenia, and hyperchloremic acidosis from large crystalloid infusions increases coagulopathy. Ongoing hemorrhage affects all 3 components of the "triad of death" and increases coagulopathy.

The complications of resuscitating a patient with large volumes of crystalloid has led to a "hemostatic resuscitation" approach: resuscitating the patient with blood and blood products that will help mitigate the coagulopathy of trauma until definitive control of the bleeding is achieved.

The **goal of a hemostatic resuscitation is to replace the patient with products that approximates the blood that they have lost.** This hemostatic resuscitation is often referred to as a "**massive transfusion**" as it includes large volumes of PRBCs, fresh frozen plasma, and platelets. There is no one single definition of what constitutes a massive transfusion, but several definitions have been proposed. These include:

1. Replacement of 1 entire blood volume within 24 hours.
2. Transfusion of >10 U of PRBCs in 24 hours.
3. Transfusion of >20 U of PRBCs in 24 hours.

Also, there are definitions of "**dynamic massive transfusion**" including

1. Transfusion of >4 U of PRBCs in 1 hour when ongoing need is foreseeable.
2. Replacement of 50% of total blood volume within 3 hours.

When patients receive a blood transfusion, they are actually receiving a transfusion of PRBCs. This is the end product of whole blood (taken from a donor) that has been centrifuged so that the heavier components (the red blood cells) can be separated from the lighter components (the plasma and platelets). The coagulation factors remain in the plasma component. When a patient is transfused, they receive red blood cells to increase oxygen-carrying capacity, but do not receive any coagulation factors. Multiple transfusions of PRBCs without addition of coagulation factors will lead to a dilutional coagulopathy. Thus, during **massive transfusions, when patients are given large volumes of PRBCs, they should also be given fresh frozen plasma (FFP) to provide hemostatic factors.** The exact ratio of PRBCs to FFP to provide the perfect hemostatic scenario is not known. However, **most experts would agree that a 1:1:1 ratio of PRBCs:FFP:platelets** is the best formula for a hemostatic resuscitation. One unit of plateletpheresis is approximately 6 to 10 random platelet concentrates, so **1 U of single donor plateletpheresis is transfused after 6 U of PRBCs and FFP**.

Coagulopathy Following Massive Transfusions

Up to one-third of trauma patients with significant injury will present to the trauma bay with a coagulopathy already in progress. This is in part due to loss of coagulation factors from bleeding, as well as tissue injury and hypoperfusion. To understand the conditions that affect coagulopathy after massive transfusions, it is first important to understand the normal process of coagulation. The major physiologic events that occur during coagulation are **vasoconstriction, platelet plug formation, fibrin formation, and fibrinolysis.** During platelet plug formation, the coagulation factors interact with the surface of the platelets to form a fibrin lattice that provides support to the platelet plug.

During and after massive transfusion, many of the factors associated with normal coagulation are altered. **Thrombocytopenia** limits the amount of platelet plug that can be formed at the site of injury. Initially, this is caused by absolute loss of platelets from hemorrhage and dilution from crystalloid administration. The infusion of large volumes of crystalloid contributes to coagulopathy during massive transfusions. Therefore, **crystalloid infusion should be limited during massive transfusions.** Then, during the massive transfusion, PRBCs and FFP are administered, both of which contain minimal amounts of platelets. This can lead to further drop in the platelet count. Often, hospitals have a limited supply of platelets, due to their short shelf life. This can lead to a delay in the administration of platelets, even during massive transfusions given by protocol.

The storage solution for blood products contains citrate as a preservative to keep the products from clotting during storage. Citrate is a strong binder of calcium, so **when large volumes of PRBCs are given, intravascular stores of calcium can be depleted.** Coagulation defects can be seen when calcium levels drop below 0.7 mmol/L.

Despite administration of all blood components (RBCs, FFP, platelets), coagulopathy can still be seen in some patients during massive transfusion. It is thought that administration of specific clotting factors can help the coagulation process. Factor VII can be made in a recombinant fashion and administered intravenously. The administration of recombinant activated Factor VII (rFVII) is still controversial. In a randomized controlled trial, rFVII was shown to decrease the PRBCs use by 20% in trauma patients who required massive transfusions. The administration of rFVII contributes to a prothrombotic state, which could increase the risk of venous thromboembolic events. In recent studies, there does not appear to be an increased risk for thromboembolic events in trauma patients.

Other life-threatening problems that exacerbate coagulopathy are hypothermia and acidosis. These 3 problems combined are often referred to as the "triad of death" and each problem compounds the other. Hypothermia often begins in the trauma bay and continues to progress through the operating room and even into the ICU. Hypothermia directly affects the coagulation cascade by inhibiting the initiation of clot formation and increasing the time it takes for thrombin levels to reach normal. It is extremely important in all trauma patients to keep them warm by warming the fluids administered (including blood products) and keeping the patient covered with warm blankets or other warming devices. Acidosis is often started by hypoperfusion of tissue after blood loss, but can be exacerbated by administration of large volumes of normal saline. The chloride content of normal saline (154 mEq/L) can lead to a hyperchloremic acidosis. Acidosis impairs the ability of thrombin to participate in hemostasis and severely inhibits the activity of enzyme complexes on lipid surfaces.

Laboratory Studies

Current management of patients undergoing massive transfusions include frequent laboratory monitoring of arterial lactate to assess adequacy of resuscitation, ionized calcium, and electrolytes. The laboratory values that are used to determine the coagulation status of the patient are the prothrombin time (PT), partial thromboplastin time (PTT), and international normalized ratio (INR). These tests are problematic in trauma patients in that the trauma patient's actual coagulopathic state is in constant flux as they are continuously receiving large volumes of blood, plasma, and platelets. The standard coagulation lab examinations take time to analyze, so the result reported does not necessarily reflect the patient's coagulation state when the results are returned. Also, in order to run the PT/PTT tests, the patient's blood sample is warmed to 37°C and mixed with platelet-poor plasma. Trauma patients are often hypothermic, so this analysis again does not reflect the patient's actual coagulation status, nor does it reflect the cellular interactions of clotting.

Evidence is starting to show that **rotational thromboelastometry (ROTEM) or thromboelastograms (TEGs) are superior to standard coagulation measurements in trauma patients.** These lab tests can be performed in a near real-time analysis and return rapid results. This allows for immediate analysis and goal-directed therapy of the coagulation disorder. The thromboelastogram (Figure 41–1) is measured on a

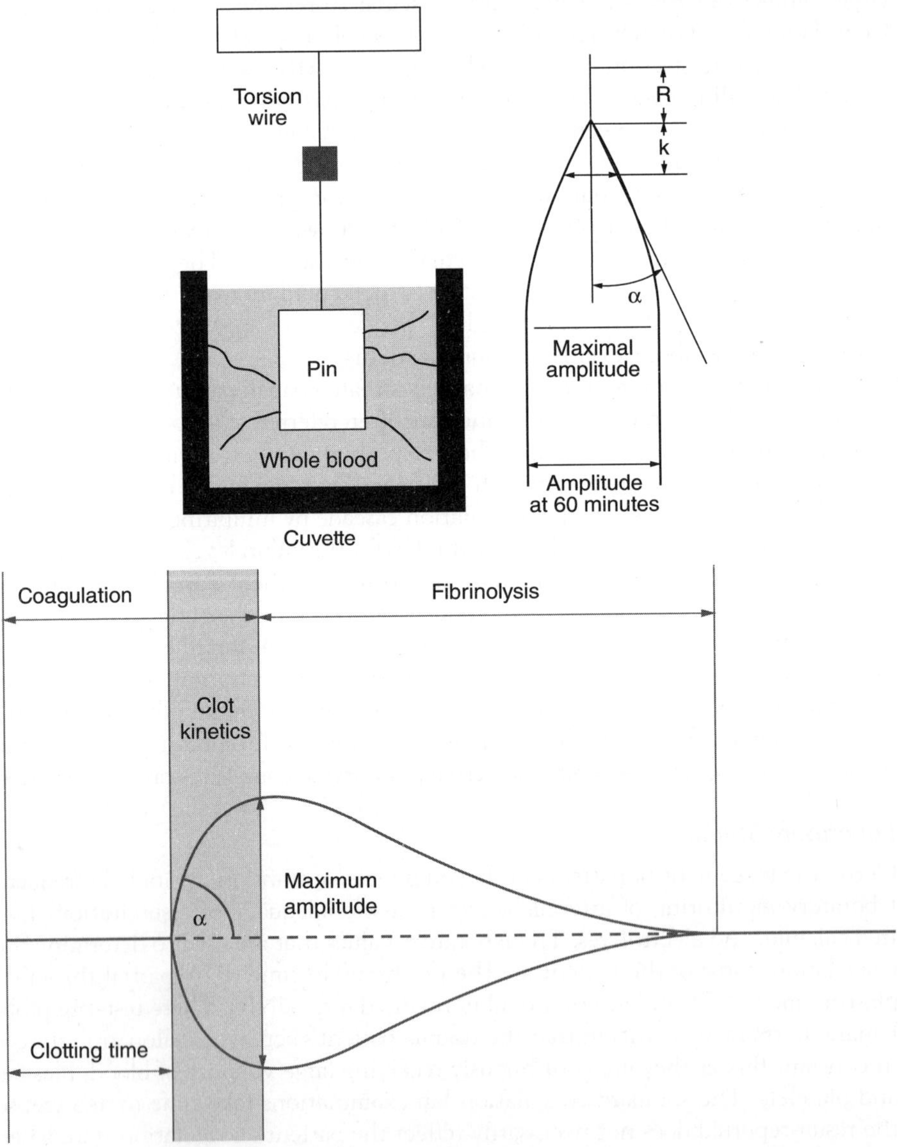

Figure 41–1. A sample of Celite-activated whole blood (0.4 mL) is placed into a prewarmed cuvette. A pin suspended from a torsion wire is then lowered into the cuvette. The cuvette is rotated backward and forward in a small arc. As the fibrin strands interact with the activated platelets on the surface of the pin, the rotational movement of the cuvette is transmitted to the pin. The stronger the clot, the more the pin moves.

small aliquot of whole blood and measures the clotting time (R value), clot formation (α-angle), clot strength (MA, maximum amplitude), and clot lysis (LY 30). The clotting time measures the time to onset of clot formation. An increase in the clotting time represents a deficiency of coagulation factors. The kinetics of the clot formation is represented by the α-angle. This represents the rate of fibrin build-up and cross-linking. The maximum amplitude is a measurement of the overall clot strength. The clot strength is a representation of platelet and fibrin interactivity. The use of TEG has shown to decrease the mortality rate and improve transfusion practices in patients receiving massive transfusions.

CLINICAL CASE CORRELATION

- **See also Case 4 (Hemodynamic Monitoring), Case 5 (Vasoactive Drugs and Pharmacology), Case 21 (GI Bleeding), Case 26 (Fluid and Electrolyte Abnormalities), and Case 28 (Blunt Trauma).**

COMPREHENSION QUESTIONS

41.1 A 20-year-old man is shot in the right upper quadrant of his abdomen. On admission to the trauma bay, the paramedics inform you that he has 2 large bore IVs and has been given 2 L of normal saline en route to the hospital. His airway is patent, he is breathing spontaneously with oxygen saturations of 99% on 2 L/min by nasal cannula. His blood pressure is 80/40 mm Hg and his heart rate is 120 beats/minute. He has a missile wound to the right upper quadrant of the abdomen. His abdomen is very tender and he is cold and diaphoretic. The best next step in treatment for this patient is:

A. Administer 500 mL of 5% albumin.

B. Administer 2 L of lactated Ringer solution.

C. Give 2 U of type-specific blood.

D. Give 2 U of non–type-specific blood (O negative).

E. Warm the patient and send for coagulation labs.

41.2 A 37-year-old woman is brought in by paramedics after sustaining a severe crush injury of her right lower extremity. She is taken to the operation room (OR) where her lower extremity is explored, washed out, has an external fixation device placed, and a wound vacuum device placed over the open wound. The surgery takes several hours, and she is admitted to the ICU after the surgery. Her wound vacuum output is 1.5 L of frank blood over the next 4 hours. She received 2 U of PRBCs during the surgery and has received 3 more units since arriving in the ICU, and 1 more unit is being transfused now. Her heart rate is 120 beats/minute and her blood pressure is 90/60 mm Hg. Her current hemoglobin concentration is 7 g/dL and platelet count is 475,000. Her INR is 1.9. Her temperature is 35°C. The best next step in management of this patient is:

A. Transfuse platelets.

B. Transfuse FFP and recheck INR in 2 hours.

C. Take patient to OR for continued bleed from wound.

D. Decrease the wound vacuum suction.

E. Transfuse 2 more units of blood and recheck hemoglobin.

41.3 A patient is undergoing a massive transfusion during an operation for a Grade IV liver laceration. He has received 9 U of PRBCs and 8 U of FFP. The best next step in treating this patient is:

A. 4 more units of PRBCs

B. 2 L of crystalloid

C. 1 U of plateletpheresis

D. 6 U of plateletpheresis

E. 1 U of cryoprecipitate

41.4 A 63-year-old woman is undergoing colectomy for severe diverticulitis. During the operation, there is a significant amount of bleeding from an unidentified mesenteric vessel. The surgeons have stated that they are having difficulty getting control of the vessel and have called for a vascular surgeon. While the surgeons are working to get surgical control of the bleeding, she has been transfused 6 U of PRBCs in the last hour. She is still bleeding and intermittently hypotensive. The next step in management is:

A. Continue to transfuse red blood cells based on whether she is still hypotensive.

B. Continue to work on surgical control of bleeding and begin a massive transfusion protocol.

C. Check her INR and transfuse FFP only if INR >2.0.

D. Administer rFVII and normal saline intravenously

ANSWERS TO QUESTIONS

41.1 **D.** This patient has a gunshot wound to the right upper quadrant and is hypotensive and tachycardic. His appearance is consistent with high grade of shock. He is breathing and has normal saturations, so it is unlikely that he has an injury to his chest. His abdomen is tender and he most likely has blood in his abdomen. In this patient who has already received 2 L of normal saline before reaching the hospital and is still hypotensive, it is appropriate to start giving the patient blood. In the initial trauma setting, it is inappropriate to wait for type-specific blood. The first blood transfusions should be non-type and crossed blood (Type O). A sample of the patient's blood should be sent for analysis so that future transfusions can be cross-matched. While it is important to start warming the patient as soon as possible, immediate resuscitation with blood and blood products predicates the warming and evaluation of coagulation status.

41.2 **C.** This patient suffered a significant injury to her lower extremity that required an operation, fixation device, and wound vacuum placed over her open wound. After being admitted to the ICU, she continues to have several problems. Her bleeding has not stopped, she has low blood concentrations, her coagulation has elevated, and she is cold. The most concerning aspect of this patient is her continued bleeding as noted by the high output of blood in her wound vacuum. When faced with a patient who does not respond appropriately to resuscitation, it is important to consider that the cause is inadequate "source control." In this case the acute surgical bleeding must be stopped so that she can be adequately resuscitated. It is likely that she will need more blood, FFP, and possibly platelets while the bleeding is being controlled, but the first step is to control surgical bleeding.

41.3 **C.** During a massive transfusion, the goal is to achieve a hemostatic resuscitation. Although this is best achieved in a 1:1:1 ratio of blood products. One pack of plateletpheresis equal to 6 to 10 packs of pooled platelet packs. Thus, after 6 to 8 U of PRBCs and FFP are given, 1 U of platelets should be administered.

41.4 **B.** This patient has required 6 U of PRBCs in the last hour and there is anticipation that the she will have ongoing transfusion requirements. This meets the definition of a dynamic massive transfusion needs. While the surgeons are gaining surgical control of the bleeding, a massive transfusion should begin so that hemostatic resuscitation can be started to decrease the probability that the patient will become coagulopathic.

CLINICAL PEARLS

- Up to one-third of all trauma patients who arrive to the emergency department are already coagulopathic.
- The "triad of death" is the presence of coagulopathy, acidosis, and hypothermia. Each of these detrimental conditions exacerbates the other and should be preempted by active warming of the patient and the use of hemostatic resuscitation.
- The current recommendation for massive transfusions is that it should be done in a 1:1:1 ratio of PRBCs:FFP:platelets.
- The standard coagulation laboratory studies lag behind in severely injured trauma patients undergoing massive transfusions. TEG or ROTEM analysis is likely a better representation of the patient's actual coagulation status.
- One unit of single pool plateletpheresis is equivalent to 6-10 units of randomly donated platelets and is given for every 6 units of packed RBC in the massive transfusion protocol.

REFERENCES

Boffard KD, Riou B, Warren B, et al. Recombinant factor VIIa as adjunctive therapy for bleeding control in severely injured trauma patients: two parallel randomized, placebo-controlled, double-blind clinical trials. *J Trauma.* 2005;59:8-15.

Sihler KC, Napolitano LM. Complications of massive transfusion. *Chest,* 2010;137:209-220.

Johansson PI, Ostrowski SR, Secher NH. Management of major blood loss: an update. *Acta Anaesthesiol Scand.* 2010;54(9):1039-1049.

Perkins JG, Schreiber MA, Wade CE, et al. Early versus late recombinant factor VIIa in combat trauma patients requiring massive transfusion. *J Trauma.* 2007;62(5):1095-1099; discussion 1099-1101.

Sihler KC, Napolitano LM. Massive transfusion: new insights. *Chest.* 2009;136(6):1654-1667.

Tieu BH, Holcomb JB, Schreiber MA. Coagulopathy: its pathophysiology and treatment in the injured patient. *World J Surg.* 2007;31(5):1055-1064.

CASE 42

A 46-year-old man was admitted to the ICU for the management of severe acute pancreatitis. The patient developed acute respiratory insufficiency requiring intubation and mechanical ventilator support. His respiratory status remains unimproved on hospital day 4. At this point, his hemodynamic status has improved, and he no longer requires vasoactive agents for support of his blood pressure.

- How would you initiate nutritional support for this patient?
- What are the potential limitations in your ability to deliver nutritional support?
- What are the factors that contribute to the increase in this patient's nutritional requirements?

ANSWERS TO CASE 42:
Nutritional Issues in the ICU

Summary: A 46-year-old man is hospitalized in the ICU with severe acute pancreatitis. He is now hemodynamically stable, but is still requiring ventilatory support on hospital day 4.

- **Initiating nutritional support:** Begin appropriate enteral nutritional support based on his nutritional status and projected needs. This nutrition plan needs to take into account his ongoing severe inflammatory response and his associated respiratory dysfunction.
- **Potential limitations to deliver nutritional support:** For this patient with severe acute pancreatitis requiring mechanical ventilator support and large-volume fluid resuscitation, traditional nutritional intake by mouth may not be possible. In addition, the intestinal edema associated with his resuscitation may contribute to impaired intestinal motility and absorption.
- **Factors contributing to increased nutritional requirements:** Hypermetabolism and increased catabolism from his pancreatitis will contribute to marked increase in amino acid requirement and decreased ability to utilize glucose.

ANALYSIS

Objectives

1. To learn the approaches to nutritional assessments and strategies of monitoring responses to nutritional support.
2. To learn the nutritional management of patients with pancreatitis and renal insufficiency (with and without concurrent hemodialysis).
3. To learn the principles of nutritional support specifically designed for the modulation of host inflammatory and immune responses.

Considerations

This is a 46-year-old man who has been in the hospital for 4 days. The severe inflammatory response in pancreatitis can generate large fluid shifts between the intravascular and extravascular space leading to hemodynamic instability as well as edema and respiratory failure. Patients with severe pancreatitis require aggressive fluid resuscitation to maintain adequate intravascular volume to support end-organ perfusion. This patient's hypotension did not respond initially to fluid resuscitation alone and required pressor support, but now his BP has improved. Typically, these patients will have large net positive fluid balance, to which the lungs are most sensitive, especially in the setting of ARDS. This type of lung injury requires prolonged mechanical respiratory support beyond the initial resuscitation phase. In addition, his initial hypotension may have decreased his end-organ perfusion, which can lead to acute kidney injury. This patient's source of acute pancreatitis is unknown, but based on statistics, alcoholic pancreatitis is highly probable. If his pancreatitis is due to alcohol, he may also have a poor baseline nutritional status due to chronic excess alcohol consumption. Additionally, he may have deficiencies that would benefit from specific vitamin and mineral supplementation in addition to caloric and protein provision. Enteral nutritional support will target the delivery of 25 to 30 kcal/kg of nonprotein calories and 1.5 to 2.0 g/kg of proteins per day. Close monitoring to avoid hyperglycemia (glucose >140-160) should be implemented. Similarly, if nasogastric feeding is initiated, the patient should be closely monitored for signs of intolerance such as abdominal distension, and/or high gastric residual volumes (>500 mL).

APPROACH TO:
Nutritional Issues in the ICU

DEFINITIONS

ENTERAL NUTRITION: Nutrition provided through the gastrointestinal tract via a tube, catheter, or stoma that delivers nutrients distal to the oral cavity.

PARENTERAL NUTRITION: The intravenous administration of nutrition, either via central or peripheral access.

PROTEIN-CALORIE MALNUTRITION: A recent weight loss of >10% to 15% or actual body weight <90% of ideal body weight.

TROPHIC FEEDING: Low-volume enteral feeding (usually 10-30 mL/h) meant to prevent mucosal atrophy but insufficient to provide adequate calorie and protein requirements.

CLINICAL APPROACH

Critical illness is associated with a catabolic response because of changes in the hormonal milieu related to cytokine responses that occur following major physiological insults. The increased metabolic response continues into a later anabolic phase of tissue healing. Both of these increase the patient's nutritional requirements. **The goals of nutrition therapy are to modify (most cases down-regulate) the metabolic response to stress, to prevent oxidative cellular injury, and to up-regulate the host immune responses.** Initiation of early nutritional support, primarily enteral nutrition, is a proactive strategy directed at reducing some of the deleterious effects produced by the host's hypermetabolic responses, which in turn should reduce complications, ICU length of stay, and mortality.

In the majority of critically ill patients, it is practical, safe, and less expensive to utilize **enteral** nutrition over parenteral nutrition. Results from the various clinical trials comparing enteral versus parenteral nutrition in critically ill patients have shown that **enteral nutrition is associated with the reduction in infectious complications,** specifically central-line infections and pneumonia. Enteral nutrition is also associated with cost savings from reduced adverse events and savings from reduced hospital length of stay. **It appears that critically ill ICU patients with hemodynamic**

compromise and requiring high doses of vasoactive agents and large volume of blood products may have an increased risk of intolerance to enteral nutritional support and increased risk of gut-related complications. Therefore, it is generally advisable to **withhold enteral feeding until the patients are fully resuscitated.**

Enteral nutrition utilizes the gut barrier to control water and electrolyte absorption. It also supports the functional integrity of the gut by maintaining tight junctions between the intraepithelial cells, stimulating blood flow, and inducing the release of trophic endogenous agents (ie, cholecystokinin, gastrin, bombesin, and bile salts). Furthermore, the structural integrity of the gut, including villous height and mass of secretory IgA-producing immunocytes, is better maintained with enteral nutrition. Loss of functional integrity can adversely affect gut permeability producing increase in bacterial challenge, perpetuation of systemic inflammatory response syndrome (SIRS), increase in the risk for systemic infection, and increase in the likelihood of multiorgan dysfunction syndrome (MODS) development.

In a previously healthy patient with **no evidence of malnutrition, the use of parenteral nutrition may be withheld until after 7 to 10 days of hospitalization without nutrition.** This is mostly due to concerns with infectious complications associated with parenteral nutrition. If, however, there is preexisting protein-calorie malnutrition and enteral nutrition support is not feasible, it is appropriate to initiate parenteral nutrition much earlier after adequate resuscitation has taken place. Parenteral nutrition is indicated primarily for patients in whom enteral nutrition is not feasible or not tolerated, and in severely malnourished patients who are about to undergo major upper GI surgery.

Initiating nutritional therapy first requires an assessment of the patient's nutritional status by determining weight loss and previous nutrient intake prior to admission, level of disease severity, comorbid conditions, and function of the gastrointestinal (GI) tract. Estimates of calorie requirement of the patient's **basic metabolic rate is done with the Harris-Benedict equation.** This can also be measured via indirect calorimetry with the aid of a respiratory therapist. Protein requirements are estimated from the patient's degree of illness and monitored with 24-hour nitrogen-balance measurements. **Traditional markers (albumin, pre-albumin, transferrin, retinol-binding protein) are a reflection of the acute phase response and do not accurately represent nutrition status in the ICU patient.** These markers by themselves have too low specificity, but may, together along with body weight changes, provide an estimate of general nutrition status.

Enteral nutrition should be started within 24 to 48 hours following admission, or as soon as fluid resuscitation is completed and the patient is hemodynamically stable. Feeding started within this time frame is associated with less gut permeability and diminished activation and release of inflammatory cytokines; early enteral feeding has also been shown to reduce infectious morbidity and hospital length of stay. Either gastric or small bowel feeding is acceptable in the ICU patient but small bowel is preferable in patients with high risk of aspiration and patients with severe brain injury (intracranial hypertension is associated with decreased gastric emptying).

The use of **"trickle" or trophic feeds** may prevent mucosal atrophy, but has **not been shown to improve outcomes** from the standpoint of immune modulation. Feedings should be increased toward goal or at least to >50% to 65% of caloric goal over the first 48 to 72 hours following initiation for maximal benefits. Gastric residuals <500 mL in the absence of other signs of intolerance are acceptable and do not increase the risk of aspiration or pneumonia. **In critically ill patients, protein is the most important macronutrient for supporting immune function and wound healing.** Assessment of the adequacy of protein nutrition is estimated from nitrogen balance (needs to be 1.2-2.0 g/kg/d) or nonprotein calorie:nitrogen ratio (70:1 to 100:1). Phosphate levels should be monitored closely and replaced when needed in respiratory failure patients for optimal pulmonary function.

Many enteral formulations are available to meet the needs of different patients. In patients with ARDS or lung injury, enteral formulations characterized by an anti-inflammatory lipid profile and antioxidants should be used (ie, omega-3 fish oils, borage oil) for they have been shown to reduce ICU length of stay, duration of mechanical ventilation, organ failure, and mortality. Patients with respiratory failure can receive calorically dense formulations if fluid restriction is needed. Antioxidant vitamins (including vitamin E and ascorbic acid) and trace minerals (including selenium, zinc, and copper) may also improve ICU patient outcomes. Thiamine and folate supplementation for individuals with history of chronic alcohol abuse is important. Formulations with low glucose concentrations are available for diabetics as well to improve glycemic control.

Special considerations regarding enteral nutrition should be made for patients with renal failure. Acute kidney injury (AKI) usually develops in the setting of multiple organ failure in the critically ill individual. These patients also require the standard enteral formulations described previously with continued adherence to the protein and calorie provisions as before. If significant electrolyte abnormalities develop, formulations with appropriate electrolyte profiles may be considered. **In AKI patients receiving renal replacement therapy (RRT), increased protein provision should be considered. RRT results in amino acid loss of approximately 10 to 20 g/d depending on the method, length of time, and type of filters used. These patients require formulations with 1.5 to 2.0 g/kg/d of protein, and some studies suggesting as high as 2.5 g/kg/d of protein to preserve a positive nitrogen balance.**

Patients with severe acute pancreatitis should have a nasogastric (NG) tube placed on admission and enteral nutrition started as soon as fluid volume resuscitation is complete. Three meta-analyses showed that use of **enteral nutrition compared to parenteral nutrition reduces infectious morbidity, hospital length of stay, need for surgical interventions, multiple organ failure, and mortality**. Outcome benefits are seen in patients with acute pancreatitis when enteral nutrition is initiated within 24 to 48 hours. There has been no significant difference seen in outcomes of feeding by the gastric versus jejunal route; however, jejunal feeding may be better tolerated in these patients as severe pancreatitis can be associated with poor gastric emptying. To improve tolerance to enteral nutrition higher in the GI tract, low-fat elemental formulations in continuous infusion rather than bolus feeding should be used.

CLINICAL CASE CORRELATION

- **See also Case 26 (Fluid/Electrolyte Abnormalities) and Case 40 (Postoperative Care in ICU).**

COMPREHENSION QUESTIONS

42.1 You are making your nutritional rounds in the ICU. Which of the following patients is the best candidate for enteral rather than parenteral nutrition?

A. A 72-year-old woman on her eighth ICU day with sepsis from a ventilator-associated pneumonia requiring 2 vasoactive agents for support of her blood pressure.

B. A 62-year-old malnourished man with an obstructing esophageal cancer about to undergo an Ivor-Lewis esophagectomy.

C. A 75-year-old healthy man who underwent an uncomplicated right hemicolectomy for a malignancy 7 days ago. He is ambulating but still has abdominal distension and has not had flatus yet.

D. A 26-year-old man with multiple gunshot wounds to the abdomen and extensive small bowel injury who has just undergone extensive small bowel resection and now has only 45 cm of small bowel left and no ileocecal valve.

E. A 60-year-old woman who underwent a subtotal gastrectomy for stage 2 adenocarcinoma of the stomach 8 days ago and has developed an anastomotic leak.

42.2 Which of the following methods is the best for assessing nutritional status in a critically ill patient?

A. History and physical examination

B. Albumen, pre-albumin, and retinol-binding protein

C. Triceps skin fold

D. Harris-Benedict equation

E. Percent body fat estimation

42.3 Which of the following is the most accurate statement regarding enteral and parenteral nutrition?

A. Both enteral and parenteral nutrition help preserve structural integrity of the gut.

B. The cost savings of enteral over parenteral nutrition is from the direct cost of the cheaper generic enteral solutions versus the more expensive parenteral nutrition solutions.

C. There is a clear mortality benefit of using enteral nutrition versus parenteral nutrition in the ICU patient.

D. In patients with severe acute pancreatitis, enteral rather than parenteral nutrition is the preferred method of nutrition.

E. Peripheral TPN administration is associated with lower complications than enteral nutritional support.

42.4 A 57-year-old woman who weighs 132 lb (60 kg) is admitted to the ICU for acute pancreatitis complicated by acute kidney injury. She is requires hemodialysis every other day. Which of the following is the best nutrition regimen for this patient?

A. Place a nasojejunal (NJ) tube and feed continuous enteral 2000 kcal/d solution containing 120 g of protein daily.

B. Place a NG tube and feed continuous enteral 2000 kcal/d solution containing 80 g of protein daily.

C. Place a surgical jejunostomy tube and feed enteral 2000 kcal/d solution containing 115 g of protein daily in bolus fashion.

D. Place a peripherally inserted central line and give parenteral 2000 kcal/d solution containing 120 g of protein daily.

E. Place a NG tube and begin feeding to deliver 1800 kcal/d and 60 g of protein a day.

42.5 A-56-year-old man is admitted to the ICU for respiratory failure due to acute lung injury after a motor vehicle accident. The patient is placed on the ventilator. Which of the following is the most accurate management principle in this patient?

A. Calorie-dense, low volume enteral solutions should be used.

B. Anti-inflammatory lipid profile and antioxidants such as omega-3 fish oils and borage oil are typically avoided.

C. Uric acid supplementation is needed to help with ventilation.

D. High caloric intake and hyperglycemia are usually not issues in this type of patient.

E. Close aspiration monitoring and cease enteric feeding if gastric residuals are >100 mL.

ANSWERS TO QUESTIONS

42.1 **C. The best candidate for enteral nutrition is patient (C), because he underwent a right hemi-colectomy 7 days ago. Candidate (A) is still requiring 2 vasopressor agents which is a relative contraindication. Patient (B) is about to undergo major GI surgery and parenteral nutrition is a better option. Patients (D) and (E) have functional issues with their GI tract: (D) had small bowel surgery and possibly a short gut, and patient (E) has an anastomotic leak of his stomach.** In a previously healthy patient with no evidence of malnutrition, parenteral nutrition should not be given until after 7 to 10 days of hospitalization without nutrition if the duration of parenteral nutrition is expected to be >5 to 7 days. This can be started earlier if there is an evidence of malnutrition. Enteral nutrition should be given unless patients do not have a functioning GI tract or if they have hemodynamic compromise, specifically those requiring high-dose catecholamine agents, large volume, or blood products. Parenteral nutrition is also recommended in patients in whom enteral nutrition is not feasible and who are about to undergo major upper GI surgery under the following conditions: (1) if the patient is malnourished, give parenteral nutrition 5 to 7 days preoperatively and continue postoperatively; (2) if nutrition is normal, delay parenteral nutrition 5 to 7 days postoperatively, should enteral nutrition continue not to be feasible and duration of parenteral nutrition is expected to be >5 to 7 days. Special circumstances such as short bowel syndrome and high-output proximal GI enterocutaneous fistulas would also be indications for parenteral nutrition.

42.2 **A.** Assessment of nutritional status is done best by evaluating patient's weight loss and previous nutrient intake prior to admission, level of disease severity, comorbid conditions, and function of the gastrointestinal tract. Albumin, pre-albumin, trasnferrin, and retinol-binding protein are a reflection of the acute-phase response and do not accurately represent nutrition status in the ICU. Triceps skin fold and other anthropometry may be affected by edema. The Harris-Benedict equation is an estimation of basal metabolic caloric requirements based on weight, not an assessment tool for nutritional status.

42.3 **D.** Even in severe acute pancreatitis, initiation of enteral nutrition after acute resuscitation is the preferred method of nutrition delivery. Only enteral nutrition helps preserve villous height and structural integrity of the gut. The majority of cost savings from enteral nutrition is from its decreased infection rate and hospital stay. There is a clear infectious benefit with enteral nutrition, but no clear mortality benefit has been found.

42.4 **A.** The ideal regimen for a renal failure patient undergoing renal replacement therapy in the ICU is one with 1.5 to 2.0 g/kg/d of protein. In severe acute pancreatitis, enteral nutrition is preferred and there is no outcome difference between using gastric versus jejunal feeding but placing surgical jejunostomy tubes carry their own inherent risks. Furthermore, patients tolerate continuous feeds easier than they tolerate bolus feeding in this situation.

42.5 **A.** The feedings should be calorie-dense, low-volume enteral solutions. Enteral solutions characterized by an anti-inflammatory lipid profile and antioxidants such as omega-3 fish oils and borage oil are desirable. Phosphate supplementation (not uric acid) are needed to help with ventilation. Excess caloric intake and hyperglycemia should be avoided to decrease infectious complications. Gastric residuals <500 mL in the absence of other signs of intolerance are acceptable and do not increase the risk of aspiration or pneumonia.

CLINICAL PEARLS

- Enteral nutrition is practical, safe, less expensive, and leads to fewer infections than parenteral nutrition.
- Enteral nutrition should be started within 24 to 48 hours following admission or as soon as fluid resuscitation is completed and the patient is hemodynamically stable.
- In patients receiving renal replacement therapy (RRT), increased protein should be considered.
- Markers such as albumin, pre-albumin, trasnferrin, and retinol-binding protein are a reflection of the acute-phase response and do not accurately represent nutrition status in the ICU patient; however, the serial measurements can help determine progress with nutritional therapy.

REFERENCES

Latifi R. Nutritional therapy in critically ill and injured patients. *Surg Clin N Am.* 2011;91:579-593.

McClave SA, Martindale RG, Vanek VW, et al. Guidelines for the provision and assessment of nutrition support therapy in the adult critically ill patient: Society of Critical Care Medicine and American Society for Parenteral and Enteral Nutrition. *Crit Care Med.* 2009;37:1-30.

SECTION III

Listing of Cases

Listing by Case Number

Listing by Disorder (Alphabetical)

INDEX

Note: Page numbers followed by a *t* or *f* indicate that the entry is included in a table or figure.

B

C

F

I

N

O

T